Hazardous Waste: Evaluating Environmental Risks

Hazardous Waste: Evaluating Environmental Risks

Edited by Victor Bonn

SYRAWOOD
PUBLISHING HOUSE

New York

Published by Syrawood Publishing House,
750 Third Avenue, 9th Floor,
New York, NY 10017, USA
www.syrawoodpublishinghouse.com

Hazardous Waste: Evaluating Environmental Risks
Edited by Victor Bonn

International Standard Book Number: 978-1-68286-482-1 (Hardback)

Cataloging-in-Publication Data

Hazardous waste : evaluating environmental risks / edited by Victor Bonn.
p. cm.
Includes bibliographical references and index.
ISBN 978-1-68286-482-1
1. Hazardous wastes. 2. Factory and trade waste. 3. Environmental health.
4. Hazardous wastes--Environmental aspects. I. Bonn, Victor.
TD1030 .H39 2017
628.42--dc23

Printed in China.

TABLE OF CONTENTS

PREFACE

The world is advancing at a fast pace like never before. Therefore, the need is to keep up with the latest developments. This book was an idea that came to fruition when the specialists in the area realized the need to coordinate together and document essential themes in the subject. That's when I was requested to be the editor. Editing this book has been an honour as it brings together diverse authors researching on different streams of the field. The book collates essential materials contributed by veterans in the area which can be utilized by students and researchers alike.

This book on hazardous waste discusses the diverse aspects of hazardous waste removal and its impact on human and environmental health. Hazardous waste is a primary concern of environmentalists across the globe. Environmental monitoring has various tools to sample, survey and assess environmental damage and toxicity levels. This book addresses varied topics such as assessments of toxic waste management and the tools and technologies that are used for the same purpose. Different approaches, evaluations, methodologies and advanced studies on evaluation and mitigation of hazardous waste and its impacts have been included in this book. It is a compilation of chapters that discuss the most vital concepts and emerging trends in this area of study. For all those who are interested in this field, this book can prove to be an essential guide.

Each chapter is a sole-standing publication that reflects each author´s interpretation. Thus, the book displays a multi-facetted picture of our current understanding of applications and diverse aspects of the field. I would like to thank the contributors of this book and my family for their endless support.

Editor

1

Bioavailability and bioaccumulation characterization of essential and heavy metals contents in *R. acetosa, S. oleracea and U. dioica* from copper polluted and referent areas

Biljana Balabanova[1†], Trajče Stafilov[2,3*] and Katerina Bačeva[2,3†]

Abstract

Background: Bioavailability of metals occurring in soil is the basic source of its accumulation in vegetables and herbs. The impact of soil pollution (due to urban and mining areas) on the food chain presents a challenge for many investigations. Availability of metals in a potentially polluted soil and their possible transfer and bioaccumulation in sorrel (*Rumex acetosa*), spinach (*Spinacia oleracea*) and common nettle (*Urtica dioica*), were examined.

Methods: Microwave digestion was applied for total digestion of the plant tissues, while on the soil samples open wet digestion with a mixture of acids was applied. Three extraction methods were implemented for the bioavailable metals in the soil. Atomic emission spectrometry with inductively coupled plasma was used for determination of the total contents of 21 elements.

Results: Significant enrichments in agricultural soil for As, Pb and Zn (in urban area), Cd, Cu and Ni (in a copper mine area), compared with the respective values from European standards were detected. On the basis of three different extraction methods, higher availability was assumed for both lithogenic and anthropogenic elements. Translocation values >1 were obtained for As, Cd, Cu, Ni, Pb and Zn. Higher bioconcentrating value was obtained only for Cd, while the bioaccumulation values vary from 0.17 for Cd to 0.82 for Zn.

Conclusions: The potential availability of hazardous metals in urban and mining soils is examined using DTPA-TEA-$CaCl_2$ (urban) and HCl (Cu-mines areas). Our results suggested that *S. oleracea* and *R. acetosa* have a phytostabilization potential for Cd, Cu, Ni and Pb, while *U. dioica* only for Cu. *R. acetosa* has a potential for phytoextraction of Cd in urban and copper polluted areas.

Keywords: Metals, Bioaccumulation, *Rumex acetosa*, *Spinacia oleracea*, *Urtica dioica*, ICP-AES

Background

Since food contamination is one of the major routes for entry of metals into the humans and animals, monitoring the bioavailability pools of metals in contaminated vegetables has generated a great interest [1-5]. Pertaining to this awareness, a lot of studies have been conducted for determining the metals contents in the vegetables and herbs that are included in human diet [6-8]. Vegetables/herbs contamination with heavy metals derives primarily from contaminated soil [4]. The uptake of metals from the soil depends on different factors such as their soluble content, soil pH, plant growth stages, types of species, etc. [9-11]. Plants have developed different strategies to grow on agricultural soils rich in heavy metals [1,4,5]. In this way, the food presents the main source of human exposure to toxic metals [12,3]. Different plant parts accumulate different levels of these metals. For example, higher metal concentrations were observed in the

* Correspondence: trajcest@pmf.ukim.mk
†Equal contributors
[2]Institute of Chemistry, Faculty of Science, Ss. Cyril and Methodius University, Arhimedova 5, 1000 Skopje, Macedonia
[3]Research Center for Environment and Materials, Macedonian Academy of Sciences and Arts, Krste Misirkov 2, 1000 Skopje, Republic of Macedonia
Full list of author information is available at the end of the article

edible and inedible parts of vegetable species as reported by many authors [13-15]. Considering this, sorrel (*Rumex acetosa L.*), spinach (*Spinacia oleracea*) and common nettle (*Urtica dioica L.*) were used as vegetable/herb samples for investigating the possible toxic metals bioaccumulation and transferring ability from reference and polluted agricultural lands (mines and urban areas). Appropriately, mines' surroundings and urban areas were selected as investigation areas to determine the anthropogenic impact on the agricultural land and food quality (in terms of pollution with toxic metals). Previous investigation shows that the "Bučim" copper mine and the former "Damjan" iron mine have a significant impact on air and soil pollution in their close environs [16-19]. However, the environmental impact on the food chain has been very poorly investigated. Most frequent leaf vegetables and herbs in the investigated area were sorrel, spinach and common nettle. The sorrel and spinach as vegetables, and the common nettle as herb and food additive, are commonly used in the local population's diet and globally, they are numbered among the most popular foods for their high content of vitamins and minerals [20].

The main goal of this work is to assess the complex phenomenon of essential and toxic metals distribution in the food chain in the old mining areas. As main markers of pollution in agricultural land and vegetables two types of markers were used: simple markers, represented by the elements contents in the contaminated soils and by the elements contents in the vegetables consumed by the population in the polluted and unpolluted areas. Sorrel (*Rumex acetosa L.*), spinach (*Spinacia oleracea*) and common nettle (*Urtica dioica L.*) have been cultivated in the contaminated agricultural land of the local settlements for a long period of time now, and this is why their phytostabilization and phytoextraction ability were also examined.

Methods

Sampling and sampling site characterization

Plant species and soil samples were collected from four localities (Figure 1, Table 1). The first locality (site 1) - village Topolnica was the most polluted region, affected by the activities of "Bučim" copper mine and flotation tailings [16-18]. The second locality (site 2) is village Damjan, air-distanced 4 km from the flotation tailings dam and 2 km from the ore wastes dam of "Bučim" copper mine. This settlement is also affected by the former iron mine "Damjan", as given by Balabanova et al. [18]. The third sampling location (site 3), village Lakavica, was 12 km distanced from the pollution source. Previous investigation of air distribution (using plant species moss and lichens) determined no significant distribution of air transported metals from the copper mine. Therefore, this area can be used as a reference area. The fourth sampling locality (site 4), the town of Štip, was used for measuring the impact in the urban environment. A total of 10 plant samples including roots, stems and leaves of each species, were collected from each site, mixed together to form a composite sample, and placed in labeled bags for further analysis. Soil samples (5 replicates), at 0–20 cm depth from the rhizosphere of each plant, were taken from each site where from the plant sample was found. Soil samples (a composite mixture) were air dried at room temperature for two weeks, crushed and pulverized to pass through a 2-mm sieve.

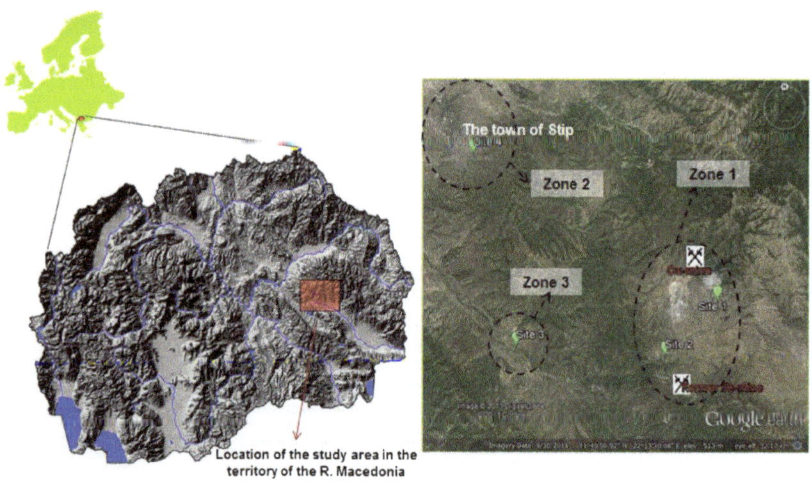

Figure 1 Locality of the study area on the territory of the R. Macedonia divided in zones. Zone 1 – polluted area; Zone 2 – urban area; Zone 3 – control area, non-contaminated area.

Table 1 Geographical coordinates of sampling locations

Site	Locality	Site characterization	E	N
1	Village Topolnica	Cu-mine environ	22°22'47.00"	41°39'41.73"
2	Village Damjan	Former Fe mine environ	22°20'33.91"	41°37'57.03"
3	Village Lakavica	Reference area	22°14'7.95"	41°38'13.91"
4	Town of Štip	Urban area	22°12'16.23"	41°44'16.90"

Sample pre-treatment for elements contents analysis

Soil digestion (total and extractability forms)

For total digestion, an open wet digestion method with a mixture of acids was applied. Precisely measured masses of soil samples (0.2500 g) were placed in a Teflon digestion vessel and were digested on a hot plate at temperature 150-180°C. At first, HNO_3 was added to remove all organic matters, then a mixture of HF and $HClO_4$ was added, followed by a third step where HCl and water were added to dissolve the residues. The solution was quantitatively transferred to a 25 mL volumetric flask [18].

Three methods were applied for the study of the plant-availability of the elements: (1) Extraction with deionized H_2O that provides information on the actual availability of the elements in the soil solution; (2) Extraction with 0.1 M HCl for 1 h and filtering through an acid-resistant filter, displacing potentially available forms that are not easily extracted. The immobilization of the heavy metals in the contaminated soil is carried out through chelating and washing with mineral acids. In this way the efficiency in the extraction of heavy metals from the soil is determined. An effective pH level is required to enable remediation of heavy metals from contaminated soils. Because of the differences in the affinities of heavy metals with soil and soil constituents the effective pH levels are likely to vary depending on the type of the heavy metals and the strength of their bonding with the soil. (3) Extraction of the soluble species of trace elements in a mixed buffered solution (pH = 7.3) of triethanolamine (TEA, 0.1 mol L^{-1}) with $CaCl_2$ (0.01 mol L^{-1}) and diethylenetriaminepentaacetic acid (DTPA, 0.005 mol L^{-1}), which is often recommended for extraction of toxic or biogenic metals. The DTPA extracting solution was prepared in the following way: 0.005 mol L^{-1} DTPA, 0.01 mol L^{-1} $CaCl_2$ and 0.1 mol L^{-1} TEA was adjusted to pH to 7.30 ± 0.05 with 1:1 HCl [21].

Plants digestion

The plants collected from the agricultural soils were washed with water and rinsed with distillated water, to ensure that they are thoroughly cleaned and any outside contamination has been removed. Every plant species was separated root from shoot. Plant samples were dried at room temperature for almost two weeks, pulverized and passed through a 2 mm stainless steel sieve. In this way representative samples were prepared.

For digestion of the plant tissue samples, a microwave digestion system (CEM, model Mars, USA) was applied. 0.5 g of plant tissue samples were precisely (with accuracy of 0.0001) measured, then 5 mL concentrated nitric acid, HNO_3 (69%, 108 *m/V*, trace pure) and 2 mL hydrogen peroxide, H_2O_2 (30%, *m/V*, trace pure) were added. The Teflon vessels were carefully closed and a microwave digestion method was applied. The digestion method was performed in two steps for total dissolution of the plants tissue at 180°C and pressure of 600 psi applying 100% of 1600 W power energy [16,17,21]. When the digestion was completed, the digests were quantitatively transferred into 25 mL volumetric flaks. The digests from plant tissue prepared in this way were then analysed for the total elements contents.

Spectroscopic analysis

The total contents of 21 elements were analyzed: (1) macro biogenic elements (Ca, K, Na, Mg, and P), (2) elements that have the essential functionality in micro-contents (Ba, Cr, Li, Cu, Fe, Mo, Mn, Sr and Zn), and elements that are toxic even in traces (Ag, Al, As, Cd, Ni, Pb and V). The elements contents were determined using atomic emission spectrometry with inductively coupled plasma, ICP-AES (Varian, model 715-ES, USA) with application of an ultrasonic nebuliser CETAC (ICP/U-5000AT+) for improved sensitivity for the elements contents in the plants digest.

In addition, quality control was assured by standard reference materials (moss as plant species), M2 and M3 moss plant tissue (for the plant species) and JSAC 0401 as soil reference material. The difference between measured and certified values for all analyzed elements was satisfactory, ranging within 10%. The internal standard addition method was applied to all measured elements, and the recoveries of all elements were in the range of 96.6-103%. The method sensitivity in regard to the lower limit of detection of the elements contents in the plants digest was improved using an ultrasonic nebuliser: 0.001 mg kg^{-1} for Mn and Li; 0.0125 mg kg^{-1} for Al, Cu; 0.002 mg kg^{-1} for Fe; 0.003 mg kg^{-1} for Zn; 0.005 mg kg^{-1} for Cd; 0.01 mg kg^{-1} for Ag, Mo, V; 0.025 mg kg^{-1} for Ba, Ca, Mg, Sr; 0.05 mg kg^{-1} for Cr; 0.25 mg kg^{-1} for Ni; 0.25 mg kg^{-1} for As, P, Pb; 2.5 mg kg^{-1} for Na; 5 mg kg^{-1} for K. The values for the soil digest are maximized for 10% using a standard nebuliser.

Data processing

The values obtained for the contents of the investigated elements were statistically processed using basic descriptive statistics. Box–Cox transformation was used for data transformation [22,23]. Bivariate statistic method was applied to check the data about the correlations between elements contents. Multivariate statistic methods (principal component analysis-PCA and factor analysis-FA) were used to reveal the associations of the chemical elements [24-26]. Biological Concentration Factor (BCF) was calculated as metal concentration ratio of plant roots to soil as given by Malik et al. [3] and Yoon et al. [6]. Translocation Factor (TF) was described as ratio of heavy metals in plant shoot to that in plant root [7,27]. Biological Accumulation Factor (BAF) was calculated as ratio of heavy metal in shoots to that in the soil [3,7,27].

Results and discussion

Soil analysis

Characterization of metals contents in soils

The total contents of the analyzed elements in the soil were analyzed in order to characterize possible soil pollution and to determine the transfer efficiency from the soil. The distribution of the macro elements varies among the localities in the investigated area, yet the median values are in line with certain European standards [28]. The maximum contents for Ca and P were obtained in the agricultural land from the urban site (3.5 and 0.2%, respectively, Table 2). The maximum contents for K and Mg were obtained from the agricultural land in the Cu-mine environ (2.3 and 1.1%, respectively). This occurrence is due to the intensive use of organic fertilizers on the rural agricultural land. The most enriched Al content was obtained in the Fe-mine environs, due to geochemistry of the soil minerals [18]. The median values for the total contents of As, Cd, Cr, Cu, Fe, Ni, Pb, and Zn in the soil showed that these elements are found in higher contents compared to the European average values (Table 2). Thus, the European mean values for As, Cd, Cr, Cu, Fe, Ni, Pb and Zn are 11.6, 0.28, 94.8, 17.3, 38 000, 21.8, 32.6, 68.1 mg kg^{-1} respectively, as given by Salminen et al. [28]. Comparing these values with the respective values obtained in this study, enrichment ratios (ER) were calculated: $ER_{As} = 2.5$, $ER_{Cd} = 3.1$, $ER_{Cu} = 4.01$, $ER_{Ni} = 1.33$, $ER_{Pb} = 1.46$, $ER_{Zn} = 1.48$. It can be noticed that there are no significant enrichment considering the Cr and Fe contents [28]. However, the total Cr contents quantified in the agricultural land can be considered as not contaminated. The iron contents shows enrichment only in the agricultural land in the Cu-mine environ, $ER_{Fe} = 1.13$, compared to the European average for Fe contents in soil [28]. Despite the detected

Table 2 The contents of the analyzed elements in soil (total and extractability contents), given in mg kg^{-1}, n = 4

Element	Extraction in H_2O	Extraction in 0.1 mol L^{-1} HCl	Extraction in DTPA-$CaCl_2$-TEA	Total contents			
				Copper mine environ (site 1)	Former iron mine environ (site 2)	Reference area (site 3)	Urban area (site 4)
Ag	<0.01	0.02 ± 0.01	<0.01	0.47	0.76	0.46	1.09
Al	23.9 ± 16.5	**62.9 ± 46.2**	0.78 ± 0.88	58992	61061	59467	59643
As	<0.25	**<0.25**	<0.25	**26.9**	23.4	18.9	**48.7**
Ba	0.18 ± 0.05	**10.9 ± 5.81**	0.71 ± 0.40	311	403	343	437
Ca	104 ± 47.7	**3421 ± 430**	1222 ± 197	22677	20447	21954	35394
Cd	0.01 ± 0.001	0.05 ± 0.03	0.05 ± 0.03	**1.06**	0.96	0.86	0.59
Cr	0.04 ± 0.02	0.06 ± 0.03	0.01 ± 0.003	**63.6**	41.9	55.8	54.2
Cu	0.30 ± 0.06	1.57 ± 1.97	**8.60 ± 6.65**	**100**	63.7	34.3	79.0
Fe	27.9 ± 18.1	4.43 ± 4.84	28.0 ± 33.4	**43025**	32629	32646	31242
K	56.2 ± 15.6	**155 ± 47.2**	81.6 ± 26.6	23716	19805	16173	20290
Li	0.01 ± 0.004	0.04 ± 0.006	0.006 ± 0.005	7.79	5.70	7.74	9.81
Mg	21.7 ± 6.15	**305 ± 79.6**	103 ± 28.7	10676	6583	8956	8629
Mn	0.47 ± 0.31	**44.4 ± 28.5**	10.6 ± 2.82	521	577	575	567
Mo	0.04 ± 0.04	0.04 ± 0.02	0.03 ± 0.03	4.0	3.2	2.8	2.5
Na	6.91 ± 4.67	9.73 ± 5.94	6.06 ± 5.35	8582	**9248**	8506	7956
Ni	0.18 ± 0.05	**0.84 ± 0.54**	0.55 ± 0.22	19.6	**39.0**	23.9	34.0
P	16.6 ± 3.75	**177 ± 24.8**	5.19 ± 1.41	1385	931	995	**2104**
Pb	0.25 ± 0.07	0.38 ± 0.26	**1.71 ± 1.15**	24.4	44.8	36.8	**83.9**
V	0.08 ± 0.03	0.10 ± 0.08	0.06 ± 0.04	**93.8**	72.2	82.7	67.9
Zn	0.28 ± 0.11	**6.02 ± 5.34**	5.02 ± 5.10	78.8	72.9	73.2	**181**

Bold values indicated the maximum extracted content of current element under specific extraction reagents.

enrichments, the respective level of its content in the soil is not considered as toxic to the plants, according to Marschner [11]. Considering this, it can be concluded that the analyzed agriculture soils are polluted with As, Cd, Cu and Pb. The maximum values for Cd (1.06 mg kg^{-1}) and Cu (100 mg kg^{-1}) were obtained from the soil samples from the very close surroundings of the copper mine (marked as bold values in Table 2). The maximum values for As and Pb were obtained from the urban area soil samples (49 and 84 mg kg^{-1}, respectively). In the same agricultural land the nutritive mineral Zn contents reaches to 181 mg $kgkg^{-1}$ (Table 2). For almost all analyzed elements no significant variations were detected between the total contents in the soil sampled from site 2 and site 3.

Different levels of availability can be estimated depending on the extracting power of the extraction reagent that was used. Very low variations were identified between the extraction solutions for Cd, Cr and Ni. It was found that 1.6% of arsenic were extracted using 0.1 mol L^{-1} HCl ranging from 0.07 mg kg^{-1} in the reference area (Site 3) to 0.35 mg kg^{-1} in the urban area agricultural soil- site 4 (Table 2). The sequestering reagent was much more effective in the case of Cu and Pb (extracted contents of 12.4% and 3.6%, respectively) as presented in Table 2. Despite the median values for the Zn extraction contents, the maximum extraction was obtained using the sequestering reagent at site 4 (soil from urban area). This is probably a result of the Cd-Pb-Zn enrichments in the urban agricultural land. Similar results were obtained for Fe extraction with H_2O and with DTPA–$CaCl_2$–TEA, where the efficiency was not significant (<1%). The acid reagent (0.1 mol L^{-1} HCl) is a very efficient extractability agent in the case of Ba, Ca, K, Mg, Mn and P. Therefore, the nutritive elements are mostly extracted at lower pH values with no significant variations between the sampling locations (Table 2, Figure 1).

Multivariate component statistics

The obtained data for elements contents were processed using multivariate component statistics. In Figure 2 is presented bi-plot of principle component analysis for the metals contents in soil, their extractability power and dependence on sampling location. Two principle components (Factor 1 and Factor 2) were assumed with a total variation of 86%. The two components can separate well the anthropogenic (caused by mining activities) and lithogenic elements one from another. The anthropogenic elements (As, Cd, Cu, Pb, Zn) including Ca, Mg, Ba and Mn as naturally enriched, are included in factor 2, which positively correlates with DTPA-TEA-$CaCl_2$ and HCl as extraction agents. Higher contents of these metals are characteristic for the soil samples from site 1 and 2, as previously reported [18]. These elements are grouped on the positive side of the PCA-plot (Figure 2). On the other hand, the typical lithogenic elements as Al, Ag, Cr, Fe, Mo, Li, V, and P-K as naturally enriched, are included in factor 1, in relation to which positive scores were established for total contents despite the water extractability (Figure 2). It can be summarized that both anthropogenic and lithogenic elements are not extracted in water solution, which means that their higher contents will be very hardly reduced by raining water or by watering the agricultural

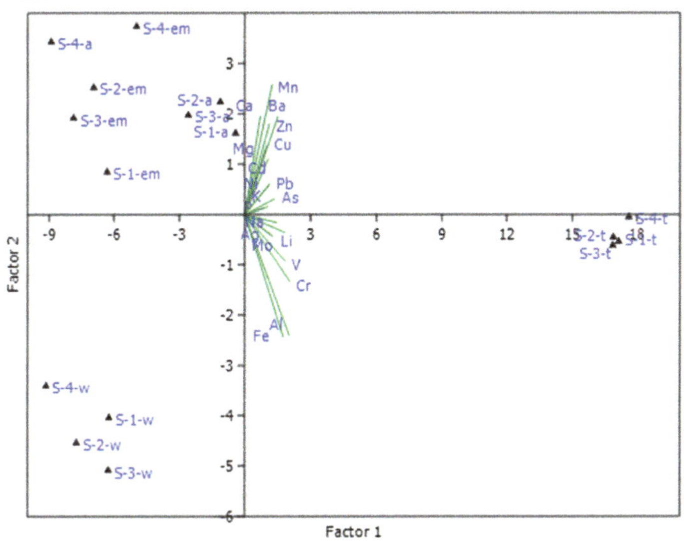

Figure 2 Biplot for PCA-soil model for dependence of elements contents from different sampling locations, and different soil extraction solutions. **w** - extraction with distilled water; **em** - extraction of elements in soil with DTPA–$CaCl_2$–TEA; **a** - extraction with 0.1 HCl; **t** - total dissolved elements; **1**-site 1, Cu-mine environ; **2**-site 2, Former Fe-mine; **3**-site 3, reference area; **4**-site 4, urban area.

Table 3 Basic statistics for elements contents in shoots and roots of plant species (contents are given in mg kg^{-1} of dried matter)

	Rumex acetosa				*Urtica dioica*				*Spinacia oleracea*			
	Shoot		Root		Shoot		Root		Shoot		Root	
Element	Range	Med	Range	Med	Range	Med	Range	Med	Range	Med	Range	Med
Ag	0.01-0.47	0.15	0.005-0.11	0.037	0.011-0.35	0.091	0.029-0.17	0.058	0.01-0.16	0.08	0.01-1.17	0.04
Al	18.8-293	55.8	174-406	328	76.0-386	223	214-1396	494	93.3-259	172	163-466	308
As	<0.25-0.94	<0.25	<0.25-1.18	0.76	<0.25-0.90	<0.25	0.53-0.94	0.89	<0.25-0.76	0.44	<0.25-0.40	<0.25
Ba	1.38-11.0	3.49	8.36-14.2	10.7	1.80-23.4	13.2	3.47-21.9	10.6	2.21-11.4	4.40	5.37-19.1	9.90
Ca	2405-5251	3777	4073-13523	5526	17689-26850	21763	4188-8798	4773	3252-9099	4049	2283-3863	2819
Cd	0.03-0.07	0.039	0.05-0.09	0.053	0.01-0.03	0.01	0.02-0.11	0.08	0.06-0.26	0.13	0.09-0.34	0.17
Cr	0.13-0.60	0.22	0.41-0.74	0.66	0.22-0.78	0.40	0.73-2.29	1.01	0.27-0.88	0.49	0.38-1.63	0.83
Cu	6.54-11.4	8.07	6.33-23.6	12.9	10.6-32.4	15.3	7.1-24.0	10.0	6.41-9.66	7.74	3.80-7.48	6.45
Fe	56.0-218	79.2	211-424	238	80.1-240	154	204-892	459	102-253	133	142-368	272
K	18945-30910	21751	5640-10711	8493	10292-17683	14800	9208-12105	10181	30197-38421	30809	19233-25846	21854
Li	0.06-0.31	0.081	0.15-0.22	0.18	0.040-0.37	0.17	0.08-0.88	0.31	0.089-0.35	0.13	0.14-0.30	0.20
Mg	1166-1783	1521	1051-1594	1192	866-1453	1237	393-1000	809	1680	1396	1058-1387	1237
Mn	11.3-30.3	17.7	6.89-16.5	11.5	16.5-77.7	23.8	18.1-48.4	31.4	12.0-70.1	23.3	10.8-33.9	19.9
Mo	0.33-1.24	0.76	0.27-1.65	0.57	0.54-2.05	1.26	0.03-0.50	0.09	0.089-0.84	0.51	0.05-0.37	0.15
Na	60.4-99.0	77.8	76.7-354	214	40.0-88.2	53.7	42.5-176	125	31.0-837	82.1	64.3-861	314
Ni	0.51-1.93	0.77	0.49-3.10	1.55	1.45-1.67	1.51	0.89-3.78	3.32	0.64-3.09	1.45	0.85-3.06	1.84
P	1540-3995	1927	1041-1766	1418	2081-3275	2506	1906-2492	2225	1962-3305	2810	2833-4507	3198
Pb	0.56-0.96	0.70	0.32-1.83	0.65	0.40-0.98	0.65	0.86-1.69	1.24	0.59-0.97	0.68	0.45-0.83	0.76
Sr	2.02-9.39	4.16	25.1-33.1	30.9	15.0-92.8	51.3	10.8-40.1	25.0	6.88-20.5	14.2	19.2-22.4	21.3
V	0.03-0.45	0.091	2.04-4.11	2.91	0.10-0.57	0.32	1.27-3.65	1.93	0.15-0.55	0.32	0.49-1.27	0.95
Zn	18.6-29.3	23.3	15.0-31.8	23.7	12.9-36.2	15.4	12.4-167	20.9	39.7-66.5	56.8	26.2-32.3	28.6

land. The potential availability of hazardous metals in urban and mining areas is recommended to be examined using DTPA-TEA-$CaCl_2$ (for urban) and HCl (for Cu-mines areas).

Plant species analysis

Characterization of metals contents-Basic descriptive statistics

Range and median values were used for presenting the data on elements contents in the plant species (Table 3). The presented values were calculated for the air-dried samples, while the moisture fraction ranges from 62.5-93%. The elements contents were analyzed separately in the edible vegetable parts (shoot) and the root. The essential macro elements (Ca, K, Mg and P) vary in their contents compared shoot to root. For example, potassium contents are enriched in *S. oleracea* (~3%). Maximum value for calcium content was obtained in the *U. dioica* shoot (2.1%) compared to the *R. acetosa* and *S. oleracea* (0.37 and 0.4%, respectively). The phosphorus content shows very low variability between shoot/root and between the analyzed vegetable species.

The content of the essential trace elements (Cu, Fe, Mn, Mo and Zn) shows higher levels than usually found [16-18]. The essential need of the plant tissue for Cu is ~0.9 mg kg^{-1} [11]. However, the determined contents of the copper in the present study is enriched to 32 mg kg^{-1} in the *U. dioica* shoot (sample collected very close to the copper mine). The essential content of Fe for the plant tissue is 18 mg kg^{-1} [11]. The determined iron content varies between shoot/root accumulation and between the species. The highest Fe content was obtained for the *U. dioica* root (892 mg kg^{-1} at the reference site location), accompanied by higher shoot content (204 mg kg^{-1}). Thus, it can be considered that the Fe-content does not depend on the anthropogenic enrichments in the mines environ. The manganese content, generally required as a cofactor in enzyme functions (2.3 mg kg^{-1}), occurs in higher contents in the analyzed vegetables, without any significant variations (ranging from 6.9-77 mg kg^{-1}). Maximum Mn values were obtained for the *U. dioica* and *S. oleracea* shoot. Molybdenum as an essential trace element required in the amount of 0.045 mg kg^{-1} as given by Gunduz et al. [4] does not occur in higher contents (ranging from 0.03-1.65 mg kg^{-1}). Zinc, as one of the most characteristic essential trace elements, is pervasive and required for several enzymes such as carboxyl peptidase, liver alcohol

Table 4 Matrix of correlation coefficients

Ag	1.00																				
Al	−0.11	1.00																			
As	0.14	0.30	1.00																		
Ba	0.18	**0.74****	0.25	1.00																	
Ca	0.06	0.20	0.17	0.27	1.00																
Cd	−0.08	0.26	0.11	0.08	**−0.50***	1.00															
Cr	−0.16	**0.92****	0.33	**0.58****	0.06	0.48	1.00														
Cu	0.32	0.03	0.32	0.14	**0.53****	**−0.66****	−0.16	1.00													
Fe	−0.10	**0.95****	0.34	**0.66****	0.07	0.33	**0.91****	0.10	1.00												
K	0.08	**−0.42***	**−0.44***	−0.36	−0.39	0.37	−0.32	**−0.47***	**−0.45***	1.00											
Li	0.08	**0.86****	0.36	**0.72****	0.16	0.30	**0.83****	0.06	**0.81****	−0.19	1.00										
Mg	−0.01	−0.17	−0.20	0.01	0.02	0.16	−0.18	−0.16	−0.21	**0.46***	0.11	1.00									
Mn	0.06	0.27	0.03	−0.01	0.31	0.13	0.32	0.04	0.24	0.24	0.25	0.09	1.00								
Mo	0.09	**−0.47***	0.00	−0.39	**0.44***	**−0.51***	**−0.54****	**0.55****	**−0.42***	−0.02	−0.34	0.26	0.07	1.00							
Na	−0.11	0.28	0.19	0.12	0.02	0.40	0.37	−0.31	0.28	−0.09	**0.41***	0.24	−0.05	−0.09	1.00						
Ni	0.07	**0.47***	0.17	0.33	0.10	0.38	**0.52****	0.01	**0.56****	−0.15	0.33	−0.22	**0.42***	−0.29	−0.05	1.00					
P	−0.10	−0.22	−0.31	−0.30	−0.38	0.18	−0.06	−0.36	−0.20	**0.54****	−0.15	−0.14	0.22	−0.17	−0.09	0.10	1.00				
Pb	0.05	**0.62****	0.36	0.38	−0.06	0.29	**0.64****	0.01	**0.64****	−0.27	**0.53****	−0.03	0.23	−0.37	0.00	**0.59****	−0.07	1.00			
Sr	0.09	**0.64****	0.30	**0.81****	**0.61****	−0.12	0.49*	0.33	**0.53****	−0.49	**0.57****	−0.11	0.02	−0.09	0.21	0.28	−0.26	0.25	1.00		
V	−0.20	**0.83****	0.37	**0.59****	0.07	0.28	**0.78****	0.08	**0.88****	**−0.66****	**0.62****	−0.28	−0.09	−0.38	0.33	**0.43***	**−0.43***	**0.50***	**0.52****	1.00	
Zn	−0.03	−0.28	−0.04	**−0.54****	−0.31	**0.56****	−0.06	−0.29	−0.16	0.40	−0.32	−0.03	0.09	−0.02	−0.03	0.26	0.22	0.08	**−0.45***	−0.15	1.00
	Ag	Al	As	Ba	Ca	Cd	Cr	Cu	Fe	K	Li	Mg	Mn	Mo	Na	Ni	P	Pb	Sr	V	Zn

**Correlations (Box-Cox transformed values), the marked correlations are significant at $p < 0.01000$. $N = 24$.
*Correlations (Box-Cox transformed values), the marked correlations are significant at $p < 0.05000$. $N = 24$.

dehydrogenase, and carbonic anhydrase with nominal needs of 11 mg kg^{-1} [11]. There was enriched accumulation of Zn in the vegetables, ranging from 12.4-167 mg kg^{-1}. The maximum Zn content was obtained for the *U. dioica* root from site 2.

The other trace elements (As, Cd, Cr and Pb) in higher contents can produce toxic effects on the vegetables, or negative effects on humans consuming them as food. As regards arsenic, half of the values found were below the limit of detection, for all three vegetable species. Only in the urban area the arsenic content was found as potentially hazardous (0.21-0.34 mg kg^{-1}), especially in the *U. dioica* root and the *R. acetosa* root and shoot. The maximum permitted values for Cd and Pb content in fresh vegetables are regulated by established standard rules in the Republic of Macedonia, considering 0.2 and 0.3 mg kg^{-1}, respectively, as the highest permitted contents [29]. Higher values for Cd contents in the *U. dioica* and *R. acetosa* were obtained from the urban site location. The maximum value for Cd content was obtained from the *S. oleracea* root (0.34 mg kg^{-1}, values for dried mass fraction) in the urban area. However, the Cd content in these species, including the moisture mass fraction, alleviates the situation, because the obtained value was below 0.3 mg kg^{-1}. Lead was also analyzed as a potentially toxic metal, due to the copper anthropogenic enrichment in the investigated area, as previously considered [16,17]. The values for Pb contents range from 0.4 to 2 mg kg^{-1} for dried mass, while for the fresh matter (including the moisture fraction mass) they range 0.05-0.41 mg kg^{-1}, pointing to partial contamination (maximum permitted contents - 0.3 mg kg^{-1} in fresh matter). Hazardous Pb contents were obtained from *U. dioica* and *R. acetosa.* The maximum value for Pb content (0.41 mg kg^{-1}) was obtained from the former Fe mine environ (site 2) in the *R. acetosa* root, while as regards the shoot and root of the *U. dioica* shoot and root, higher values were obtained from the Cu-mine environ and from the urban area.

Chromium belongs to the group of essential micronutrients. The Cr contents ranges from 0.13 mg kg^{-1} to 2.29 mg kg^{-1}. However, the inorganic chromium absorption is quite low i.e. 1-2% of the available content in the soil. The Cu contents were in the range of 6.33-32 mg kg^{-1} (for dried vegetables). Considering the Cu-mine at site-1, the maximum value for Cu-content was obtained from the *U. dioica* root (8.65 mg kg^{-1} for fresh plant tissue). There is no established permitted value for Cu, but compared with the Cu content in the *U. dioica* from the reference area (7.45 mg kg^{-1}), there is a slight enrichment. Significant enrichments were established for the Fe content in plant tissues for the *R. acetosa* < *S. oleracea* < *U. dioica* roots. However, this occurrence was expected, especially regarding the location (2), where a former Fe-mine is located. Soil analysis has shown Fe contents ~3%. For the rest of the elements there is no significant variation in the metals contents between the plant species and the sampling locations.

Metals correlations and associations in vegetables/herbs

Correlations between the elements contents in the investigated vegetables were established using bivariate statistics. The significant correlations are marked in bold in Table 4. The correlations of Fe-Al (r = 0.95), Fe-Cr (r = 0.91), Cr-Al (0.92) were selected as significant relations for the lithoogenic elements accumulation. The lithogenic impact of the region is related with the Eocene flysh and molase as well as the impact of oldest formation: Pleistocene sediments and Proterozoic gneisses, as given by Balabanova et al. [18] and Stafilov et al. [19]. The correlation Cu-Cd, relies on the anthropogenic influence of the copper mine as previously was found using moss and lichen plant species as sampling media [16,17].

The multivariate data processing method was also applied to reduce and optimize the numerous data matrix. Factor analysis was used to minimize the elements distribution. Using the *engine-values screening* in data correlation (>1.00), the distribution was reduced to two factors (associations of elements). The matrix for factor loadings is given in Table 5. Elements associations

Table 5 Factor loadings for elements contents (F > 0.50)

	F1	F2	Initial communality	Final communality	Specific variance
Ag	**−0.076**	0.058	0.844	0.009	0.991
Al	**0.955**	0.090	0.990	0.919	0.081
As	**0.392**	−0.234	0.852	0.209	0.791
Ba	**0.683**	−0.309	0.990	0.562	0.438
Ca	0.119	**−0.688**	0.964	0.487	0.513
Cd	0.122	**0.787**	0.989	0.635	0.365
Cr	**0.882**	0.380	0.982	0.923	0.077
Cu	0.155	**−0.680**	0.917	0.486	0.514
Fe	**0.934**	0.121	0.988	0.887	0.113
K	−0.486	**0.507**	0.946	0.493	0.507
Li	**0.860**	0.070	0.986	0.745	0.255
Mg	**−0.223**	0.028	0.977	0.051	0.949
Mn	**0.127**	0.124	0.878	0.031	0.969
Mo	−0.336	**−0.514**	0.955	0.378	0.622
Na	0.071	**0.430**	0.954	0.190	0.810
Ni	**0.516**	0.293	0.906	0.352	0.648
P	−0.219	**0.400**	0.937	0.207	0.793
Pb	0.165	**0.662**	0.959	0.465	0.535
V	**0.700**	−0.043	0.883	0.492	0.508
Zn	−0.108	**0.323**	0.972	0.116	0.884

F1, F2 -factor loadings, values in bold correspond for each variable to the factor for which the squared cosine is the largest, (Box-Cox transformed values).

Table 6 Factor loadings for vegetable species in relation to factors obtained for elements associations

Code	Plant species/part	F1	F2
RA 1	*Rumex acetosa* shoot	**−1.120**	−0.171
	Rumex acetosa root	−0.398	**1.489**
UD 1	*Urtica dioica* shoot	−1.129	**0.945**
	Urtica dioica root	**1.226**	0.483
SO 1	*Spinacia oleracea* shoot	**−1.044**	−0.712
	Spinacia oleracea root	**−0.608**	−0.593
RA 2	*Rumex acetosa* shoot	**−1.170**	−0.100
	Rumex acetosa root	**0.864**	0.171
UD 2	*Urtica dioica* shoot	**−1.154**	0.392
	Urtica dioica root	0.427	**−0.799**
SO 2	*Spinacia oleracea* shoot	−0.255	**−0.834**
	Spinacia oleracea root	0.225	**−0.698**
RA 3	*Rumex acetosa* shoot	**−1.250**	−0.382
	Rumex acetosa root	**0.237**	0.290
UD 3	*Urtica dioica* shoot	0.024	**2.142**
	Urtica dioica root	**3.410**	0.230
SO 3	*Spinacia oleracea* shoot	**−0.410**	−0.765
	Spinacia oleracea root	0.434	**−0.798**
RA 4	*Rumex acetosa* shoot	−0.087	**−0.208**
	Rumex acetosa root	0.212	**1.039**
UD 4	*Urtica dioicashoot*	0.208	**1.969**
	Urtica dioica root	**0.426**	0.426
SO 4	*Spinacia oleracea* shoot	0.085	**−1.371**
	Spinacia oleracea root	0.848	**−2.145**

Values in bold correspond for each observation to the factor for which the squared cosine is the largest; RA-*Rumex acetosa*, UD-*Urtica dioica*, SO-*Spinacia oleracea*, Site 1- copper mine environ and Site 2 – Former Fe-mine environ; Site 3 – reference area, non-contaminated area; Site 4 – urban area.

depend on their geogenic and anthropogenic origins. Two significant components were identified: F1 (Ag-Al-As-Ba-Cr-Fe-Li-Mg-Mn-Ni-V) and F2 (Ca-Cd-Cu-K-P-Mo-Na-Pb-Zn), as given in Table 5. The correlations of elements contents in different plant parts (shoot and root) were analyzed. The factor patterns were also examines for possible correlation with the elements' factor associations (Table 6). *R. acetosa* significantly correlates with the F1 association, which means that this species shows affinity for geogenic elements. From the other side, *U. dioica* and *S. oleracea* differ in their factor correlations, primarily depending on the environmental conditions, which mean that a specific accumulation does not occur (Table 6). Considering the sampling locations, for site 1 and 2 most of the patterns loading have significance for Factor 1, while the vegetables and herbs sampled from the urban area (site 4) have significance for Factor 2. The samples collected from the reference area (site 3) differ between F1 and F2 (Table 6).

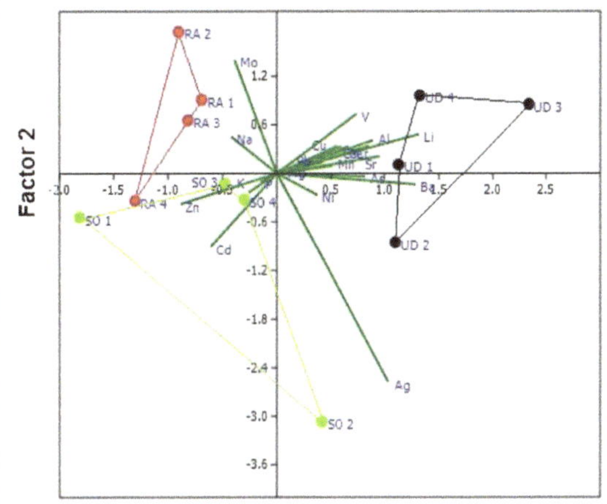

Figure 3 Principle components of vegetable species and its elements contents. RA - *Rumex acetosa;* UD - *Urtica dioica;* SO - *Spinacia oleracea;* Site 1 and 2 – polluted areas; Site 4 – urban area; Site 3 – control area, non-contaminated area.

Screen plot and PC loadings for PCA2 - plant model are presented in Figure 3. It is obvious from this model that the first two PCs explain only 64.4% of the variance. Graphical representation of the PCA2 - plant model is given on Figure 3. The two factors can well separate the three vegetables/herbs species in relation to their elements accumulation. The *R. acetosa* species occupies an area strongly correlated with higher contents of Na and Mo; there are certain natural phenomena that control the specific trend in their accumulation. The first quartile in the PCA graph confirms the specific trends in the correlation of Cd and Zn accumulation from sorrel in urban areas (Figure 3). *Spinacia oleracea* species are mainly correlated with higher contents of Zn and Cd, as given previously in Table 4, the significant correlations Cd-Zn (0.56). Common nettle (*U. dioica*) shows particular specificity for accumulation of certain elements. Some of the lithogenic elements such as Al, Cr, Li, Mn, Sr and V show specific correlation with the *U. dioica* accumulation. The samples of *S. oleracea* and *U. dioica* collected from the former Fe mine area (site 2) are characterized with specific accumulation of Ag, As, Ba and Ni. This certainly relies on the geology of the area and the specific ability of these certain species to accumulate the respective contents, despite their lower contents in the soil.

Bioavailability and translocation metals in R. acetosa, S. oleracea and U. dioica

TF, BCF and BAC values >1 had been used to evaluate the potential of plant species for phytoextraction and phytostabilization of metals in soil [7]. For the macro biogenic elements TF values were in the order of K > P

Table 7 Estimation of analyzed elements from plant species

Elements		Ag	Al	As	Ba	Ca	Cd	Cr	Cu	Fe	K	Li	Mg	Mn	Mo	Na	Ni	P	Pb	V	Zn
Translocation factor-TF																					
R. acetosa	1	2.05	0.11	0.92	0.15	0.18	0.61	0.43	0.48	0.26	**2.85**	0.66	0.91	0.88	0.75	0.21	0.57	**3.84**	**2.12**	0.01	0.92
	2	0.34	0.17	0.49	0.21	0.63	0.36	0.35	0.50	0.23	**2.01**	0.29	**1.07**	**1.43**	**1.39**	0.27	0.16	**1.04**	0.39	0.05	0.85
	3	6.20	0.11	**1.05**	0.43	**1.05**	0.90	0.21	**1.03**	0.23	**2.89**	0.34	**1.21**	**1.72**	**1.13**	0.75	0.41	**1.18**	0.41	0.01	**1.38**
	4	1.07	0.92	0.21	0.77	0.90	**1.35**	0.87	0.75	1.03	**3.90**	**1.86**	**1.70**	**2.98**	**1.23**	0.79	3.94	**1.38**	**1.39**	0.16	**1.08**
U.dioica	1	7.00	0.22	0.26	0.61	**3.49**	0.07	0.21	**1.18**	0.17	**1.46**	0.26	**1.68**	**1.60**	**4.06**	0.56	0.49	**1.12**	0.45	0.05	0.58
	2	0.05	0.35	0.58	0.52	**4.22**	0.05	0.31	**1.12**	0.39	**1.66**	0.51	**1.84**	**1.54**	**9.47**	0.94	0.44	**1.72**	0.26	0.07	0.21
	3	3.66	0.23	0.29	**1.07**	**2.93**	0.05	0.25	**4.56**	0.23	**1.34**	0.42	0.76	0.38	**1.30**	0.32	0.46	**1.03**	0.50	0.14	0.77
	4	1.16	0.81	0.98	**1.87**	**6.03**	**1.83**	0.81	**1.14**	0.80	**1.06**	0.97	0.83	0.98	**5.01**	0.56	**1.76**	0.91	**1.13**	0.45	**1.26**
S.oleracea	1	2.33	0.57	**1.01**	0.41	**1.56**	0.68	0.71	**1.35**	0.72	**1.59**	0.73	**1.09**	**1.11**	**1.52**	0.25	0.75	**1.16**	**1.31**	0.31	**2.49**
	2	0.03	0.38	**2.56**	0.60	**1.50**	**1.05**	0.46	**1.04**	0.40	**1.32**	0.53	**1.42**	**1.13**	**1.57**	0.59	**1.28**	0.98	**1.16**	0.27	**1.33**
	3	0.32	0.55	0.62	0.28	**1.23**	0.59	0.67	**1.29**	0.69	**1.17**	0.53	0.86	**1.20**	**1.93**	0.24	**1.11**	0.80	**1.09**	0.44	**1.76**
	4	1.61	0.72	**3.04**	0.67	**2.36**	0.75	0.54	**1.68**	0.59	**1.89**	**1.50**	**1.30**	**2.06**	**3.71**	0.97	0.48	0.44	**1.07**	0.39	**2.05**
Bioaccumulation factor - BAF																					
R. acetosa	1	0.49	<0.01	0.03	<0.01	0.11	0.03	<0.01	0.11	<0.01	*0.91*	0.01	0.11	0.02	0.31	0.01	0.05	**2.88**	0.02	<0.01	0.37
	2	0.01	<0.01	0.01	<0.01	0.16	0.03	0.01	0.11	<0.01	*0.96*	0.01	0.26	0.04	0.37	0.01	0.02	**1.97**	0.02	<0.01	0.37
	3	0.13	<0.01	<0.01	0.02	0.19	0.05	0.00	0.19	<0.01	**1.91**	0.01	0.15	0.02	0.12	0.01	0.01	**2.03**	<0.01	<0.01	0.28
	4	0.43	<0.01	<0.01	0.03	0.15	0.11	0.01	0.12	0.01	**1.08**	0.03	0.21	0.05	0.13	0.01	0.06	*0.71*	0.01	0.01	0.10
U.dioica	1	*0.75*	<0.01	<0.01	0.02	*0.78*	<0.01	<0.01	0.28	<0.01	*0.75*	0.01	0.11	0.15	*0.51*	0.01	0.07	**2.01**	0.02	<0.01	0.16
	2	0.01	<0.01	<0.01	0.00	*0.87*	<0.01	0.01	0.16	<0.01	*0.77*	0.01	0.13	0.05	0.38	<0.01	0.07	**3.52**	0.01	<0.01	0.49
	3	0.23	0.01	<0.01	0.07	**1.17**	<0.01	0.01	*0.94*	0.01	**1.91**	0.05	0.16	0.03	0.20	0.01	0.04	**2.24**	0.02	0.01	0.21
	4	0.07	0.01	0.02	0.05	*0.76*	0.06	0.01	0.15	0.01	**1.08**	0.03	0.15	0.03	*0.52*	0.01	0.05	*0.95*	0.01	0.01	0.10
S.oleracea	1	0.26	<0.01	0.01	0.01	0.21	0.06	<0.01	0.08	<0.01	**1.29**	0.01	0.12	0.02	0.14	0.01	0.03	**2.39**	0.02	<0.01	*0.82*
	2	0.04	<0.01	0.03	0.03	0.17	0.17	0.01	0.10	<0.01	**1.56**	0.02	0.23	0.03	0.03	<0.01	0.13	**2.99**	0.03	<0.01	*0.54*
	3	0.01	<0.01	0.01	0.01	0.12	0.12	0.01	0.28	0.01	**1.87**	0.02	0.13	0.05	0.17	<0.01	0.04	**2.85**	0.02	0.01	*0.66*
	4	0.15	<0.01	0.02	0.01	0.11	0.43	0.02	0.18	<0.01	**1.89**	0.04	0.19	0.12	0.34	0.11	0.04	*0.90*	0.01	0.01	0.36
Bioconcentrating factor (BCF)																					
R.acetosa	0.24	<0.01	0.04	0.03	*0.60*	0.05	0.01	0.24	0.01	0.32	0.02	0.12	0.02	0.41	0.03	0.09	*0.75*	0.01	0.02	*0.40*	0.24
	0.04	0.01	0.02	0.02	0.25	0.09	0.02	0.21	0.01	0.48	0.04	0.24	0.03	0.26	0.04	0.13	**1.90**	0.04	0.04	*0.42*	0.04
	0.01	<0.01	0.01	0.04	0.19	0.06	0.01	0.18	0.01	*0.66*	0.02	0.12	0.01	0.11	0.02	0.04	**1.73**	0.02	0.05	0.20	0.01
	0.04	<0.01	0.02	0.03	0.17	0.09	*0.42*	0.15	0.01	0.28	0.02	0.12	0.02	0.11	0.01	0.01	*0.51*	0.01	0.04	0.09	0.04

Table 7 Estimation of analyzed elements from plant species *(Continued)*

U.dioica	0.11	0.01	0.04	0.03	0.22	0.07	0.02	0.24	0.01	*0.51*	0.04	0.07	0.09	0.13	0.01	0.18	**1.80**	0.04	0.03	0.28	0.11
	0.23	<0.01	0.02	0.01	0.20	0.11	0.02	0.15	0.01	0.46	0.01	0.06	0.03	0.04	<0.01	0.16	**2.05**	0.03	0.02	**2.30**	0.23
	0.06	0.02	0.05	0.06	0.40	0.11	0.04	0.21	0.03	*0.66*	0.11	0.11	0.08	0.02	0.02	0.08	**2.17**	0.05	0.04	0.27	0.06
	0.06	0.01	0.02	0.02	0.13	0.03	0.02	0.13	0.01	0.48	0.03	0.10	0.03	0.01	0.02	0.03	**1.05**	0.01	0.02	0.07	0.06
S.oleracea	0.11	<0.01	0.01	0.02	0.13	0.09	0.01	0.17	0.00	*0.81*	0.02	0.11	0.02	0.09	0.06	0.04	**2.06**	0.02	0.01	*0.33*	0.11
	0.54	<0.01	0.01	0.05	0.11	0.16	0.02	0.10	0.01	**1.18**	0.03	0.16	0.03	0.02	0.01	0.10	**3.04**	0.02	0.01	*0.41*	*0.54*
	0.07	0.01	0.02	0.03	0.12	0.21	0.02	0.22	0.01	**1.60**	0.04	0.15	0.04	0.09	0.02	0.03	**3.56**	0.02	0.02	*0.37*	0.07
	<0.01	<0.01	0.01	0.02	0.11	*0.57*	0.03	0.15	0.01	**1.00**	0.02	0.15	0.06	0.01	0.11	0.09	**2.06**	0.01	0.01	0.18	<0.01

Values >1 are bolded, indicating significant efficiency; values in range of 0.50-0.99 for BAF and BCF are italic, indicating potential efficiency; 1-site 1, Cu mine environ, 2-site 2, former Fe mine environ, 3 – site 3 reference area, 4-site 4, urban area.

> Mg > Na > Ca for *R. acetosa*. For *S. Oleracea* and *U. dioica* the following order applies Ca > K > Mg > P > Na (Table 7). Regarding the lithogenic elements there are no significant variations in the TF values among all three plants species: Al (0.11-0.92); Ba (0.15-1.87); Cr (0.21-0.87); Li (0.34-1.86); Ni (0.16-1.76) and V (0.01-0.45) as given in Table 7. For molybdenum higher TF values were obtained ranging from 0.75-9.47, with emphasis on *U. dioica*. For copper, as the main anthropogenic element in the investigated area, significant TF values were obtained: for *R. acetosa* ranging from 0.48-1.30; for *U. dioica* from 1.12-4.56; and for *S. oleracea* from 1.04-1.68 (Table 7). For Cd contents in *R. acetosa* and *S. oleracea* similar TF values were obtained for all four location sites. *Urtica dioica* varies in TF for Cd, with a significant value (1.83) obtained from the urban area. The translocation factor for Pb was higher in the *R. acetosa* as plant species (2.12), considering the location site as the most polluted from the Cu mine, where As, Cd, Pb and Zn were found in higher contents in soil. Considering this, the TF values for almost all of the analyzed elements are in range from 0.1-9.5. Higher root to shoot translocation of these metals indicated that these plants have vital characteristics to be used for phytoextraction of these metals as indicated by Ghosh and Singh [12]. According to Marschner [11] and Overesch et al. [13] *R. acetosa* has the highest translocation efficiency for Ni and Cr. In the present study *R. acetosa* had higher TF values for Cd, Cu, Ni and Pb. Thus, this species could have the potential to be used for phytoextraction of the mentioned metals in potentially polluted areas. *Urtica dioica* showed potential to be used for phytoextraction only for Cu but not much specific potential for Pb, as previously investigated by Grubor [30].

The bioaccumulation factor (BAF) of the studied plant species was in the lower range (<1) for almost all of the analyzed metals (Table 7). The macro-biogenic elements for all three species had significant BAF values; for Ca in the range of 0.11-1.17, for K: 0.75-1.91, for Mg: 0.11-0.33, and for P: 0.71-2.99). The bioaccumulation factors for Cu and Zn were in the range from 0.10-0.94 and 0.10-0.84, respectively. For the other potentially hazardous metals such as As, Cd and Pb, the bioacummulation ratios ranged <0.01-0.06; <0.01-0.43 and 0.01-0.03, respectively. The maximum BAF_{Cd} and BAF_{As} for all plant species were obtained from the urban area (site 4). While the metal contents ratio root/soil for Cu, Ni, and Pb varies, no specific variations related to the sampling location were established.

Root/soil ratio (bioconcentration factor -BCF) was used for qualification of plant species for phytostabilization of contaminated soils. Regarding the bioconcentration ratios, for the majority of the elements values smaller than 1 were obtained (Table 7). The BCF values in the range of 0.1-0.50 (as potential phytostabilization) and values from 0.5-1.0 (as partial phytostabilization) should not be neglected. The BCF values for Cu were in the range from 0.10-0.24, for Zn in the range from 0.07-2.30 (the max. value was obtained for *U. dioica* at location 2). For Cd a BCF value of 0.57 was obtained for *S. oleracea* and for Cr a BCF value of 0.42 for *R. acetosa* in the urban area (Table 7). Despite the heavy metals, S. *oleracea* shows higher BCF values for K and P (1.60 and 3.56, respectively), which means that from soils that are fertilized without control, higher contents of P and K can be phytostabilized.

Conclusions

This study shows that even in lower contents in partially contaminated soil As, Cd, Cu, Ni and Pb are very extractible and available from cultivated plants. Many authors suggested that common nettle (*U. dioica*) and spinach (*S. oleracea*) are very suitable phytoextraction plants in very polluted areas, but this study revealed that common nettle (*U. dioica*), spinach (*S. oleracea*) and sorrel (*R. acetosa*) are mostly efficient for bioaccumulation of Cd and Pb in potentially polluted areas. None of the species was specified as a hyper accumulator; nevertheless all three species show potential for phytoextraction and phytostabilization of Cd, Cu, Pb and Zn. In addition, further studies are required to determine the growth performance, biomass production and metal accumulation of these species in metal contaminated soils for their better management, conservation and assurance of better food quality when growing on urban, industrial and agricultural land near mines.

Competing interests

The authors declare that they have no competing interests.

Authors' contributions

The three authors have had equal contribution to the realization of all the steps included in this scientific paper. All authors read and approved the final manuscript.

Acknowledgements

The authors would like to thank the Laboratory of Atomic Spectroscopy at the Institute of Chemistry, Faculty of Science, Ss. Cyril and Methodius University, Skopje, Republic of Macedonia, where the analysis were conducted.

Author details

[1]Faculty of Agriculture, Goce Delčev University, Krste Misirkov bb, 2000 Štip, Macedonia. [2]Institute of Chemistry, Faculty of Science, Ss. Cyril and Methodius University, Arhimedova 5, 1000 Skopje, Macedonia. [3]Research Center for Environment and Materials, Macedonian Academy of Sciences and Arts, Krste Misirkov 2, 1000 Skopje, Republic of Macedonia.

References

1. Intawongse M, Dean JR. Uptake of heavy metals by vegetable plants grown on contaminated soil and their bioavailability in the human gastrointestinal tract. Food Addit Contam A. 2006;23:36–48.

2. Mishra A, Tripathi BD. Heavy metal contamination of soil, and bioaccumulation in vegetables irrigated with treated wastewater in the tropical city of Varanasi. India Toxicol Environ Chem. 2008;90(5):861–71.
3. Malik RN, Husain SZ, Nazir I. Heavy metal contamination and accumulation in soil and wild plant species from industrial area of Islamabad, Pakistan. Pak J Bot. 2010;42:291–301.
4. Gunduz S, Uygur FN, Kahramanoğlu I. Heavy metal phytoremediation potentials of *Lepidum sativum* L., *Lactuca sativa* L., *Spinacia oleracea* L. and *Raphanus sativus* L. Her J Agric Food Sci Res. 2012;1(1):1–5.
5. Kothe E, Varma A. Bio-geo interactions in metal-contaminated soils. Berlin, Heidelberg: Springer Verlag; 2012. Springer Press.
6. Yoon J, Cao X, Zhou Q, Ma LQ. Accumulation of Pb, Cu, and Zn in native plants growing on a contaminated Florida site. Sci Total Environ. 2006;368:456–64.
7. Li MS, Luo YP, Su ZY. Heavy metal concentrations in soils and plant accumulation in a restored manganese mine land in Guangxi, South China. Environ Pollut. 2007;147:168–75.
8. Nordin N, Selamat J. Heavy metals in spices and herbs from whole sale markets in Malaysia. Food Addit Contam B. 2013;6(1):36–41.
9. Mench M, Vangronsveld J, Didier V, Clijsters H. Evaluatingof metal mobility, plant availability and immobilization by chemical agents in a limed-salty soil. Environ Pollut. 1994;86:279–86.
10. Hammer D, Keller C. Changes in the rhizosphere of heavy metal accumulating plants as evidenced by chemical extractants. J Environ Qual. 2002;31:1561–9.
11. Marschner H. Mineral nutrition of higher plants. London, UK: Elsevier Academic Press; 2002.
12. Ghosh M, Singh SP. A review on phytoremediation of heavy metals and utilization it's by products. Appl Ecol Env Res. 2005;3:1–18.
13. Overesch M, Rinklebe J, Broll G, Neue HU. Metals and arsenic in soils and corresponding vegetation at Central Elbe River flood plains (Germany). Environ Pollut. 2007;145:800–12.
14. Alloway BJ. Trace metals and metalloids in soils and their bioavailability: heavy metals in soils. London: Springer Press; 2012.
15. Ismail A, Riaz M, Akhtar S, Ismail T, Amir M, Zafar-ul-Hye M. Heavy metals in vegetables and respective soils irrigated by canal, municipal waste and tube-well waters. Food Addit Contam B. 2014. doi:10.1080/19393210.2014.88878.
16. Balabanova B, Stafilov T, Bačeva K, Šajn R. Biomonitoring of atmospheric pollution with heavy metals in the copper mine vicinity located near Radoviš, Republic of Macedonia. J Environ Sci Heal A. 2010;45:1504–18.
17. Balabanova B, Stafilov T, Šajn R, Bačeva K. Characterisation of heavy metals in lichen species *Hypogymnia physodes* and *Evernia prunastri* due to biomonitoring of air pollution in the vicinity of copper mine. Int J Environ Res. 2012;6:779–94.
18. Balabanova B, Stafilov T, Šajn R, Bačeva K. Spatial distribution and characterization of some toxic metals and lithogenic elements in top soil and sub soil from copper mine environs. Inter J Environ Protec. 2013;3:1–9.
19. Stafilov T, Balabanova B, Šajn R, Bačeva K, Boev B. Geochemical atlas of Radoviš and the environs and the distribution of heavy metals in air. Skopje: Faculty of Natural Science and Mathematics; 2010.
20. Manara A. Plant responses to heavy metal toxicity. In: Furini A, editor. Plants and heavy metals. London: Springer; 2012.
21. Bačeva K, Stafilov T, Matevski V. Bioaccumulation of heavy metals by endemic Viola species from the soil in the vicinity of the As-Sb-Tl mine "Allchar", Republic of Macedonia. Int J Phytoremediat. 2013;16:247–365.
22. Box GEP, Cox DR. An analysis of transformations. J R Stat Soc B. 1964;26(2):211–52.
23. Zhang CS, Zhang SA. Robust-symmetric mean: a new way of mean calculation for environmental data. Geo J. 1996;40:209–12.
24. Filzmoser P, Garrett RG, Reimann C. Multivariate outlier detection in exploration geochemistry. Comput Geo Sci. 2005;31:579–87.
25. Žibret G, Šajn R. Hunting for geochemical associations of elements: factor analysis and self-organizing maps. Math Geosci. 2010;42:681–703.
26. Gergen I, Harmanescu M. Application of principal component analysis in the pollution assessment with heavy metals of vegetable food chain in the old mining areas. Chem Cent J. 2012;6:156–69.
27. Cui S, Zhou Q, Chao L. Potential hyper-accumulation of Pb, Zn, Cu and Cd in endurant plants distributed in an old smelter, northeast China. Environ Geo. 2007;51:1043–8.
28. Salminen R, Batista MJ, Bidovec M, Demetriades A, De Vivo B, De Vos W, et al. Geochemical atlas of Europe. Part 1 – Background information, methodology and maps. Espoo, Finland: Geological survey of Finland; 2005. p. 526. ISBN 951-690-921-3.
29. Official gazette of the R. Macedonia, No. 118, 2005. Rules on general requirements for food safety. Skopje: Sluzben vesnik na R.M; 2005. p. 30. in Macedonian.
30. Grubor M. Lead uptake, tolerance, and accumulation exhibited by the plants *Urtica dioica* and *Sedum spectabile* in contaminated soil without additives. Arch Biol Sci 2008. 2008;60(2):239–44.

Hydrodynamic and kinetic study of a hybrid detoxification process with zero liquid discharge system in an industrial wastewater treatment

Mohammad Fadhil Abid*, Amir Aziz Abdulrahman and Noor Hussein Hamza

Abstract

This work focused on the degradation of toxic organic compounds such as methyl violet dye (MV) in water, using a combined photocatalysis/low pressure reverse osmosis (LPRO) system. The performance of the hybrid system was investigated in terms of the degradation efficiency of MV, COD and membrane separation of TiO_2. The aim of the present study was to design a novel solar reactor and analyze its performance for removal of MV from water with titanium dioxide as the photocatalyst. Various operating parameters were studied to investigate the behavior of the designed reactor like initial dye concentration (C = 10-50 mg/L), loading of catalyst (C_{TiO2} = 200-800 mg/L), suspension flow rate (Q_L = 0.3-1.5 L/min), pH of suspension (5–10), and H_2O_2 concentration (C_{H2O2} = 200-1000 mg/L). The operating parameters were optimized to give higher efficiency to the reactor performance. Optimum parameters of the photocatalysis process were loading of catalyst (400 mg/L), suspension flow rate (0.5 L/min), H_2O_2 concentration (400 mg/L), and pH = 5. The designed reactor when operating at optimum conditions offered a degradation of MV up to 0.9527 within one hours of operation time, while a conversion of 0.9995 was obtained in three hours. The effluent from the photocatalytic reactor was fed to a LPRO separation system which produced permeate of turbidity value of 0.09 NTU which is closed to that of drinking water (i.e., 0.08 NTU). The product water was analyzed using UV-spectrophotometer and FTIR. The analysis results confirmed that the water from the Hybrid-System could be safely recycled and reuse. It was found that the kinetics of dye degradation was first order with respect to dye concentration and could be well described by Langmuir-Hinshelwood model. A power-law based empirical correlation was developed for the photocatalysis system, related the dye degradation (R) with studied operating conditions.

Keywords: Solar photocatalysis, Membrane separation, Hybrid system, Zero liquid discharge, Titanium dioxide photocatalyst, Dye synthetic wastewater, Falling-film slurry reactor

Introduction

Pollution of ground water and rivers by organic pollutants is a constant concern and a common problem throughout the world. Some of these organic pollutants are; herbicides, pesticides, and fungicides used in agricultural activities, which can be carried away by rain and polluted water resources, hydrocarbons from wastewater discharges from oil production activities and synthetic dyes from textile industry's waste processing fluids [1]. Textile dyes and other commercial colorants have become as toxic organic compounds the focus of environmental remediation efforts because of their natural biodegradability is made increasingly difficult owing to the improved properties of dyestuffs [2]. Color interferes with penetration of sunlight into the water, retards photosynthesis, inhibits the growth of aquatic biota and interferes with solubility in water bodies [3]. Various physical, chemical and biological pretreatment and post-treatment techniques have been developed over the last two decades to remove color from dye contaminated wastewater in order to cost effectively meet environmental regulatory requirements. Chemical and biological treatments have been conventionally followed till now but these treatment methods have their own disadvantages. The aerobic treatment process is associated with production and disposal of large amounts of biological sludge, while wastewater treated by, anaerobic treatment method does not bring down the pollution parameters the satisfactory level [4]. As international environmental standards are

* Correspondence: dr_mfa@uotechnology.edu.iq
Chemical Engineering Department, University of Technology, Baghdad, Iraq

becoming more stringent, (ISO 14001, 1996), a technological system for the removal of organic pollutants, such as dyes has to be developed. Heterogeneous photocatalysis is one of the advanced oxidation process (AOP) that has proven to be a promising method for the elimination of toxic and bio-resistant organic and inorganic compounds in wastewater by transforming them into innocuous species [5,6]. Advanced oxidation process (AOP) is a chemical oxidative process, which can be applied to wastewater treatment to oxidize pollutants. It generates hydroxyl radicals which considered as the second strongest known oxidant (2.8 V vs. standard hydrogen electrode). It is able to oxidize and mineralize almost every organic molecule, yielding CO_2 and inorganic ions [7]. AOPs not only oxidized the organic compounds, but also a complete mineralization is achievable, and the processes are not specific and therefore are capable of destroying a broad range of organic compounds. The process is very powerful, and is immune to organic toxicity. In the eighties and nineties, water reuse started to become a popular means to reduce freshwater intake and reduce treatment costs. A concept that refers to closed circuits of water, such that disposal is eliminated. Advantages and disadvantages of zero discharge facilities are currently being seriously considered and discussed. Zero liquid discharge minimizes the consumption of freshwater to that of make-up; therefore, it should help relieve freshwater availability limitations in places where it is scarce or expensive [8]. In photocatalytic degradation of dyes in wastewaters, the main operating parameters which affect the process are pH of the solution to be degraded, oxidizing agent, catalyst loading, and contaminant concentration [9]. Photocatalytic reactions are the result of the interaction of photons having the appropriate wavelength with a solid semiconductor [10]. Recent studies have been devoted to the use of photocatalysis in the removal of dyes from wastewaters, particularly, because of the ability of this method to completely mineralize the target pollutants [11].

The general mechanism of photocatalysis could be represented elsewhere [12-14]. Many semiconductors have been tested so far as photocatalysts, although only TiO_2 in the anatase form seems to have the most interesting required attributes; such as high stability, good performance and low cost [15]. In this respect, the photodecomposition power of TiO_2, for a wide variety of organic compounds present in water, has been reported in the literature [16].

Photocatalytic reactors for water treatment can generally be classified into two main configurations, depending on the deployed state of the photocatalysts: (1) reactors with suspended photocatalyst particles and (2) reactors with photocatalyst immobilised onto continuous inert carrier [17]. Various types of reactors have been used in the photocatalytic water treatment, including the annular slurry photoreactor [18], cascade photoreactor [19], downflow contactor reactor [20] and, etc. The disparity between these two main configurations is that the first one requires an additional downstream separation unit for the recovery of photocatalyst particles while the latter permits a continuous operation. Vincenzo et al. [21] carried out a photodegradation of two common and very stable azo-dyes, in aqueous suspensions of polycrystalline TiO2 irradiated by sunlight using a plug flow reactor in a total recirculation loop. They reported that Complete decolourization was obtained in few hours for both dyes but mineralisation occurred after longer times with the formation of CO2, nitrates and sulphates. Damszel et al. [22] investigated the possibility of application of the hybrid photocatalysis/membrane processes system for removal of azo dyes (Acid Red 18, Direct Green 99 and Acid Yellow 36) from water. The photocatalytic reactions were conducted in the flow reactor with immobilized photocatalyst bed and in the suspended system integrated with ultrafiltration (UF). They found that the solutions containing the model azo dyes could be successfully decolorized during the photocatalytic processes applied in the studies. The application of UF process results in separation of photocatalyst from the treated solutions whereas during the (NF) and membrane distillation (MD) high retention of degradation products was obtained.

The main objectives of this work were the evaluation and testing of a novel photocatalytic reactor for the degradation of methyl violet (MV) dye which is selected as a model organic toxic pollutant in water using a commercial TiO_2 catalyst. And also to study the possibility to couple a membrane separation system with the reaction system, to remove TiO_2 particles from product stream of the solar photocatalytic reactor to achieve a zero liquid discharge.

Materials and methods

Chemicals

Methyl violet 6B (MV) dye (commercial grade, $C_{24}H_{28}N_3Cl$, λmax (nm) = 586, Sigma Aldrich Co., USA.), Titanium dioxide powder (antase type, ≥99.5% trace metals basis, particle size ~ 21 nm, specific surface area (35–65 m^2/g), particle density (4.26 g/mL (at 25°C)), Sigma Aldrich Co.) were used as received. Reagent-grade hydrogen peroxide (H_2O_2) (50% v/v solution), was used as oxidant. Technical grade hydrochloric acid (35%) and sodium hydroxide (98% flakes) were used to adjust the pH of synthetic wastewater (to around 5–10). Distilled water (conductivity <10 μS cm^{-1}, Cl^- = 0.7–0.8 mg L^{-1}, $NO3^-$ = 0.5 mg L^{-1}, organic carbon <0.5 mg L^{-1}).

Analytical determinations

Mineralization was followed by measuring, the color which is a function of concentration was determined spectrophotometrically at a dominate wave length by method no. 2120 Standard Method, using a Shimadzu UV -Visible spectrophotometer (UB_1201 PC). COD was determined by open reflux method 5220 Standard Method (ET 108). FTIR (Bruker Tensor 27) system was used to identify the functional groups in product solutions with aid of (Figure 1). Turbidity of water treated by membrane system (LPRO) was measured by Turbid Direct meter (Lovibond). The sunlight intensity was measured by using Davis 6152C Vantage Pro2 Weather Station radiometer. Table 1 shows a sample of incident solar radiation measurements. Calibration curves of dye concentration vs. light absorbency and TiO_2 concentration vs. turbidity were illustrated in (Figures 2 and 3), respectively.

Experiment set-up

The hybrid process setup consists of two treatment systems connected together. Figure 4 shows the schematic view of the (photocatalysis reaction/LPRO membrane) system. The photocatalytic reactor was operated as a batch process. The system consists of a solar reactor (no.5), wastewater preparation tank (no.1) made of 5 L-PVC, a circulation pump (no.2), Type: In–line centrifugal pump (Wtg204), Head (H) = (25–40) m, variable impeller speed (750, 1200, 1850 min^{-1}), V = 220 volt). The solar reactor was mounted on a fixed platform tilted 37° (local latitude) and directed south-east. It was made up of a flat-plate colorless glass of dimensions 1000 × 750 × 4 mm. The base of the reactor was made of aluminum. This geometry enables the light entering the liquid film from almost any direction to be reflected and can also be employed for the photocatalytic reaction. The circulating pump was used to feed the water from the tank to the reactor via a calibrated flow meter (no.3). The aqueous solution was allowed to trickle down freely from a pipe (no.6) pierced by several openings placed at the top of the reactor. The water and reagents added to the tank from openings in the lid. A thermocouple type (pt-100) was placed into the water preparation tank to measure the mixture temperature. A mechanical mixer was used to obtain homogeneous conditions in the water tank. In the present work, the pH of the effluent from the photocatalytic reactor was neutralized in a 5 L vessel (no.7) and then left for 4 hours. The sediment was washed with H_2O_2, dried, and weighted for further use. The neutralized solution was fed to a 5 L PVC tank (no.8) which served as a feeding tank to the low pressure reverse osmosis membrane (LPRO) type (RE1812-CSM Co.) which was used to separate the TiO_2 nanoparticles from the photoreactor effluent via a diaphram pump (no.14), (type CR50-N-N-2, single phase: 50 Hz, 220 V). The (LPRO) was a spiral wound module made of composite polyamide with an effective area of 0.7 m^2. The separation system also contained two holding tanks, all are made of PVC, these are the concentrate tank (no.18), and the permeate tank (no.17). Each tank is supplied with suitable fittings and connections to serve the process. Laboratory portable conductivity and pH meters from Hanna-USA were used for further check and quick measurements.

Experimental design

Photocatalytic reactor experiments were aimed to study the effect of operating parameters (catalyst loading, hydrogen peroxide concentration, flow rate, pH, and dye concentration) on the degradation efficiency and COD removal of organic pollutant. Table 2 shows the range of operating variables that used in photocatalytic experiment.

Results and discussion

Effect of operating parameters on dye degradation and COD removal in photocatalytic reactor

Effect of pH

pH is an important parameter for the photocatalytic process, and it is of interest to study its influence on the degradation rate of the MV dye. (Figures 5 and 6) illustrate the variation of dye degradation rate against

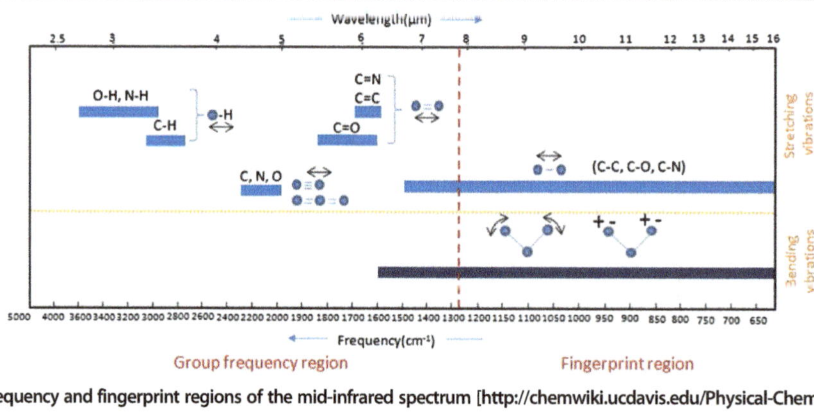

Figure 1 Group frequency and fingerprint regions of the mid-infrared spectrum [http://chemwiki.ucdavis.edu/Physical-Chemistry/Spectroscopy].

Table 1 Average daily incident solar radiation (kWh m^{-2}) on 37° inclined surface at University of Technology-Baghdad

No.	Average daily global incident solar radiation, kWh. m^{-2}	Average daily UV incident solar radiation, kWh.m^{-2}	Month
1	5.7	0.456	May
2	6.8	0.544	June
3	5.7	0.456	July
4	4.5	0.36	August
5	5.9	0.472	September

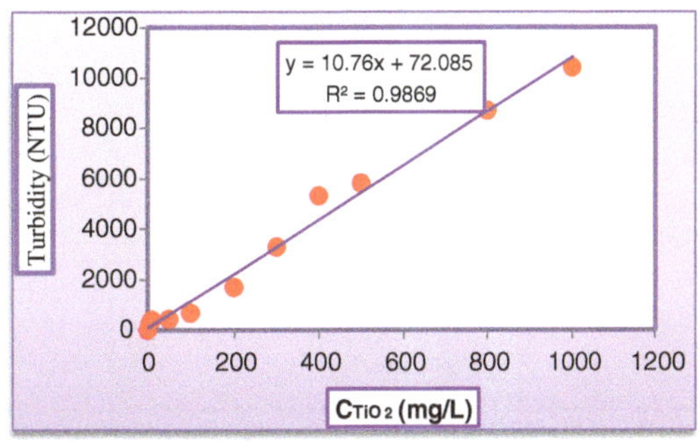

Figure 3 Calibration curve of Turbidity for various TiO_2 loadings in water.

illuminated time and the variation of COD in reactor effluent against pH after 180 min, respectively. Results obtained experimentally by varying initial pH of polluted solution from 5 to 10 with keeping all other parameters unchanged at (C_{MV} = 30 mg/L, $C_{TiO2=}$ 400 mg/L, Q_L = 0.5 L/min) clearly indicated a neat decrease in dye degradation. It could be noticed from (Figure 5) that the final degradation obtained in acidic solution at pH equal 5 was 99.95% and at pH = 6 it was 95.22% while at pH = 7, pH = 9, and pH = 10, the final degradation efficiency were 72.2%, 60.98%, and 48.2%, respectively. At the same condition, Figure 6 indicated that COD removal was 99.9% after 180 min of operation. This could be explained from the surface charge of TiO_2 point of view. In acidic pH, the surface of TiO_2 acquires a positive charge thereby attracting the anionic MV dye, leading to a greater adsorption and hence increasing the degradation rate and COD removal in the acidic media. However, the reverse image is observed in the basic medium where the TiO_2 surface was negatively charged which repels the dye molecules away from the surface of the catalyst thereby decreasing the degradation rate. The adsorption is maxima at pH 5 and so is the degradation rate and COD removal. The change of the surface properties of TiO_2 with the change of pH values around its point of zero charge (pH_{pzc}) is according to the following reaction [23]:

$$TiOH + H^+ \rightleftarrows TiOH_2^+ \quad pH < pH_{pzs} \tag{1}$$

$$TiOH + OH^- \rightleftarrows TiO^- \quad pH > pH_{pzs} \tag{2}$$

pH changes can thus influence the adsorption of dye molecules onto the TiO_2 surface, an important step for the photooxidation to take place. For Degussa P25, the pH_{pzc} is around 5.8 to 6.9. So, when pH <6 a strong adsorption of MV on the TiO_2 particles is observed as a result of the electrostatic attraction of the positively charged TiO_2 with the dye. In our case the highest degradation efficiency was achieved at pH = 5. In alkaline solution, the MV molecules are negatively charged and their adsorption is also expected to be affected by an increase in the density of TiO^- groups on the semiconductor surface. Thus, due to Coulombic repulsion, substrate is scarcely adsorbed. At high pH values, hydroxyl radicals are so rapidly scavenged that they do not have the opportunity to react with dyes [24,25]. For the above reasons the photocatalytic activity of anionic dyes reached a maximum in acidic conditions followed by a decrease in the pH range 7–10 [26].

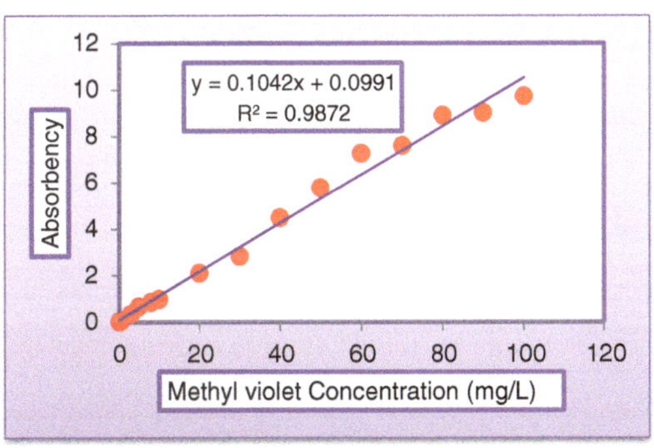

Figure 2 Calibration curve of methyl violet dye.

Effect of hydrogen peroxide (H_2O_2)

The addition of H_2O_2 may play an important role in the limitation rate of photogenerated hole–electron pairs which had been attributed to degradation rate and COD removal of the MV dyes. (Figures 7 and 8) plot the variation of dye degradation against H_2O_2 concentration in solution keeping all other parameters unchanged and COD removal in reactor effluent after 180 min at the same operating conditions, respectively. Different concentrations of H_2O_2 (300 to 1000 mg/L) were added to study the effect of H_2O_2 concentration on the decolorization rate and COD removal. As can be seen, the removal rate increased with increasing initial concentration of H_2O_2. The decolorization rate was slow at low H_2O_2 concentration, as the formation of

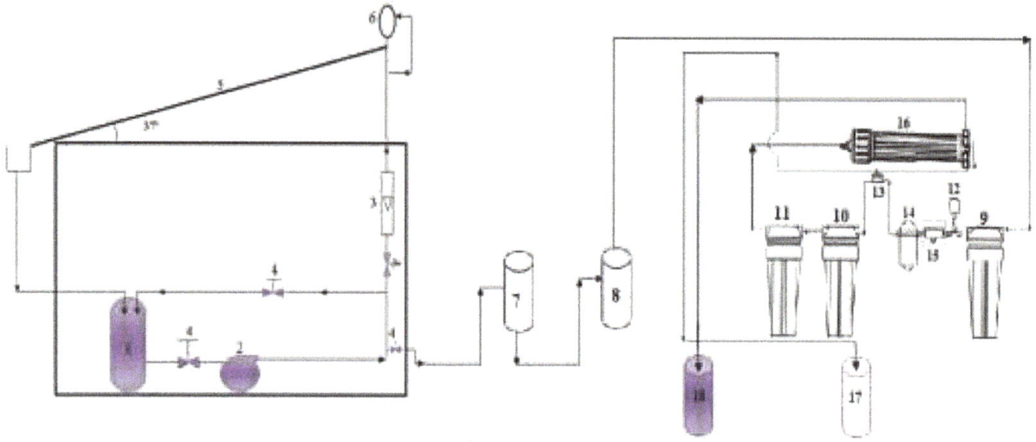

Figure 4 **1- Feed tank to reactor; 2- Feeding pump; 3- Rotameter; 4- Valve; 5- Flate plate reactor; 6- Liquid distributo; r 7- Neutralization tank; 8- Feed tank to membrane; 9- 5micron PP filter; 10&11- Buffer vessels; 12- Low pressure switch 13- Auto shut off 14- Booster pump; 15- Inlet solenoid valve; 16- LPRO membrane; 17- Permeate tank; 18- Concentrate tank.**

hydroxyl radicals was insufficient, this may be explained the ability of H_2O_2 to trapping the electrons preventing the electron–hole recombination and hence increasing the chance of formation of $OH^{\bullet}$ radicals on the surface of the catalyst [27]. However, as the initial concentration of H_2O_2 increased beyond a certain value (400 mg/L, the increasing in decomposition rate becomes less. This because at higher H_2O_2 concentration, more $OH^{\bullet}$ was produced leading to a faster oxidation rate. However, these excess free radicals preferred to react with the excess of H_2O_2 rather than with the dye [28]. As shown in Figure 8, the addition of H_2O_2 (400 mg/L) to the dispersed solution resulted in a significant increase on the removal of COD. At the end of 180 min. of irradiation, almost total removal (99.5%) was obtained. When H_2O_2 concentration was increased to 1000 mg/L, COD reduction was only 87.4%. It seems that Hydrogen peroxide played a dual role in photocatalytic reaction, it is acting as an electron acceptor and could decompose to produce $OH^{\bullet}$ radicals [6]. It is clear from Figure 9 that the rate of degradation goes on increasing with increased concentration of H_2O_2 and approached maxima at 400 mg/L and then started to decrease with further increase in concentration of H_2O_2. The optimum hydrogen peroxide concentration for the

Table 2 Range of operating variables in photocatalytic experiment

Operating parameter	Range
Catalyst loading (TiO_2), mg/L	200, 300, 400, 500, 800
Hydrogen peroxide concentration, mg/L	300, 400, 500, 800, 1000
Flow rate, L/min	0.3, 0.5, 1, 1.5
pH	5, 6, 7, 9, 10
Dye concentration, mg/L	10,20, 30, 40, 50

degradation of MV dye is 400 mg/L. This amount of H_2O_2 will be employed into all experiments. (Figure 5) through (Figure 9) depict that the decolourization rates under UV/H2O2 decreased with increasing pH. In alkaline condition, H2O2 will decompose into water and oxygen rather than hydroxyl radicals. This causes the lower decolourization rates of azo dyes at higher pH values because the concentration of OH- is reduced under these conditions. The decolourization rate was increasingly less effective at pH values higher than 8, while acidic conditions achieve a more effective decolourization These results were confirmed by the findings of [29-32].

Effect of liquid flow rate

Falling–film reactors characterized by a high ratio of exposure (surface area to liquid volume), which positively impact the performance of such type of reactors. Flow rate of synthetic wastewater is another important parameter which must be considered. Effect of liquid flow rate on the dye degradation and COD removal was tested by taking various flow rates from (0.3 to 1.5 L/min) keeping all other parameters unchanged at (C_{MV} = 30 mg/L, C_{TiO_2} = 400 mg/L, $C_{H_2O_2}$ = 400 mg/L, and pH = 5). Figure 10 illustrates the variation of the dye degradation against illuminated time. As can be seen from Figure 10 that liquid flow rate has negative impact on degradation rate. This may be explained from the view point of shorter contact time of aqueous suspension with illumination source as the recirculation rate increased. Figure 11 illustrates the influence of liquid flow rate on the COD of the reactor effluent. It can be concluded from the graph that effluent with 0.5 L/min has undergone almost complete degradation at 180 min of solar exposure which indicated that resulted water could be recycled in the process. When the liquid

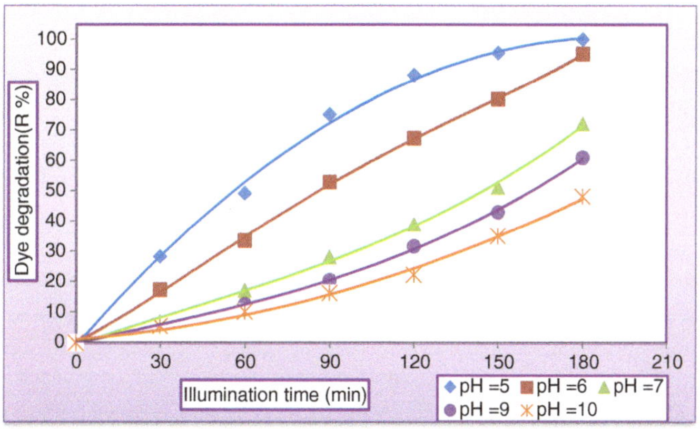

Figure 5 Variation of dye degradation against illuminated time at different pH (C_{MV} = 30 mg/L, C_{TiO2} = 400 mg/L, C_{H2O2} = 400 mg/L, and Q_L = 0.5 L/min).

flow rate increased to 1.5 L/min, COD of the reactor effluent has dropped to 241 mg/L which indicates the necessity for further light exposure. This could be firstly due to the limitation of the solar light penetration because of rise in the liquid thickness and secondly to the reduction of the residence time of substrate which lead to reduce the surface reaction efficiency. Figure 12 shows dye degradation against Reynolds number of the liquid falling–film. The liquid Reynolds number N_{Re} can be calculated from equation (3) [33].

$$N_{Re} = 4Q_L\rho_L/W\mu_L\cos\beta \tag{3}$$

where Q_L = Liquid flow rate (m^3/s), ρ_L = Density of water (kg/m^3), W = Width of reactor, μ_L = Dynamic viscosity of water (kg/m. s), and β = altitude angle. As can be seen, the impact of liquid Reynolds number on dye degradation shows a positively increasing trend to a point where all the surface of the photocataytic reactor was covered with a thin falling–film of synthetic wastewater, where dye degradation reported 99.95% at N_{Re} = 69.2 after then dye degradation started to decrease with further increasing of liquid flow rate at N_{Re} = 138.4, N_{Re} = 207.6, and N_{Re} = 276.6 the dye degradation were 82.3%, 64.4%, and 40.32%, respectively. This may be attributed to decreasing the residence time of reactants as the liquid flow rate increased.

Effect of initial dye concentration

The effect of initial concentration of dye solution on dye degradation efficiency has been investigated by varying the dye concentrations from (10 to 50 mg/L). Figure 13 plots the variation of dye degradation against (MV) dye concentration in the presence of 400 mg TiO_2/L under solar light by keeping all other parameters unchanged. As can be seen from Figure 13 that after 180 min of irradiation time the degradation rate was 99.99%, 99.97%, 99.95%, 93.2%, and 91.52% at concentration of MV equal

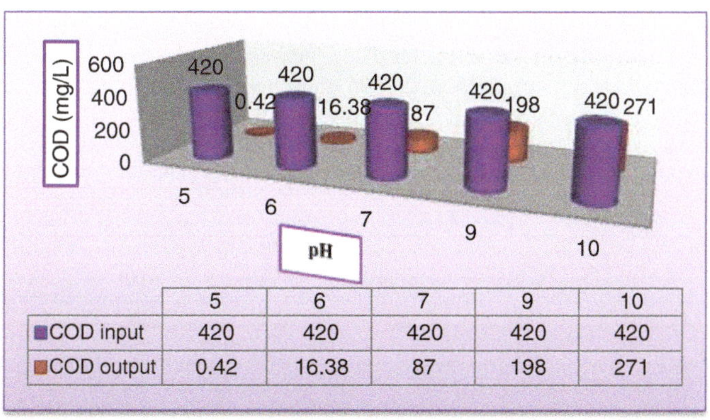

Figure 6 Effect pH on COD removal (C_{MV} = 30 mg/L, C_{TiO2} = 400 mg/L, C_{H2O2} = 400 mg/L, and Q_L = 0.5 L/min) after 180 min.

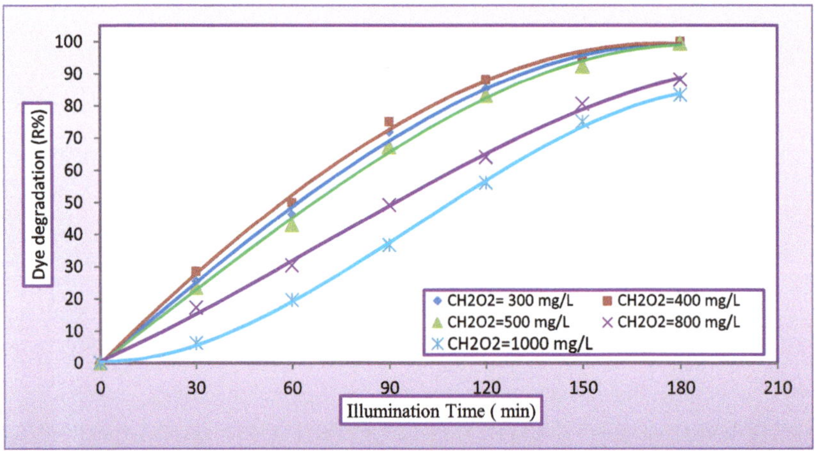

Figure 7 **Variation of dye degradation with illuminated time at different concentration of H_2O_2 (C_{MV} = 30 mg/L, C_{TiO2} = 400 mg/L, pH = 5, and Q_L = 0.5 L/min).**

to (10, 20, 30, 40, and 50 mg/L), respectively. Dye degradation was observed to decrease as initial concentration increased. It could be concluded from the present experiments that as the dye concentration increases, the fraction of un-adsorbed dye in the solution increases, leading to lesser penetration of light through the solution onto the surface of TiO_2, thereby decreasing the rate of formation of OH radicals, consequently the degradation efficiency decreased. However, the reverse image is observed at lower substrate concentration, where the light intensity and time of irradiation is same but interception of the photons to the catalyst surface is increased leading to the formation of more numbers of OH radicals, thereby increasing the rate of reaction. This concludes that as the initial concentration of the dye increases, the requirement of catalyst surface needed for the degradation also increases. Our results were confirmed by the findings of many researchers [25,26].

Effect of catalyst loading

The amount of catalyst is one of the main parameters for the degradation studies from economical point of view. To investigate the effect of the photocatalyst, its loading in the dispersion was varied between (200 to 800 mg/L) under UV light. Figure 14 shows the variation of dye degradation (R %) against illuminated time for various photocatalyst loading by keeping all other parameters unchanged. As can be seen, at a specified catalyst loading the degradation efficiency appeared to increase rapidly at the first part of experimental period while the rate of increase seems to be slower at the second part. This may be due to the concentration of the

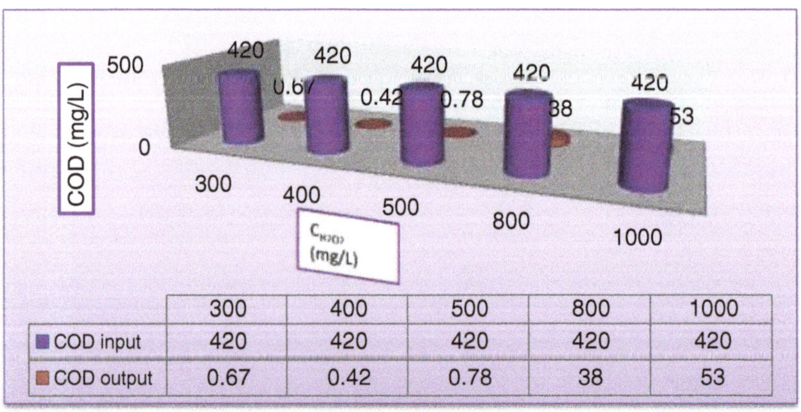

	300	400	500	800	1000
COD input	420	420	420	420	420
COD output	0.67	0.42	0.78	38	53

Figure 8 **Variation of COD removal in reactor effluent at different concentration of H_2O_2 (C_{MV} = 30 mg/L, C_{TiO2} = 400 mg/L, pH = 5, and Q_L = 0.5 L/min) after 180 min.**

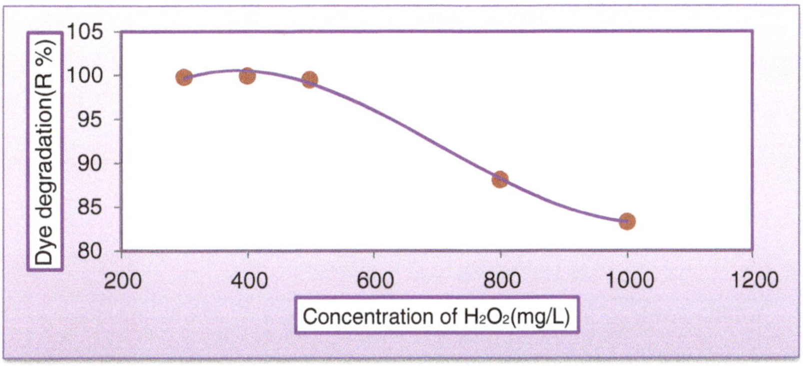

Figure 9 Variation of dye degradation with concentration of H_2O_2 (C_{MV} = 30 mg/L, C_{TiO2} = 400 mg/L, pH = 5, and Q_L = 0.5 L/min) after 180 min.

dye which is higher at the beginning of the photo-degradation process resulted in high rate of reaction and dye concentration decreases as the reaction proceeds. Figure 14 demonstrates a positive impact of catalyst concentration on dye degradation; this trend was almost due the increase of active site with absorption and dye adsorption. Our results were in agreements with the findings of [25,34]. In order to avoid the use of excess catalyst it is necessary to find out the optimum loading for efficient removal of dye. Figure 15 illustrates the optimum catalyst concentration for the degradation of MV dye after 180 min of treatment process. From Figure 15 it was observed that as catalyst concentration increased from (200 to 400 mg/L) the degradation rate increases correspondingly, this can be explained by the fact that there was an increased in the photon adsorption with increased concentration. The degradation rate decreased as the catalyst loading increased from (400 to 800) mg/L, this phenomenon may be explained by the light scattering, caused by the lightproof suspended catalyst [25,28].

Photocatalysis kinetics

The photocatalytic oxidation kinetics of many organic compounds has often been modeled with the Langmuir–Hinshelwood equation, which also covers the adsorption properties of the substrate on the photocatalyst surface. This model, developed by [35,36], is expressed as equation (4):

$$r = -dC/dt = k_r KC/(1 + KC) \quad (4)$$

where r is the reaction rate (mg/L.min), k_r the reaction rate constant (mg/L.min), K the adsorption equilibrium constant (L/mg) and C the concentration of dye (mg/L).

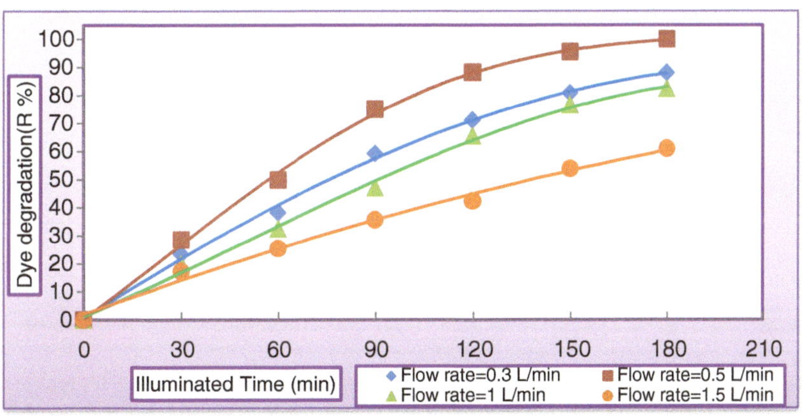

Figure 10 Variation of dye degradation with illuminated time at different liquid flow rate (C_{MV} = 30 mg/L, C_{TiO2} = 400 mg/L, pH = 5, and C_{H2O2} = 400 mg/L).

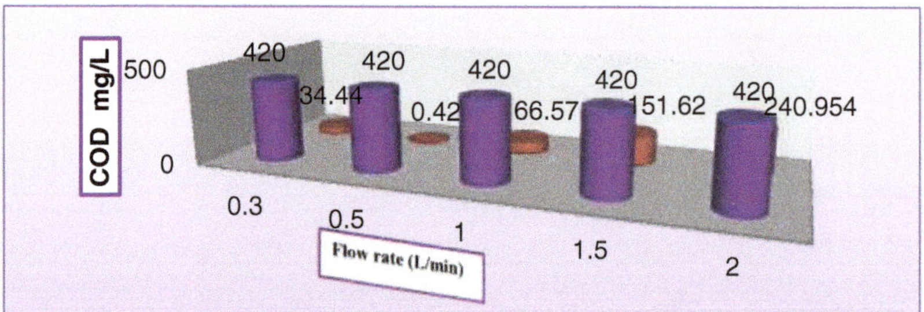

	0.3	0.5	1	1.5	2
COD input	420	420	420	420	420
COD output	34.44	0.42	66.57	151.62	240.954

Figure 11 Effect of liquid flow rate on COD removal in reactor effluent (C_{MV} = 30 mg/L, C_{TiO2} = 400 mg/L, pH = 5, and C_{H2O2} = 400 mg/L) after 180 min.

The degradation rate of dye was studied as a function of the initial dye concentration in the range (10 to 50 mg/L), for a catalyst loading of TiO_2 (0.4 mg/L). The results were illustrated in Figure 16 which shows the initial dye concentration versus reactor operating time. Equation (5) depicts a pseudo–first order reaction with respect to the methyl violet (MV) concentration. The relationship between the initial degradation rate (r_o) and the initial concentration of organic substrate for a heterogeneous photocatalytic degradation process has been described by Langmuir–Hinshelwood model and can be written as follows: if we consider that the kinetic of dye degradation is of pseudo-order, at t = 0 and $C = C_o$, equation (4) becomes:

$$r_o = k_r K C_o/(1 + K C_o) \quad (5)$$

This Equation can be rearranged into linear form:

$$1/r_o = (1/k_r K).1/C_o + 1/k_r \quad (6)$$

where $1/r_o$ and $1/C_o$ are the dependent and independent variables, respectively, $1/k_r$ is the intercept and $(1/k_r K)$ is the slope of the straight line shown in Figure 17. The L-H adsorption constant and the rate constant were obtained using initial rate method [37] by plotting $1/r_o$ versus $1/C_o$. The values of the adsorption equilibrium constant, K and the kinetic rate constant of surface reaction, k_r were calculated. The graphical representation of equation (6) yields a straight line as shown in Figure 17 indicating a pseudo-first order reaction. The reaction rate constants k_r for photocatalytic degradation of dye

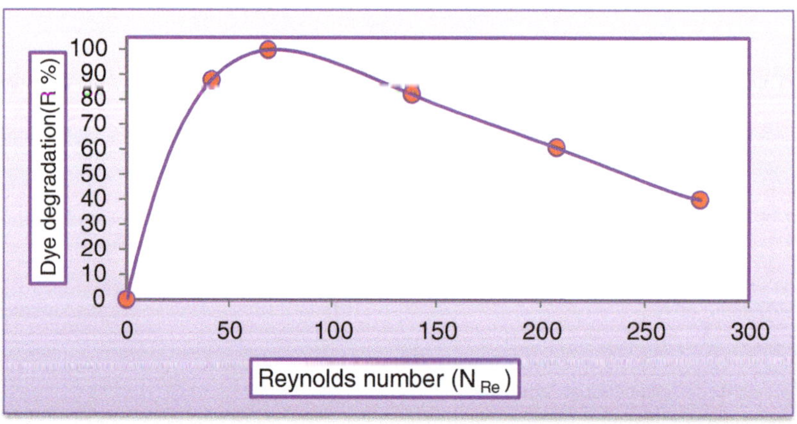

Figure 12 Variation of dye degradation with liquid Reynolds numbers (C_{MV} = 30 mg/L, C_{H2O2} = 400 mg/L, C_{TiO2} = 400 mg/L, and pH = 5) after 180 min.

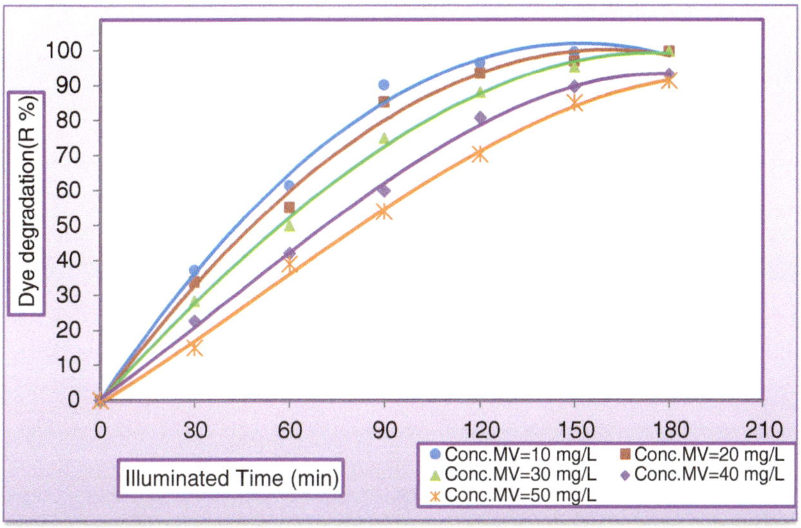

Figure 13 **Variation of dye degradation with illuminated time at different concentrations of MV dye (C_{H2O2} = 400 mg/L, C_{TiO2} = 400 mg/L, and pH = 5, Q_L = 0.5 L/min and pH = 5).**

were evaluated from experimental data Figure 17 using a linear regression. The constants k_r and K in Langmuir–Hinshelwood model were obtained as 0.791 mg/L. min and 0.0209 L/mg, respectively. The correlation coefficient R^2 was equal to 0.9892 then equation (6) will become

$$r = 0.0165C/(1 + 0.0209C) \quad (7)$$

Empirical correlation

Dye degradation at each average seasonal temperature is the result of the interaction of several parameters, namely: catalyst concentration (C_{TiO2}) Hydrogen peroxide concentration (C_{H2O2}), pH of solution, liquid flow rate (Q_L) and dye concentration (C_{MV}). A power law formula was proposed to correlate the present experimental results with dye removal of Methyl violet dye. Equation (8) represents the proposed empirical correlation:

$$R = a_o(C_{TiO2})^{a1}(C_{H2O2})^{a2}(pH)^{a3}(Q_L)^{a4}(C_{MV})^{a5} \quad (8)$$

where: a_1, a_2, a_3, a_4, and a_5 are constants, representing the magnitudes of the effect of applied catalyst concentration, hydrogen peroxide concentration, pH solution, liquid flow rate, and dye concentration, respectively on the objective function (i.e., dye degradation), while a_o is a constant which depends on the nature of the operating system.

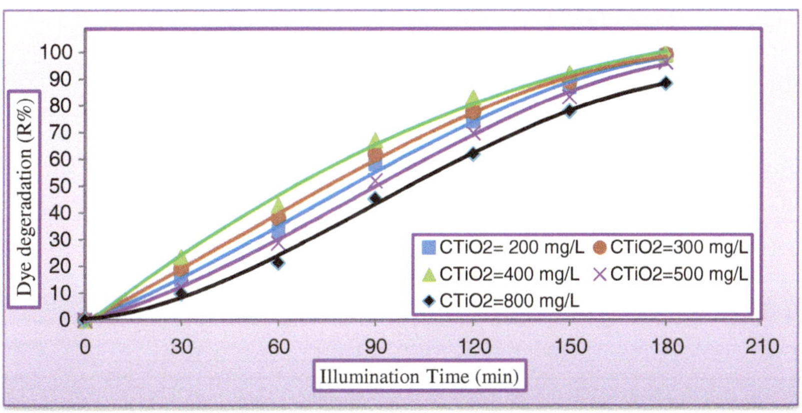

Figure 14 **Variation of dye degradation against time at different concentration of TiO_2 (C_{MV} = 30 mg/L, C_{H2O2} = 500 mg/L, pH = 5, and Q_L = 0.5 L/min).**

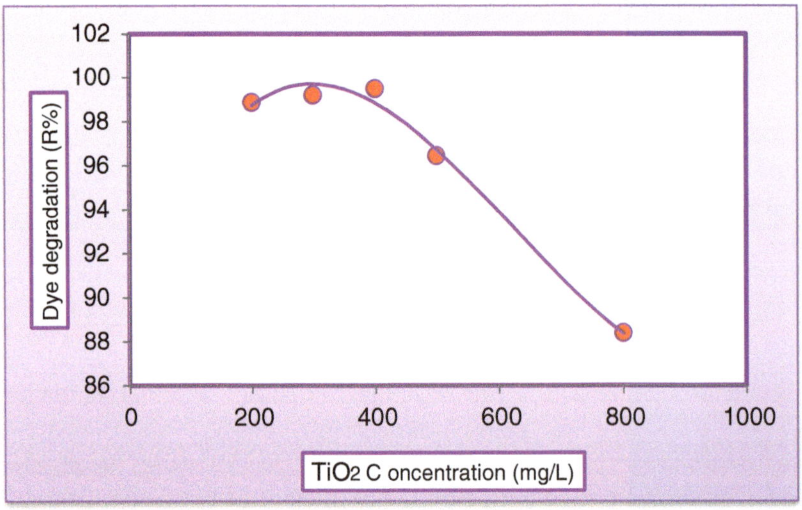

Figure 15 Variation of dye degradation against concentration of TiO_2 (C_{MV} = 30 mg/L, C_{H2O2} = 500 mg/L, pH = 5, and Q_L = 0.5 L/min) after 180 min.

Regression analysis method using STAISTICA version 6.2 software was utilized to fit the experimental data for photocatalytic reactor with the proposed model gives the following equation with correlation factor of 0.9708 and variance equal to 0.95,

$$R = 13.66(C_{TiO2})^{-0.07}(C_{H2O2})^{-0.14}(pH)^{-0.92}(Q_L)^{-0.47}(C_{MV})^{-0.04} \quad (9)$$

The coefficients of the correlation depict the predominant effect of pH on other operating variables for dye degradation. This correlation could be used as a model to predict the behavior of the dye degradation within the operating range of the studied variables.

FTIR measurements

Samples were taken after 180 min from the reactor effluent analyzed with FTIR (type: Bruker Tensor 27) after neutralization and filtration with (0.25) μm flat paper. Figure 18 shows a printout of the FTIR instrument. The Figure illustrates two curves, the red one is for the contaminated sample with dye concentration of 30 mg/L.

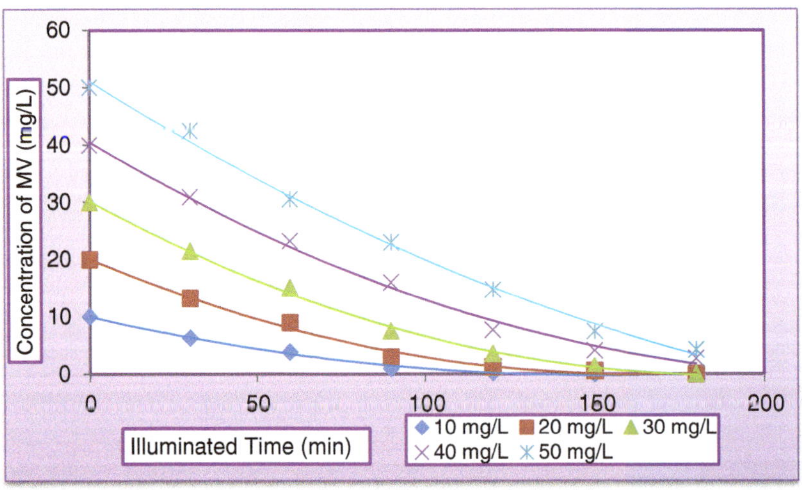

Figure 16 Effect of initial concentration of MV on the Photocatalytic degradation at optimum operating conditions.

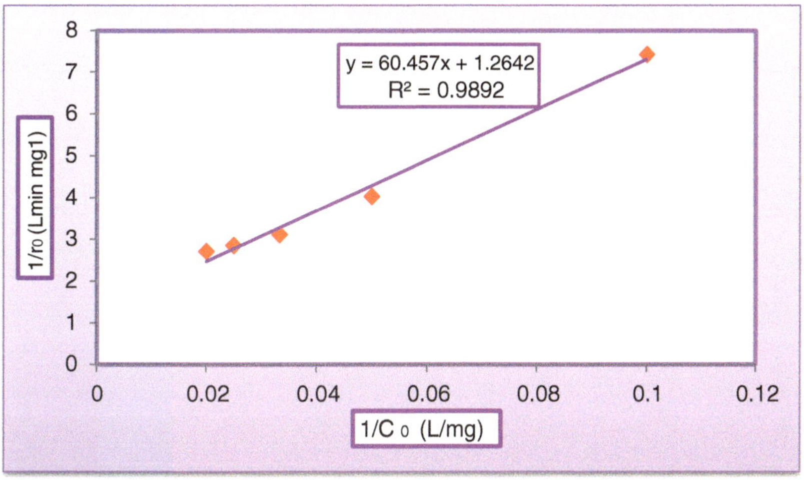

Figure 17 Linearization of Langmuir–Hinshelwood's equation of MV dye (C_{TiO2} = 400 mg/L, C_{H2O2} = 500 mg/L, pH = 5, and Q_L = 0.5 L/min).

The blue curve is for the sample taken at the reactor effluent. Three small peaks corresponding to wavenumbers of 1172.6, 1363.99, and 2348.71 cm^{-1} appeared on the red curve represent functional groups of C-C, C-O, C-N, C, N, O. These groups were not found on the blue curve which represents the sample of the reactor effluent. Comparison between the two plots confirms the disappearance of these groups. (Figure 19) plots a contrast of FTIR of MV dye compared with tap water after 180 min at optimum operating conditions The Figure at the top illustrates the functional groups in the sample taken at the outlet of the reactor after 180 min., while the Figure at the bottom shows an analysis of drinking water. Obviously the plots confirm that the degradation almost complete.

Catalyst recuperation

A neutralization process was carried out after photocatalytic treatment for sedimentation of titanium dioxide aggregate. Table 3 presents the turbidity before and after the neutralization process, and Figure 3 was used to estimate the corresponding concentration of TiO_2. The sediment was washed with H_2O_2, dried, and weighted for further use.

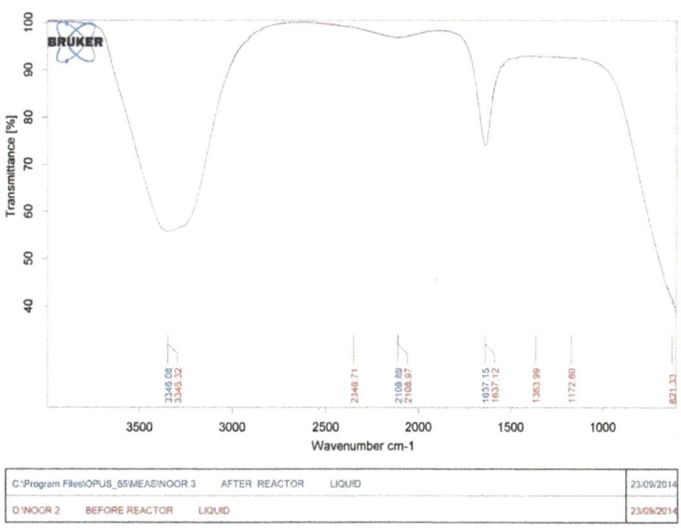

Figure 18 Printout of FTIR analysis of samples at influent and effluent of solar reactor, respectively.

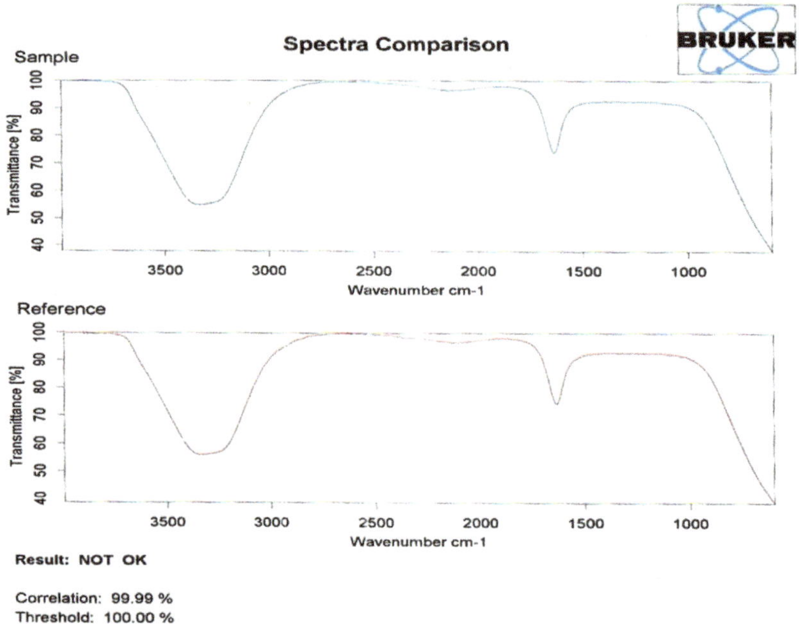

Figure 19 Contrast of FTIR of MV dye compared with tap water after 180 min at optimum operating conditions.

Membrane separation

Low pressure reverse osmosis (LPRO) membrane was used to separate TiO_2 particles from product water. The experimental results indicated that separation efficiency of LPRO was nearly 100% which suggested the use of such type of membrane for the hyper detoxification process.

Turbidity may be considered as a function of suspended solids concentration in solution. This definition could be used to estimate the separation efficiency of the membrane using equation (10).

$$\text{Seperation efficiency} = \frac{(\text{Turbidity})_{in} - (\text{Turbidity})_{permeate}}{(\text{Turbidity})_{in}} \quad (10)$$

Figure 20 represents the separation efficiency of the LPRO as a function of TiO_2 particles concentration into a neutralized solution of the photocatalytic reactor effluent. Figure 21 shows a photographic view for a sample of (a) synthetic wastewater (dye concentration = 30 mg/L), (b) after 180 min treatment by photoreactor, (c) after neutralization process, (d) after treated by LPRO membrane.

Despite the strong potential of membrane, one of the common problems encountered in applications is membrane fouling, which can significantly increase the energy consumption of the process over long- term operations [38]. Figure 22 plots the variation in permeate flux (L/min.m^2) with operating time for solutions of (400 mgTiO_2/L) and (800 mgTiO_2/L), respectively. The reduction in permeate flow rate was attributed to the deposition of suspended TiO_2 particles on the external surface of membrane at its pore openings or within its pores. This deposition became an additional barrier for water to flow through the permeate side of the membrane. Flow decline which could be originated by fouling, was a usual consequence of concentration polarization. Hence, if the feed pressure was held constant, the permeate flow will decrease. Thus, to overcome the additional barrier and to maintain constant permeate flow, the operating pressure must be increased.

Table 3 Variation of turbidity against C_{TiO2} before and after neutralization process

Exp. no.	C_{TiO_2} (mg/L)	Turbidity input (NTU)	Residual turbidity (NTU)
1	200	1710	285.133
2	300	3300	351.845
3	400	5320	416.405
4	500	5820	459.445
5	800	8690	663.885

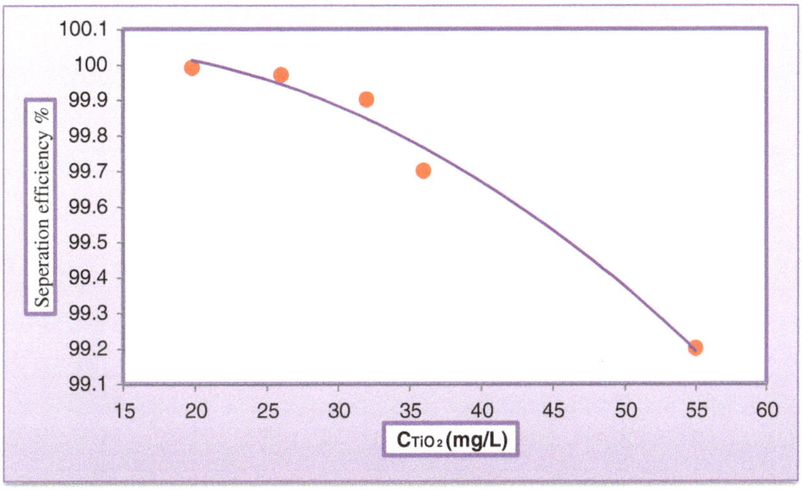

Figure 20 Variation of membrane separation efficiency against TiO_2 concentration in neutralized solution of the reactor effluent.

Conclusions

This work focused on the degradation of toxic organic compounds such as methyl violet dye (MV) in water, using a combined photocatalysis/low pressure reverse osmosis (LPRO) system. The performance of the hybrid system was investigated in terms of the degradation efficiency of MV, COD and membrane separation of TiO_2. The following conclusions have been noticed:

Photocatalysis Degradation of Dye

- It appears that the flow rate recirculation, irradiation time catalyst load, pH, H_2O_2 concentration, and concentration of dye mainly controls the rate of degradation for which optimum conditions for achieving maximum efficiency were established.
- Regarding catalyst loading, the degradation increased with the mass of catalyst up to an optimum amount. After then the degradation decreased as the catalyst loading continued to increase attributed to the UV light penetration depth which is considerably smaller than in suspension containing optimum amount of catalysts.

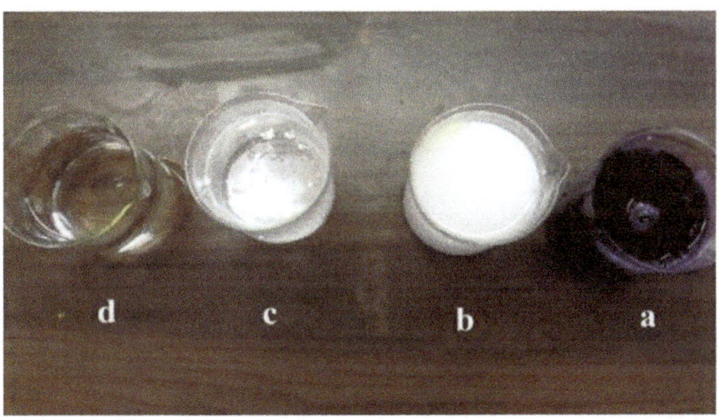

Figure 21 A sample of wastewater before and after treatment. A photographic view for a sample of **(a)** synthetic wastewater (dye concentration = 30 mg/L), **(b)** after 180 min treatment by photoreactor, **(c)** after neutralization process, **(d)** after treated by LPRO membrane.

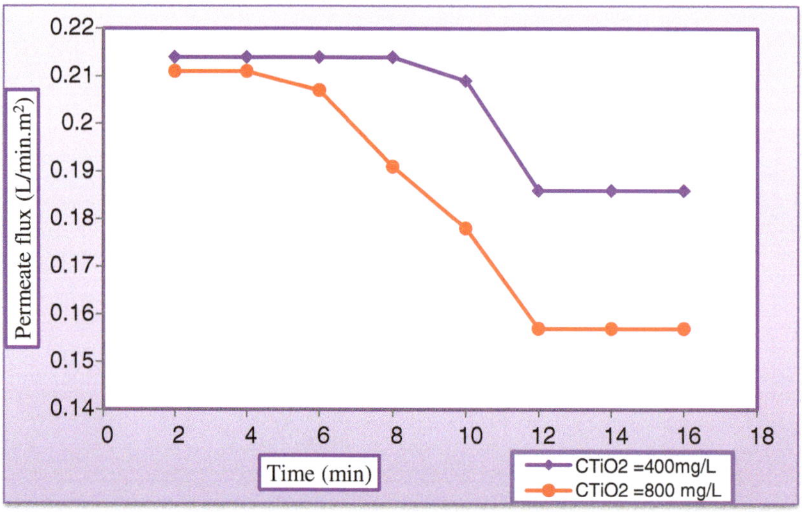

Figure 22 Variation of permeate flux of LPRO membrane against operating time at different catalyst loadings.

- The capacity of TiO_2 towards dye degradation strongly depended on pH of suspension. At basic pH, degradation was smaller than that at acidic pH where degradation of anionic dye was fast indicating that the mechanism involving complete mineralization could be achievable.
- The impact of the liquid Reynolds number on dye degradation shows a positively increasing trend to a point where all the surface of the photocataytic reactor was covered with a thin falling–film of synthetic wastewater, after then the dye degradation started to decrease with further increasing of liquid flow rate. This may be attributed to decreasing the residence time of the reactants.
- The addition of H_2O_2 to TiO_2 suspension resulted in an increase in the degradation ratio. The H_2O_2 acted as electron acceptors to make electron/hole recombination avoided and increased the concentration of $^{\bullet}OH$ radicals.
- It was found that the kinetics of dye degradation was first order with respect to dye concentration and could be well described by Langmuir-Hinshelwood model with the following rate law. The correlation coefficient (CF) was equal to 0.9892,

$$r = 0.0165C/(1 + 0.0209C)$$

Membrane separation system

To make the product water available for reuse, the TiO_2 particles in suspension must be removed. LPRO membrane was selected to perform the task. The following conclusions can be drawn from the experimental runs.

- The neutralization process of the reactor effluents seems to be feasible for reduction catalyst loading in the influent line of the membrane system.
- Increasing the catalyst loading from (400 to 800 mg/L) results in reduction of permeate flow rate by 15%.
- The TiO_2 separation efficiency of membrane could be estimated by utilizing the turbidity values of influent and effluent solutions.
- The LPRO membrane system has proved to be an efficient solution for the separation of TiO_2 suspended particles.

Competing interests

The authors declare that that they have no competing interests.

Authors' contributions

MFA gives idea of research and suggested the problem. NHH carried out the experiments under the guidance of MFA and AAA. AAA compiled the experimental data in journal format. All authors read and approved the final manuscript.

Acknowledgement

Authors are thankful to the Department of Chemical Engineering-University of Technology for providing facilities and space where the present work was carried out. Thanks are also due to the Solar Energy Research Center-Baghdad for their assistance.

References

1. Mohammed AO: **Evaluation and testing of a novel photocatalytic reactor with model water pollutants.** *MSc Thesis*. Robert Gordon University, Environmental Engineering Department, Aberdeen; 2007.
2. Chatterjee D, Patnam VR, Sikdar A, Joshi P, Misra R, Rao NN: **Kinetics of the decoloration of reactive dyes over visible light-irradiated TiO_2 semiconductor photocatalyst.** *J Hazard Mater* 2008, **156**:435–441.
3. Shahryari Z, Goharrizi AS, Azadi M: **Experimental study of methylene blue adsorption from aqueous solutions onto carbon nano tubes.** *Int J Water Resour Environ Eng* 2010, **2**:16–28.
4. Sumandeep K: **Light induced oxidative degradation studies of organic dyes and their intermediates.** *PhD Thesis*, School *of Chemistry & Biochemistry Thapar University* 2007, Patiala-India.
5. Barhon Z, Saffaj N, Albizane A, Azzi M, Mamouni R, El Haddad M: **Effect of modification of zirconium phosphate by silver on photodegradation of methylene blue.** *J Mater Environ Sci* 2012, **3**:879–884.
6. Singh C, Chaudhary R, Gandhi K: **Preliminary study on optimization of pH, oxidant and catalyst dose for high COD content: solar parabolic trough collector.** *Iranian J Environ Health Sci Eng* 2013, **10**:13.
7. Malato S, Julian B, Alfonso V, Diego A, Manuel IM, Julia C, Wolfgange G: **Applied studies in solar photocatalytic detoxification: an overview.** *Sol Energy* 2003, **75**:329–336.
8. Koppol APR, Bagajewicz MJ, Dericks BJ, Savelski MJ: **On zero water discharge solutions in the process industry.** *Adv Environ Res* 2003, **8**:151–171.
9. Akpan UG, Hammeed BH: **Parameters affecting the photocatalytic degradation of dyes using TiO_2-based photocatalysts: a review.** *J Hazard Mater* 2009, **170**:520–529.
10. Fujishima A, Zhang X, Tryk DA: **TiO_2 Photocatalysis and related surface phenomena.** *Surf Sci Rep* 2008, **63**:515–558.
11. Madhavan J, Maruthamuthu P, Murugesan S, Anandan S: **Kinetic studies on visible light-assisted degradation of acid red 88 in presence of metal-ion coupled Oxone reagent.** *Appl Catal B Environ* 2008, **83**:8–14.
12. Cassano AE, Alfano OM: **Reaction engineering of suspended solid heterogeneous photocatalytic reactors.** *Catal Today* 2000, **58**:167–197.
13. Hoffmann MR, Scot TM, Wonyong C, Bahnemann DW: **Environmental applications of semiconductor photocatalysis.** *Chem Rev* 1995, **95**:69–96.
14. Laoufi NA, Tassalit D, Bentahar F: **The Degradation of phenol in water solution by TiO_2 photocatalysis in a helical reactor.** *Global NEST J* 2008, **10**:404–418.
15. Fujishima A, Zhang X: **Titanium dioxide photocatalysis: present situation and future approaches.** *Comptes Rendus Chimie* 2006, **9**:750–760.
16. Ahmed S, Rasul MG, Brown R, Hashib MA: **Influence of parameters on the heterogeneous photocatalytic degradation of pesticides and phenolic contaminants in wastewater.** *J Environ Manag* 2011, **92**:311–330.
17. Pozzo RL, Giombi JL, Baltanas MA, Cassano AE: **The performance in a fluidized bed reactor of photocatalysts immobilized onto inert supports.** *Catal Today* 2000, **62**:175–187.
18. Chong MN, Lei S, Jin B, Saint C, Chow CWK: **Optimization of an annular photoreactor process for degradation of Congo red using a newly synthesized titania impregnated kaolinite nano-photocatalyst.** *Sep Purif* 2009, **67**:355–363.
19. Chan AHC, Chan CK, Barford JP, Porter JF: **Solar photocatalytic thin film cascade reactor for treatment of benzoic acid containing wastewater.** *Water Res* 2003, **37**:1125–1135.
20. Ochuma IJ, Fishwick RP, Wood J, Winterbottom JM: **Optimization of degradation conditions of 1,8-diazabicyclo[5.4.0]undec-7-ene in water and reaction kinetics analysis using a cocurrent downflow contactor photocatalytic reactor.** *Appl Catal B* 2007, **73**:259–268.
21. Vincenzo A, Claudio B, Alessandra BP, Elisa GL, Vittorio L, Sixto M, Giuseppe M, Leonardo P, Marco P, Edmondo P: **Azo-dyes photocatalytic degradation in aqueous suspension of TiO2 under solar irradiation.** *Chemosphere* 2002, **49**:1223–1230.
22. Grzechulska-Damszel J, Tomaszewska M, Morawski AW: **Integration of photocatalysis with membrane processes for purification of water contaminated with organic dyes.** *Desalination* 2009, **241**:118–126.
23. Poulios I, Tsachpinis I: **Photodegradation of the textile Dye reactive black 5 in the presence of semiconducting oxides.** *J Chem Technol Biotechnol* 1999, **74**:349–357.
24. Tang WZ, Zhang Z, Ann H: **TiO_2/UV Photodegradation of azo dyes in aqueous solutions.** *Environ Technol* 1997, **18**:1–12.
25. Guettaï N, Amar HA: **Photocatalytic oxidation of methyl orange in presence of titanium dioxide in aqueous suspension. Part I: parametric study.** *Desalination* 2005, **185**:427–437.
26. Konstantinou IK, Albanis TA: **TiO_2-assisted photocatalytic degradation of azo dyes in aqueous solution: kinetic and mechanistic investigations: a review.** *Appl Catal B Environ* 2004, **49**:1–14.
27. Wang Y, Hong CS: **Effect of hydrogen peroxide, periodate and persulfate on photocatalysis of 2-chlorobiphenyl in aqueous TiO_2 suspensions.** *Water Res* 1999, **33**:2031–2036.
28. Dixit A, Mungray AK, Chakraborty M: **Photochemical oxidation of phenol and chlorophenol by UV/H_2O_2/TiO_2 process: a kinetic study.** *Int J Chem Eng Appl* 2010, **1**:247–250.
29. Chen J, Rulkens WH, Bruning H: **Photochemical elimination of phenols & COD in industrial wastewaters.** *Water Sci Technol* 1997, **35**:231–238.
30. Shu HY, Huang CR, Chang MC: **Decolourization of monoazo dyes in wastewater by advanced oxidation process: a case study of Acid-Red-1 and Acid-Yellow-23.** *Chemosphere* 1994, **29**:2597–2607.
31. Galindo C, Kalt A: **UV/H2O2 oxidation of azo dyes in aqueous media: evidence of a structure degradability relationship.** *Dyes Pigments* 1999, **42**:199–207.
32. Sudarjanto G, Keller-Lehmann B, Keller J: **Photooxidation of a reactive azo-dye from the textile industry using UV/H2O2 technology: process optimization and kinetics.** *J Water Environ Technol* 2005, **3**:1–7.
33. Bird RB, Stewart WE, Lightfoot EN: *Transport phenomena*. 2nd edition. Inc. USA: John Wiley & Sons; 2002.
34. Kojima T, Gad-Allah TA, Kato S, Satokawa S: **Photocatalytic activity of magnetically separable TiO_2/SiO_2/Fe_3O_4 composite for Dye degradation.** *J Chem Eng Jpn* 2011, **44**:662–667.
35. Turchi CS, Ollis DF: **Photocatalytic degradation of organic water contaminants: mechanisms involving hydroxyl radical attack.** *J Catalysis* 1990, **122**:178–192.
36. Emeline AV, Ryabchuk V, Serpone N: **Factors affecting the efficiency of a photocatalysed process in aqueous metal-oxide dispersions, prospect of distinguishing between Two kinetic models.** *J Photochem Photobiol A Chem* 2000, **133**:89–97.
37. Wang KH, Hisieh YH, Wu CH, Chang CY: **The pH and anion effects on the heterogeneous photocatalytic degradation of o-methylbenzoic acid in TiO_2 aqueous suspension.** *Chemosphere* 2000, **40**:389–394.
38. Kennedy MD, Kamanyi J, Heijman BCJ, Amy G: **Colloidal organic matter fouling of UF membranes: role of NOM composition & size.** *Desalination* 2008, **220**:200–213.

Removal of crystal violet from water by magnetically modified activated carbon and nanomagnetic iron oxide

Soheila Hamidzadeh[1], Marzieh Torabbeigi[2*] and Seyed Jamaleddin Shahtaheri[3]

Abstract

Magnetically modified activated carbon, which synthesized by nanomagnetic iron oxide, was used for fast and effective removal of Crystal Violet from aqueous solutions. The scanning electron microscopy (SEM) images of nano-adsorbent showed that the average sizes of adsorbent are less than 100 nm. The various parameters, affecting on adsorption process, were examined including pH and temperature of dye solution, dose of adsorbent, and contact time. Then, thermodynamic parameters of sorption were calculated. Langmuir and Freundlich isotherms were used to fit the resulting data. Adsorption kinetics was consistent with a pseudo second order equation. Thermodynamic parameters of adsorption, ΔH^0, and ΔS^0 were calculated. Also, for further investigations, nano magnetic iron oxides was synthesized and used as adsorbent. Sorption capacities were depending on the temperature varied from 44.7 to 67.1 mg/g and from 12.7 to 16.5 mg/g for magnetically modified activated carbon and nanomagnetic iron oxide, respectively.

Keywords: Magnetically modified activated carbon, Crystal Violet, Langmuir isotherm, Freundlich isotherm, Nano magnetic iron oxide

Introduction

Large amounts of dyes are produced and applied in various industries. Small amounts of dyes (less than 1 ppm for some dyes) are visible in water [1,2]. As the most of the dyes in wastewater are stable to light and oxidation and also resistant to aerobic digestion, they damage to the aquatic life [3].

Crystal Violet (CV) is a synthetic basic cationic dye used for various purposes including biological stain, dermatological agent, veterinary medicine, additive to poultry feed to inhibit propagation of mold, intestinal parasites, and textile dyeing industries etc. [4,5]. It is a mutagen, mitotic poison, and also proven potent carcinogen [6,7].

Various processes were developed for the dye removal from the wastewater including adsorption and biosorption [8-10], chemical and electrochemical oxidation [11-13], membrane separation process [14], photodegradation [15], etc.

* Correspondence: torabbeigi@gmail.com
[2]Faculty of Health, Safety and Environment, Shahid Beheshti University of Medical sciences, P. O. Box 16858–116, Tehran, Iran
Full list of author information is available at the end of the article

Magnetic separation techniques have found important applications in environmental technology. In adsorption processes, the magnetic adsorbent can be easily separated from solution after adsorption process [16]. The magnetizations of adsorbents such as peanut husks [17], sawdust [18], baker's yeast cells [19], activated coconut shell carbon [20] etc. were investigated for removal dyes and other concomitances. Since Activated carbon is one of most useful adsorbent for removal of dye, in this study, it was modified by nanomagnetic iron oxide for fast and effective removal of Crystal Violet. The SEM images indicated the sizes of adsorbent particles are in nano scales. Adsorbent efficiency in removal Crystal Violet was studied. The affecting parameters on adsorption process were examined. The thermodynamic and kinetic adsorption parameters of Crystal violet onto magnetically modified activated carbon were obtained while; they have not been reported in previous studies. In order to comparative studies, nanomagnetic iron oxide (that used for magnetization of activated carbon) were synthesized and used as adsorbent.

Materials and methods

Reagents

Activated charcoal was purchased from BDH Ltd Poole England. Crystal Violet dye was from Merck Darmstadt Germany. All other chemicals used in this study were of high purity and used without further purification. Double distilled water was used for all experiments.

Adsorbent

Magnetically modified activated carbon was synthesized with slightly modified procedure described in reference [21]. 1 g of activated charcoal was placed in contact with 150 ml of sodium hydroxide 0.5 mol/l for 30 min and mixed up by stirrer thoroughly. Then, it was heated to boiling. 50 ml of solution containing Fe

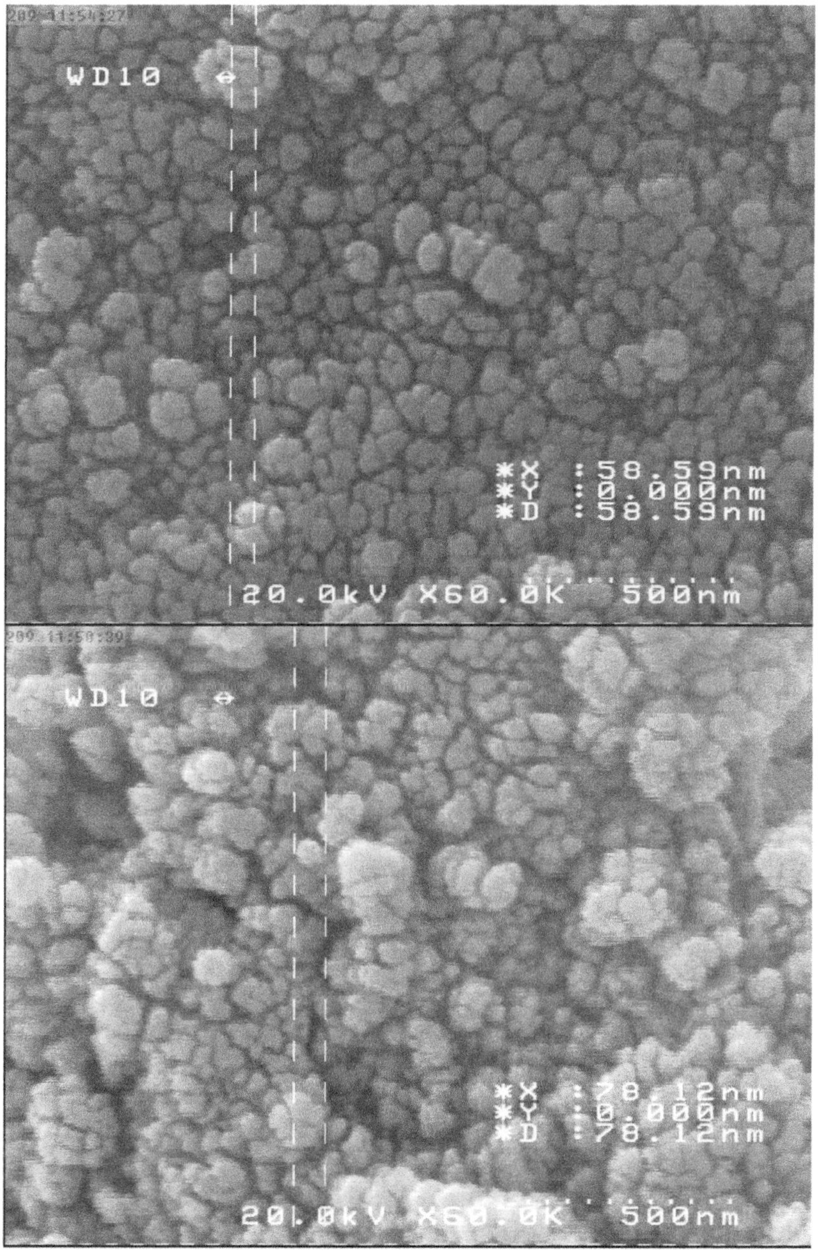

Figure 1 The SEM images of synthesized magnetically modified activated carbon.

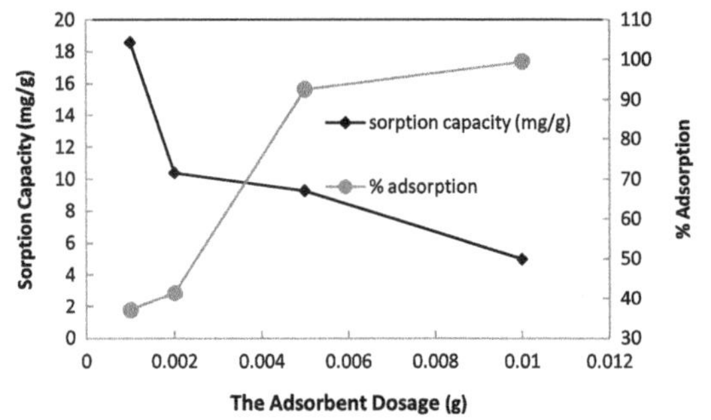

Figure 2 Effect of adsorbent dosage on adsorption percentage.

$(NO_3)_3$ 0.2 M and $FeSO_4$ 0.1 M was added quickly. The mixture was transferred into a distillation flask to reflux for two hours. Magnetically modified activated carbon was collected by magnet and then washed by water, methanol, and acetone several times to remove excess sodium hydroxide. It was then placed in oven at 80°C to drying for 12 h. The scanning electron microscopy (SEM) images of magnetically modified activated carbon have been shown in Figure 1 indicated that the sizes of synthesized magnetic particles are less than 100 nm.

Adsorption procedure

Batch adsorption experiments with 10 ml of Crystal Violet solution (5 mg/l) were done for 1–10 mg of adsorbent, 1 to 10 min contact times, 3–9 pHs, and at 20, 30 and 40°C.

pHs of solutions were adjusted by expected values of nitric acid and sodium hydroxide solutions. Analysis of

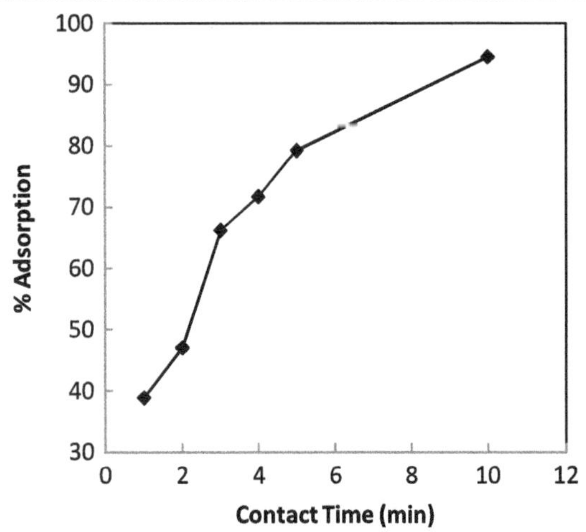

Figure 3 Effect of contact time.

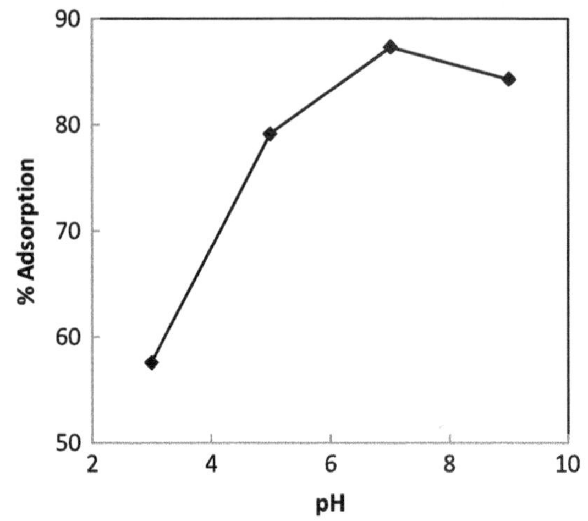

Figure 4 Effect of pH.

dye concentration was carried out by UV–vis spectrophotometer in 593 nm wavelength.

Percentage of dye removal from solution was calculated by the following equation:

$$Removal(\%) = \frac{C_0 - C_i}{C_0} \times 100 \quad (1)$$

C_0 and C_i are initial and final concentration of Crystal Violet solutions, respectively. The following formula is used to calculate the amount of dye adsorbed by the adsorbent:

$$q_e = (C_0 - C_e) \times \frac{v}{w} \quad (2)$$

Where q_e is adsorption capacity (mg of adsorbed dye per g of adsorbent), C_e is equilibrium concentration of

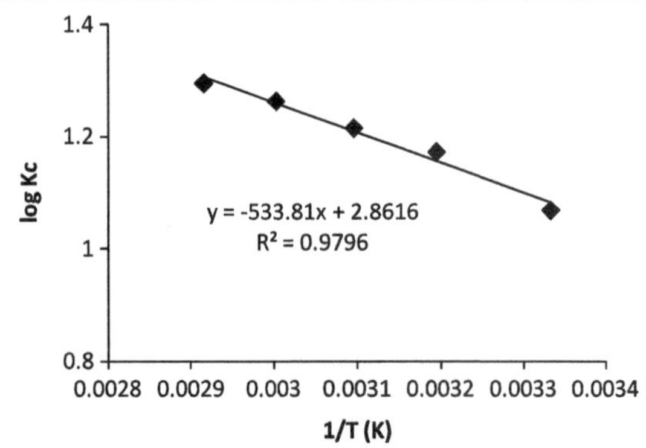

Figure 5 Eyring's plot of adsorption process.

Table 1 The thermodynamic parameters of adsorption of Crystal Violet on magnetically modified activated carbon

Temp. (K)	ΔG^0 (kJ/mol)	ΔS^0 (kJ/mol.K)	ΔH^0 (kJ/mol)
300	−6.14	0.055	10.22
313	−7.03		
323	−7.51		
333	−8.05		
343	−8.50		

dye (mg/l), v is the volume of the solution (l) and w is the mass of adsorbent (g).

Kinetic study

Pseudo-first and pseudo-second order models were applied for the adsorption kinetic studies. The first order rate equation of Lagergren was used for the adsorption:

$$\log(q_e - q_t) = \log(q_e) - \frac{k_1}{2.303}t \tag{3}$$

Where q_e and q_t are masses of dye adsorbed at equilibrium and at time t (mg g^{-1}), respectively, and k_1 is the first-order reaction rate constant (min^{-1}). Pseudo-second order equation was used based on Ho-Mckay equation:

$$\frac{t}{q_t} = \frac{1}{k_2 q_e^2} + \frac{1}{q_e}t \tag{4}$$

Where k_2 is the second order reaction rate equilibrium constant (g mg^{-1} min^{-1}).

Result and discussion

Optimization

The adsorbent dosage

As the dose of adsorbent can strongly affect the sorption capacity, the adsorption procedure was done with varied dose of adsorbent (1–10 mg). Obtained results shown in Figure 2 indicated that, increasing amount of the adsorbents increases the contact surface area and exchangeable sites, and then increases the percent removal of dye.

The contact time

The contact time is one of the important factors affecting on batch adsorption process, therefore, contact time from 1 to 10 min was studied for removal of dye. Resulting data were shown in Figure 3. This synthesized nano magnetic adsorbent removed Crystal Violet very fast, so that, more than 90 % of dye was removed in 10 min and adsorption process attains saturation at this time.

pH of Crystal Violet solution

To study the effect of pH on the adsorbent, the range of pH adjusted between 3 and 9. The experimental date indicated that, the removal of dye was so effective at pH 9. Figure 4 shows the effect of pH on removal of Crystal Violet. Cationic dyes like Crystal Violet were adsorbed on activated carbon surface at alkaline pHs [22,23].

Temperature of dye solution

Dye removal was examined at different temperatures range started from 27°C (as ambient temperature) to 70°C. 10 ml of dye solution 5 mg/l was contacted to 0.01 g of magnetically modified activated carbon for 5 min at pH 5 at 27, 40, 50, 60, and 70°C.

Thermodynamic parameters, ΔS^0 and ΔH^0 were calculated from Eyring's plot; log Kc versus 1/T (Figure 5).

$$\log K_C = \frac{\Delta S^0}{2.303R} - \frac{\Delta H^0}{2.303R}\frac{1}{T} \tag{5}$$

$$K_C = \frac{C_{ad}}{C_e} \tag{6}$$

Where K_C is the equilibrium constant, C_{ad} and C_e are the equilibrium concentrations of the dyes on the

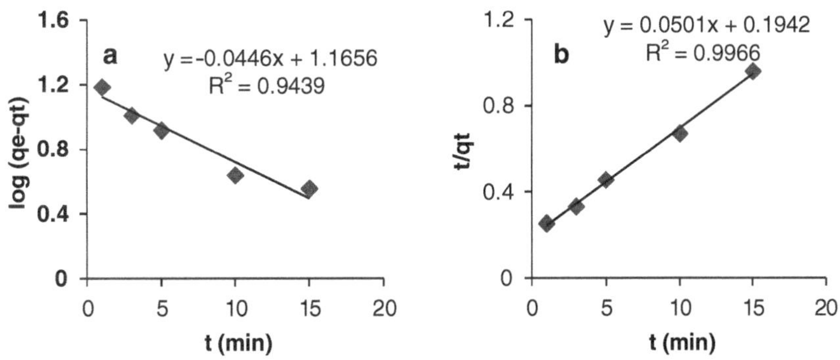

Figure 6 The fitting data of adsorption procedure by (a) pseudo-first order and (b) second order equations.

Table 2 The rate constants and linear regressions of First order and Second order for adsorption of Crystal Violet on magnetically modified activated carbon and nanomagnetic iron oxide

Adsorbent	First order		Second order	
	k_1 (min^{-1})	R^2	k_2 ($g\ mg^{-1}\ min^{-1}$)	R^2
Magnetically modified activated carbon	0.103	0.944	0.752	0.997
Nanomagnetic iron oxide	0.230	0.901	1.38×10^{-2}	0.962

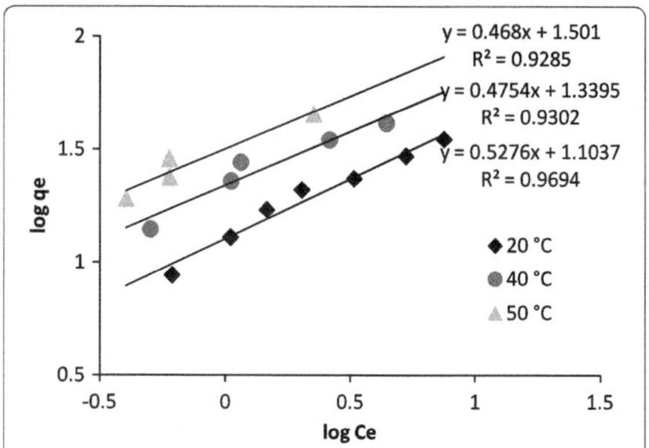

Figure 8 Freundlich isotherms in various temperatures.

adsorbent and in solution, respectively, T is the temperature in Kelvin and R is gas constant. Then, ΔG^0s in different temperature were determined by:

$$\Delta G^0 = -2.303\, R\, T\, \log K_C \tag{7}$$

Obtained thermodynamic parameters are presented in Table 1. The negative values of free energy (ΔG^0) indicate the feasibility of dye removal and spontaneous nature of adsorption process. Value of ΔH^0 confirms that the adsorption of Crystal Violet on magnetically modified activated carbon is endothermic process. The positive ΔS^0 demonstrate the affinity of Crystal Violet on to nano adsorbent.

Kinetic study

In order to determine the kinetic of adsorption, the results were evaluated by equations (3) and (4) that related to the pseudo-first order and second order kinetics, respectively. Figure 6a and b show the fitting data by pseudo-first order and second order equations. The rate constants and linear regressions (R^2) were reported in Table 2. The results indicated that, the adsorption of Crystal Violet on magnetically modified activated carbon has been described by pseudo-second order equation.

In order to perform further investigation, nanomagnetic iron oxide was synthesized as similar as described in experimental section, without any addition of activated carbon. In the same conditions, nanomagnetic iron oxide was used as adsorbent. The kinetic results shown in Table 2 indicated that, the kinetic of adsorption was the same as magnetically modified activated carbon with lower rate constant (k_2).

Adsorption isotherms

Adsorption isotherms are important to describe the adsorption mechanism and to determine the maximum adsorption capacity and also to consider the feasibility of the application process. Langmuir and Freundlich equations were used to study the adsorption isotherms. The Langmuir model is describing the monolayer adsorption onto a surface with a finite

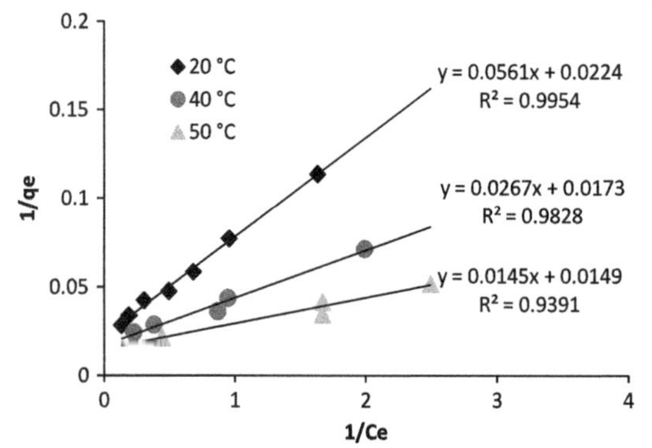

Figure 7 Langmuir isotherms in various temperatures.

Table 3 The parameters of Langmuir and Freundlich isotherms at different temperatures for adsorption of Crystal Violet on magnetically modified activated carbon and nanomagnetic iron oxide

Adsorbent	Temp. (°C)	Langmuir			Freundlich		
		q_{max}	K_L	R^2	K_F	n	R^2
Magnetically modified activated carbon	20	44.7	0.40	0.995	12.7	1.90	0.969
	40	57.8	0.65	0.983	21.9	2.10	0.930
	50	67.1	1.03	0.939	31.7	2.14	0.929
Nanomagnetic iron oxide	20	12.7	0.045	0.956	8.2	1.02	0.918
	40	14.5	0.047	0.982	10.1	1.03	0.935
	50	16.5	0.051	0.970	15.5	1.19	0.952

number of identical sites. Linear form of Langmuir isotherm is given by:

$$\frac{1}{q_e} = \frac{1}{q_{max} K_L C_e} + \frac{1}{q_{max}} \quad (8)$$

Where q_{max} (mg/g) is the maximum adsorption capacity and K_L is a constant factor related to the energy. The variations of $1/q_e$ at different temperatures are plotted versus $1/C_e$ in Figure 7.

The Freundlich model is based on the sorption onto a heterogeneous surface. The linear expression of Freundlich equation is as follow:

$$\log(q_e) = \log(K_F) + \frac{1}{n}\log(C_e) \quad (9)$$

Where K_F and n are the Freundlich constants, being indicators of adsorption capacity and adsorption intensity, respectively. Log q_e at different temperatures versus log C_e is plotted in Figure 8.

The regression coefficients and model parameters for Langmuir and Freundlich isotherms are tabulated in Table 3. The regression coefficients indicated that the data are better fitted by the Langmuir model. The maximum sorption capacity (q_{max}) and intensity of sorption (K_L) increased by arising the temperature.

In the same conditions, the experiments were performed by nanomagnetic iron oxide as the adsorbent. The obtained results listed in Table 3 show that, Langmuir and Freundlich did not well describe the adsorption isotherm model. The values of q_{max} increased by increasing the temperature and also were less than those for magnetically modified activated carbon.

Magnetically modified activated carbon is a perfect and effective adsorbent that offers a fast removal of Crystal Violet from water samples. The kinetic of the adsorption is pseudo second order. Langmuir isotherm can describe well the adsorption model. The sorption capacity and intensity of sorption are enhanced by increasing the temperature. Using nanomagnetic iron oxide as adsorbent compared with magnetically modified activated carbon showed that, it is able to sorption of Crystal Violet with less effectiveness. The previous studies on magnetic adsorbents for removal of Crystal Violet have been presented in Table 4. The time of removal in this study (10 min) was very short than the contact time in previous studies so that the minimum time of process for these studies with high sorption capacities was 90 min. Thermodynamic and kinetic parameters were not calculated in previous studies. Nanomagnetic iron oxide was not used for removal Crystal Violet previously.

Table 4 The previous studies on magnetic adsorbents to removal Crystal Violet

Adsorbents	q_{max}	Ref.
Magnetic charcoal	10 mg cm^{-3}	[23]
Magnetically labeled Baker's yeast cells	85.9 mg g^{-1}	[19]
magnetically modified *Saccharomyces cerevisiae* subsp. uvarum cells	41.7 mg g^{-1}	[24]
Ferrofluid modified sawdust	51.16 mg g^{-1}	[14]
magnetically modified *Chlorella Vulgaris* cells	42.91 mg g^{-1}	[25]
Magnetic fluid modified peanut husks	80.9 mg g^{-1}	[17]
Magnetically modified spent grain	40.2 mg g^{-1}	[26]
Magnetic carbon-iron oxide nanocomposite	81.70 mg g^{-1}	[20]
Magnetically modified spent coffee grounds	68.1 mg g^{-1}	[27]
Magnetically modified activated car bon	67.1 mg g^{-1}	Present study
Nanomagnetic iron oxide	16.5 mg g^{-1}	Present study

Conclusion

The results indicate that magnetically modified activated carbon have considerable potential for the removal of Crystal Violet, also the magnetic adsorbent can be simply removed from solution by using magnet or appropriate magnetic separator after adsorption process. The obtained results of this investigation implicate that this adsorbent was more able to remove dye in the less time with compared to some of studies listed in Table 4. Also we investigated Thermodynamic and kinetic studies for removal process more than other pervious works.

The resulting adsorption capacities demonstrate that, although nanomagnetic iron oxide can be as an adsorbent, but its efficiency is much lower than magnetically modified activated carbon.

Competing interests
The authors declare that they have no competing interests.

Authors' contributions
All of the authors have the same contribution. All authors read and approved the final manuscript.

Acknowledgments
The authors thank the staffs of Payam Noor University of Varamin, specially Mrs. Rezaiee and Mrs. Haj Husseini.

Author details
[1]Payam Noor University of Varamin, Qarchak, Varamin, Tehran, Iran. [2]Faculty of Health, Safety and Environment, Shahid Beheshti University of Medical sciences, P. O. Box 16858-116, Tehran, Iran. [3]Department of Occupational Health Engineering, School of Public Health, Institute for Environmental Research, Tehran University of Medical Sciences, Tehran 14155-6446, Iran.

References

1. Banat IM, Nigam P, Singh D, Marchant R. Microbial decolorisation of textile dye containing effluents: a review. Bioresour Technol. 1996;58:217–27.
2. Robinson T, McMullan G, Marchant R, Nigam P. Remediation of dyes in textile effluents: a critical review on current treatment technology with a proposed alternative. Bioresour Technol. 2001;77:247–55.
3. Lee CK, Low KS, Gan PY. Removal of some organic dyes by acid treat spent bleaching earth. Environ Technol. 1999;20:99–104.
4. Hao OJ, Kim H, Chiang PC. Decolorization of wastewater. Environ Sci Technol. 2000;30:449–505.
5. Eiichi I, Ogawa T, Yatome TC, Horisu H. Behavior of activated sludge with dyes. Bull Environ Contam Toxicol. 1985;35:729–34.
6. He H, Yang S, Yu K, Ju Y, Sun C, Wang L. Microwave assisted induced catalytic degradation of crystal violet in nano-nickel dioxide suspensions. J Hazard Mater. 2010;173:393–400.
7. Senthilkumaar S, Kalaamani P, Subburaam CV. Liquid phase adsorption of crystal violet on to activated carbons derived from male flowers of coconut tree. J Hazard Mater. 2006;136:800–8.
8. Garg VK, Gupta R, Yadav AB, Kumar R. Dye removal from aqueous solution by adsorption on treated sawdust. Bioresour Technol. 2003;89:121–4.
9. Mohamed MM. Acid Dye removal: comparison of surfactant modified mesoporous FSM-16 with activated carbon derived from rice husk. J Colloid Interface Sci. 2004;272:28–34.
10. Safarik I, Rego LFT, Mosiniewicz-Szablewska MBE, Weyda F, Safarikova M. New magnetically responsive yeast-based biosorbent for the efficient removal of water-soluble dyes. Enzyme Microb Technol. 2007;40:1551–6.
11. Salem IA. Activation of H_2O_2 by Amberlyst-15 resin supported with copper (II)-complexes towards oxidation of crystal violet. Chemosphere. 2001;44:1109–19.
12. Baban A, Yediler A, Lienert D, Kemerdere N, Kettrup A. Ozonation of high strength segregated effluents from a woollen textile dyeing and finishing plant. Dyes Pigments. 2003;58:93–8.
13. Vlyssides AG, Loizidou M, Karlis PK, Zorpas AA, Papaioannou D. Electrochemical oxidation of a textile dye wastewater using a Pt/Ti electrode. J Hazard Mater. 1999;B70:41–52.
14. Koyuncu I. Reactive dye removal in dye/salt mixtures by nanofiltration membranes containing vinylsulphone dyes: effects of feed concentration and cross flow velocity. Desalination. 2002;143:243–53.
15. Chen J, Liu M, Zhang J, Ying X, Jin L. Photocatalytic degradation of organic wastes by electrochemically assisted TiO2 photocatalytic system. J Environ Manage. 2004;70:43–7.
16. Safarikova M, Safarik I. The application of magnetic techniques in biosciences. Magn Electr Sep. 2001;10:223–52.
17. Safarik I, Safarikova M. Magnetic fluid modified peanut husks as an adsorbent for organic dyes removal. Physics Procedia. 2010;9:274–8.
18. Safarik I, Lunackova P, Mosiniewicz-Szablewska E, Weyda F, Safarikova M. Adsorption of water-soluble organic dyes on ferrofluidmodified sawdust. Holzforschung. 2007;61:247–53.
19. Safarik I, Ptackova L, Safarikova M. Adsorption of dyes on magnetically labeled baker's yeast cells. Eur Cells and Mater. 2002;3:52–5.
20. Singh KP, Gupta S, Singh AK, Sinha S. Optimizing adsorption of crystal violet dye from water by magnetic nanocomposite using response surface modeling approach. J Hazard Mater. 2011;186:1462–73.
21. Safarik I, Nymburska K, Safarikova M. Adsorption of water-soluble organic dyes on magnetic Charcoal. J Chem Tech Biotechnol. 1997;69:1–4.
22. Ahmad R. Studies on adsorption of crystal violet dye from aqueous solution onto coniferous pinus bark powder (CPBP). J Hazard Mater. 2009;171:767–73.
23. Porkodi K, Vasanth Kumar K. Equilibrium, kinetics and mechanism modeling and simulation of basic and acid dyes sorption onto jute fiber carbon: Eosin yellow, malachite green and crystal violet single component systems. J Hazard Mater. 2007;143:311–27.
24. Safarikova M, Ptackova L, Kibrikova I, Safarik I. Biosorption of water-soluble dyes on magnetically modified Saccharomyces cerevisiae subsp. uvarum cells. Chemosphere. 2005;59:831–5.
25. Safarikova M, Rainha Pona BM, Mosiniewicz-Szablewska E, Weyda F, Safarik I. Dye adsorption on magnetically modified Chlorella Vulgaris cells. Fresen Environ Bull. 2008;17:486–92.
26. Safarik I, Horska K, Safarikova M. Magnetically modified spent grain for dye removal. J Cereal Sci. 2011;53:78–80.
27. Safarik I, Horska K, Svobodova B, Safarikova M. Magnetically modified spent coffee grounds for dyes removal. Eur Food Res Technol. 2012;234:345–50.

4

The use of the GIS Kriging technique to determine the spatial changes of natural radionuclide concentrations in soil and forest cover

Turgay Dindaroğlu

Abstract

Background: The distribution of radionuclides occurring naturally in the earth depends on bedrock characteristics. Therefore, the spatial distribution of radionuclides is not uniform. Consequently, radionuclide information is vitally important in determining and monitoring the spatial variation of the radionuclide concentrations that are over the limits for the sustainable environment and human health.

Methods: This research was carried out using GIS methods and geostatistical analysis as Kriging techniques to reveal the spatial variation of the 226Ra, 232Th and 40 K concentrations of natural radionuclides in the Çoruh and Aras Basin. The spatial variations of the detected radionuclides were correlated with soil groups and forest cover.

Results: In the study area, 43.17% of the concentration of 40 K, 26.67% of the concentration of 226Ra and 28.16% of the 232Th concentration was determined to be over the average limits. Concentrations of radionuclides that are over the average limits have been found to be on basalt and chestnut soils. Brown and reddish brown soils have a low concentration of the spatial distribution of the radionuclides. Statistically positive correlations were detected (0.865 **) between the 226Ra and 232Th. In addition, a positive relationship between forest cover and 226Ra and a negative relationship between 232Th and 40 K were identified.

Conclusions: Excessive exposure to radiation may cause cancer and hereditary diseases. Ecological environments include the soil and the plants. Hence, the periodical monitoring of the spatial variation in concentrations of radionuclides is very important for the health of future generations.

Keywords: Natural radionuclide, Kriging technique, Soil, Forest cover

Background

Radioactive features have existed in our world since its formation. High concentrations of natural radionuclides are found in volcanic, phosphate, granite and salt rock. Rain and other water discharge crumble these rocks into very small pieces and mixes them into the groundwater. Thus, rocks increase the natural radioactivity of the soil.

The direction of the movement and the speed of the radionuclides in the soil depends on natural processes (e.g., soil structure, content of the plant species, irrigation conditions, weather conditions and accumulation) [1,2]. In some areas, the natural radionuclide concentrations are above the established limits according to UNSCEAR. If the concentration of natural radioactive elements goes over the average limits, there can be negative effects on human health [3]. Therefore, the spatial distribution of the concentrations of natural radionuclides in the soil has to be determined. It is possible to use CBS and geostatistical analysis to obtain these values.

Geostatistical techniques are a useful component of GIS applications that are frequently applied. Geostatistics involves the analysis and estimation techniques used to obtain the value of a variable dispersed in time and location.

Kriging is one of the best and most widely-known techniques used in spatial linear predictions. Kriging methods have different flexible forms, according to the survey area and data [4-7]. Kriging can also reveal the reliability of the estimated surface [8,9].

Correspondence: turgaydindaroglu@hotmail.com
Faculty of Forestry, Department of Forest Engineering, Kahramanmaras Sutcu imam University, 46100 Kahramanmaras, Turkey

Geostatistical methods also allow for examining a relationship with spatial variations of radionuclides between forest cover and soil groups. Radioactive elements in the soil do not indicate a uniform distribution in the earth. Therefore, the concentrations of radionuclides should be checked regularly as an important step in protection from the negative effects of radioactivity [10-12].

Radionuclide concentrations may be caused by the high amount of organic matter in the soil. As such, radionuclides can be absorbed by the forest soil [13,14]. Some radionuclide compounds build up in the humic acids in the soil organic layer [15,16].

Measuring the radioactivity concentration in the soil, as well as the concentrations in the plants and the water, is necessary to estimate the concentrations of radionuclides [17,18]. This study used ^{226}Ra, ^{232}Th and ^{40}K concentration values measured periodically by TAEK [19]. Spatial distributions were determined according to UNSCEAR (2000) [3], who used a kriging technique in the Çoruh and Aras Basin and the surrounding areas. The statistical relationships between the spatial variations, forest cover and soil groups were analyzed.

Materials and methods

This research was carried out in 10 provinces in eastern Turkey: Rize, Bayburt, Erzurum, Artvin, Ardahan, Kars, Iğdır, Muş, Bingöl and Erzincan. The bounding geographical coordinates of the study area are 39°50′07′′ to 39°46′ 17′′ north latitudes and 38°26′52′′ to 44°35′46′′ east longitudes (Figure 1). The study area is 9.815.000 ha in size. Forest areas were detected using local Forest Management Plan data [20].

Sampling methods and analysis

Concentrations of radioactive elements (^{226}Ra, ^{232}Th and ^{40}K) for determining soil sampling were carried out by the provincial offices of the Ministry of Environment and Urbanization. Surface soil sampling was conducted at 46 points. The concentration of radioactivity in the surface soil samples was determined by the Atomic Research Council of Turkey [19].

Risk assessment

The average natural radioactivity rate, the concentration range and the average values are presented in Table 1 [3]. To determinate the concentration of the natural radionuclides, soil samples from 10 cm thickness in 1 km^2 land were collected in the research area.

Geostatistical analysis

To conduct the geostatistical analysis, the "Kriging" interpolation technique was used within the spatial analyst extension module in ArcGIS 9.3 software. The spatial analyses were carried out with prepared maps using this technique. Concentrations of ^{226}Ra, ^{232}Th and ^{40}K were determined for the distribution area. The experimental variogram model was constructed using the Kriging method, with data obtained from the research area. The spatial transformation was performed to determine the most appropriate model to use with the parameters of the generated maps.

The ordinary Kriging formula is as follows [8,21]:

$$Z(S_0) = \sum_{i=1}^{N} \lambda_i Z(S_i)$$

where:

Z(si) is the measured value at the location (ith),

λ_i is the unknown weight for the measured value at the location (ith) and

s_0 is the estimation location.

The unknown weight (λ_p) depends on the distance to the location of the prediction and the spatial relationships among the measured values.

The statistical model estimates the unmeasured values using known values. A small difference occurs between the true value $Z(s_0)$ and the predicted value, $\Sigma\lambda_i Z(s_i)$. Therefore, the statistical prediction is minimized using the following formula:

$$\left[Z(\mathbf{S}_0) - \sum_{i=1}^{N} \lambda_i Z(\mathbf{S}_i) \right]^2$$

The Kriging interpolation technique is made possible by transferring data into the GIS environment. In this way, analysis in areas that have no data can be conducted. The following criteria were used to evaluate the model: the average error (ME) must be close to 0 and the square root of the estimated error of the mean standardized (RMSS) must be close to 1 [22]. While implementing the models, the anisotropy effect was surveyed.

Results and discussion

Anisotropic variogram models were preferred. The ^{226}Ra, ^{232}Th and ^{40}K concentration values showed a directional change. The spatial dependencies (Nugget/Sill ratio) were found to be related to the degree of autocorrelation between the sampling points. If the spatial dependence was higher between the sample points, the spatial correlation was very high. The spatially dependent variables were classified as: strongly spatially dependent if the ratio was ≤25%, mid-spatial-dependent if the ratio was 25% 75% and weakly spatially dependent if the ration was ≥75% [4,23-26].

Because the spatial dependence was strong, the variables did not differ over short distances. In this research area, spatial dependence was too high for ^{232}Th (16.91%).

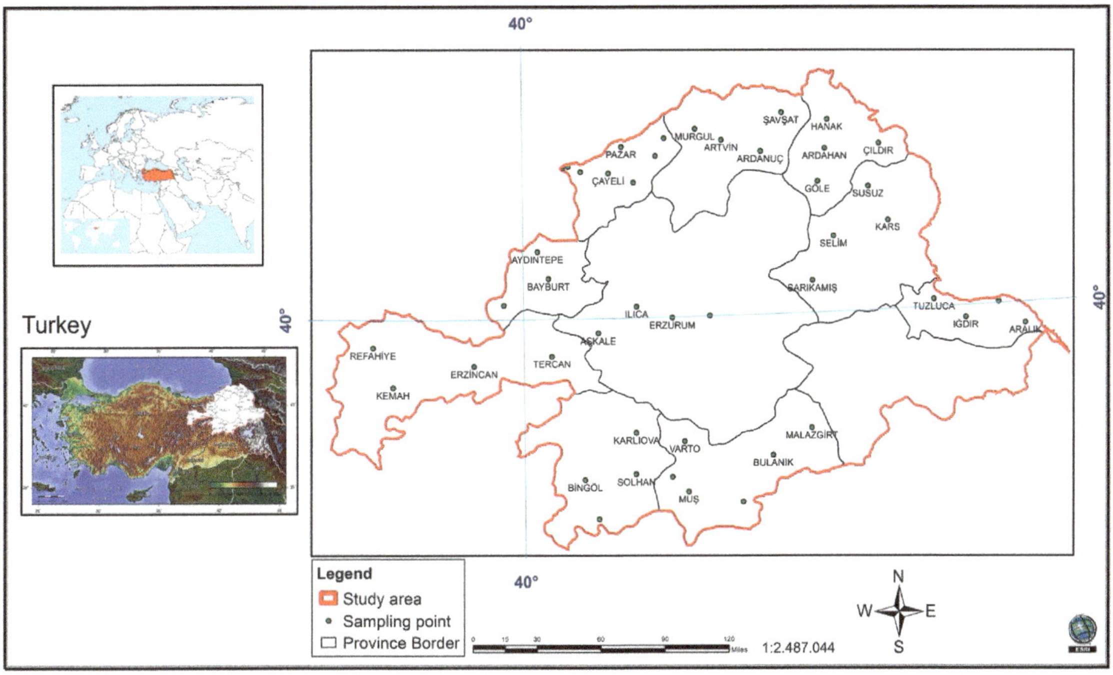

Figure 1 Location of study area.

Spatial dependence was identified as normal for ^{226}Ra and ^{40}K (25.88% and 70.60%), respectively. An effective spatial dependence distance was found between 254369.7 and 375276 meters (Table 2).

The sample point data will involve converting the spatial data of the ^{226}Ra, ^{232}Th and ^{40}K concentrations used in the interpolation for kriging. The lowest error rate models were chosen; they were the *"Exponential"* and *"Stable"* models. The maps were produced and field data were obtained in accordance with this kriging model.

Spatial distribution of ^{226}Ra:

The prediction map, according to the optimized model, was determined during the cross-validation process. The ^{226}Ra concentration prediction map shows the log ^{226}Ra. The dataset for the ^{226}Ra concentration has a high kurtosis and is positively skewed, so it is not a normal distribution. The data log transformation was applied to be closer to a normal distribution. After the log transformation was conducted, the ^{226}Ra concentrations were found to be approximately normally distributed.

The histogram of ^{226}Ra and log transformations data is presented in Figure 2. To check the data, the best model was applied to the cross-validation of the spatial correlation of the ^{226}Ra concentration of the study area. A comparison of the ME and the RMSSE for the log ^{226}Ra illustrates that the exponential model and its parameters were best for the ^{226}Ra concentration. The exponential model has the best fit with the nugget effect (C_o); it is equal to 48.35, a sill ($C_o + C$) equal to 186.83 and a range of influence equal to 254369.7. The ratio of the nugget variance to the sill is expressed in percentages equal to 25.88% (Table 2). This value is greater than 25% and less than 75%. Thus, the ^{226}Ra distribution has a moderate spatial dependence in the study area. A spatial prediction and distribution map for the ordinary kriging interpolation of ^{226}Ra is presented in Figure 3.

Table 1 Natural radioactivity the concentration range and average values

	Natural radionuclides (Bq/kg)		
	^{226}Ra	^{232}Th	^{40}K
Concentration range	17-60	11-64	140-850
Average values	35	45	400

Spatial distribution of ^{232}Th

The dataset of the ^{232}Th concentration has a high kurtosis and is positively skewed, so it is not a normal distribution. The data log transformation was applied, so could be closer to a normal distribution. After the log transformation was conducted, the ^{232}Th concentrations were approximately normally distributed. The histogram

Table 2 Model parameters

	Model	Regression function	Nugget, (C_o)	Range, A	Sill, ($C_o + C$)	Nugget/Sill, (%)	ME[1]	RMSSE[2]
^{226}Ra	Exponential	0.2695 x +18.32	48.35	254369.7	186.83	25.88	0.004	1.06
^{232}Th	Exponential	0.5063 x +15.33	50.74	304696.1	300.03	16.91	0.008	0.89
^{40}K	Stable	0.1596 x +381.99	41767.52	375276.0	59158.77	70.60	0.007	0.997

ME[1]: mean standard error.
RMSSE[2]: estimated standardized mean of error of mean square root.

of ^{232}Th and log-histogram transformation data is presented in Figure 4. To check that the best model was applied, a cross-validation of the spatial correlation of the ^{232}Th concentration of the study area was conducted. A comparison of ME and the RMSSE for log ^{232}Th shows that the exponential model and its parameters are the more appropriate for the ^{232}Th concentration. The exponential model has the best fit, with the nugget effect (C_o) being equal to 50.74, a sill ($C_o + C$) equal to 300.03 and a range of influence equal to 304696.1. The ratio of the nugget variance to the sill expressed in percentages is equal to 16.91% (Table 2). This value is smaller than 25; thus, the ^{232}Th distribution has a powerful spatial dependence in the study area. A spatial prediction and distribution map for the ordinary kriging interpolation ^{232}Th is presented in Figure 5.

Spatial distribution of ^{40}K

An optimized model determined from the cross-validation process and the ^{40}K concentration prediction map shows the log ^{40}K. The dataset for the ^{40}K concentration has a high kurtosis and is positively skewed, so it is not a normal distribution. The data log transformation was applied, so the data would be closer to a normal distribution. After the log transformation, the ^{40}K concentrations were found to be approximately normally distributed. The histogram of ^{40}K and the log transformation data is presented in Figure 6.

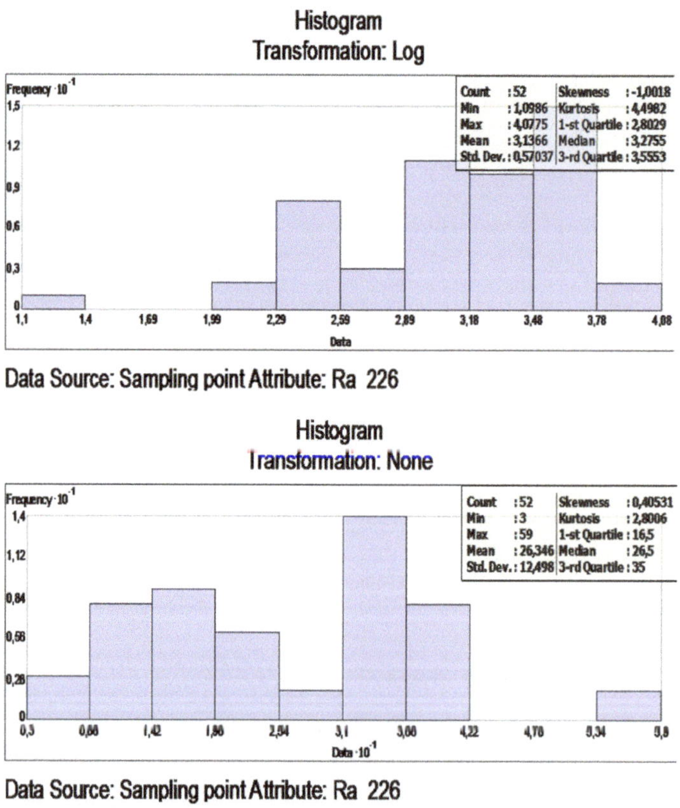

Figure 2 Frequency distribution of the ^{226}Ra and Log ^{226}Ra.

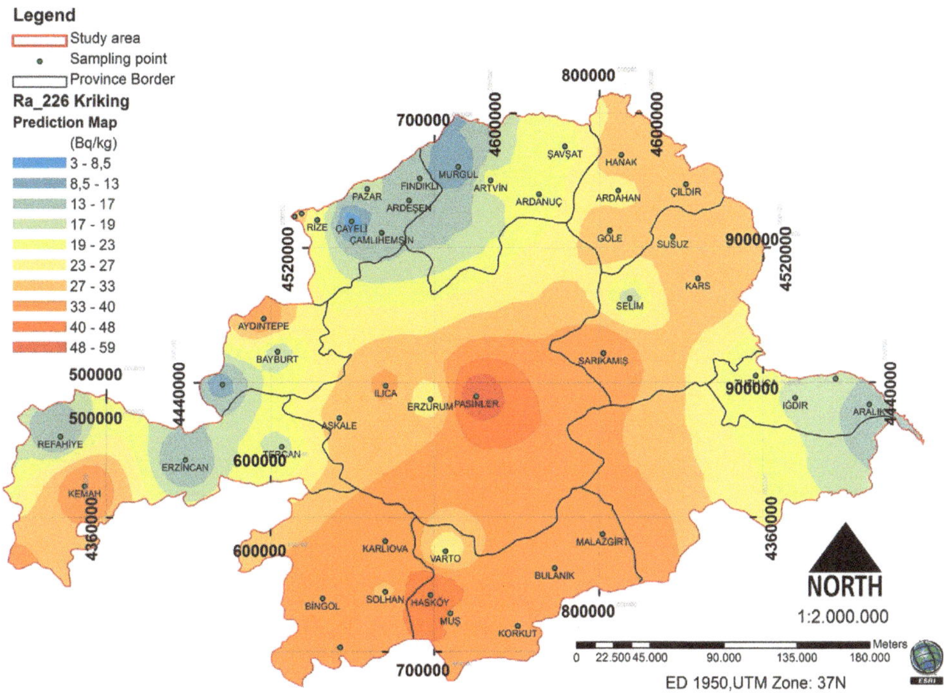

Figure 3 Spatial prediction map for the ordinary kriging interpolation of ^{226}Ra.

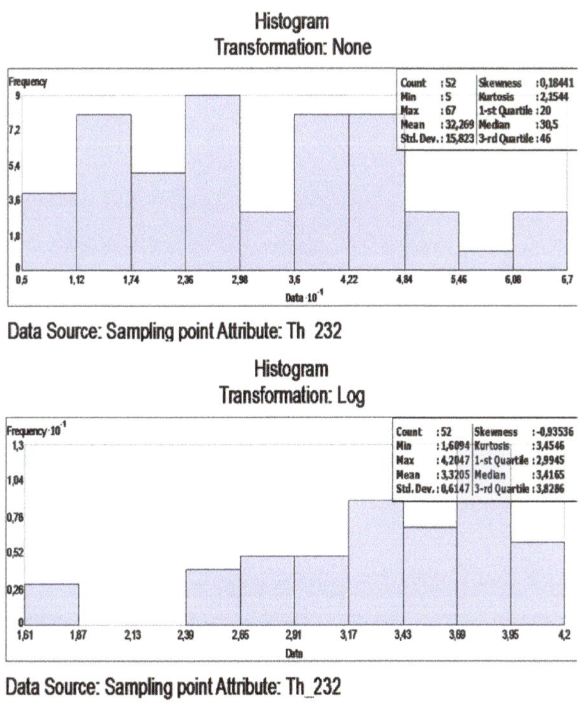

Figure 4 Frequency distribution of the ^{232}Th and Log ^{232}Th.

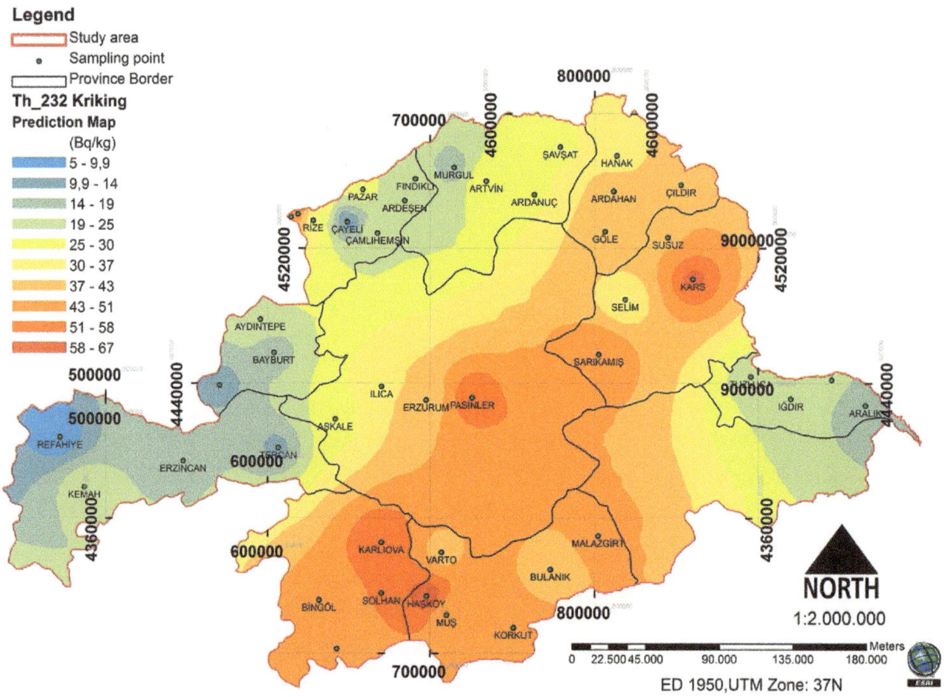

Figure 5 Spatial prediction map for the ordinary kriging interpolation of ^{232}Th.

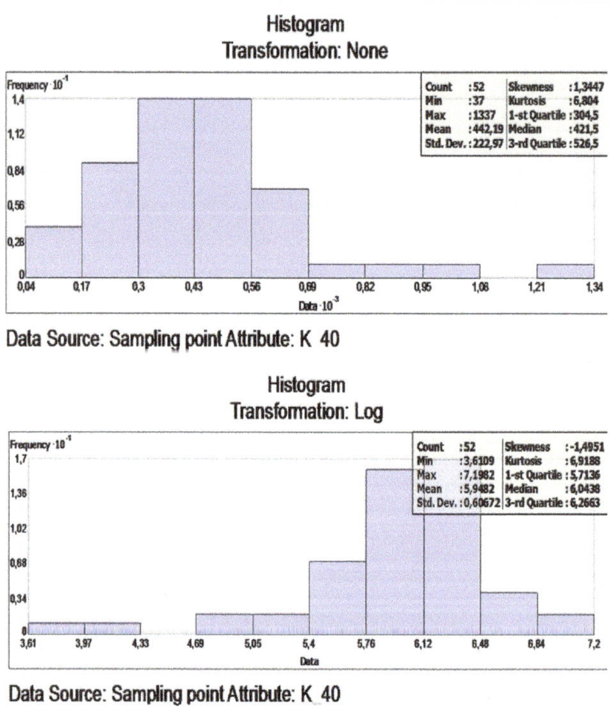

Figure 6 Frequency distribution of the ^{40}K and Log ^{40}K.

A comparison of the ME and the RMSSE for log ^{40}K shows that the stable model and its parameters is the best model that illustrates for ^{40}K concentration. The stable model has the best fit with the nugget effect (C_o) being equal to 41767.52, a sill ($C_o + C$) equal to 59158.77 and a range of influence equal to 375276. The ratio of nugget variance to sill is expressed in percentages equal to 70.60% (Table 2). This value is greater than 25 and less than 75%; thus, the ^{40}K distribution has a moderate spatial dependence in the study area. The spatial prediction and distribution map for the ordinary kriging interpolation ^{40}K is presented in Figure 7.

The relationship between forest cover and natural radionuclides

In the study area, the spatial distribution was analyzed in relation to the forest ecosystems and the radionuclides (Figures 8, 9 and 10). Between the ^{226}Ra and ^{232}Th, a positive increase in the 0.01 significance level (0.865**) was detected. Between the ^{40}K and ^{232}Th, a positive increase in the 0.05 significance level (0.718*) was detected. Between the forest cover and ^{226}Ra, a negative relationship was identified. Between the ^{232}Th and ^{40}K, a positive relationship was identified (Table 3). The radionuclide concentrations were found to depend on the soil humus content [27]. Different contents and amounts of organic matter in forest ecosystems effect the spatial variation of radionuclides in the soil.

Spatial changes of great soil groups and radionuclides in the soil

The soil group's map of the study area is presented in Figure 11. It was determined that 43.17% of the concentration of ^{40}K, 28.16% of the concentration of ^{226}Ra and 26.67% of the concentration of ^{232}Th was above the average UNSCEAR (2000) concentrations.

Within the study area, 17.49% of the Basaltic soils and 11.51% of the Chestnut soils had above average concentrations of the ^{40}K radionuclides. In addition, 10.8% of the Basaltic soils and 9.59% of the Chestnut soils had above average concentrations of ^{226}Ra radionuclides. It was also determined that 10.47% of the Basaltic soils and 9.32% of the Chestnut soils had above average concentrations of ^{232}Th radionuclides (Table 4). Consequently, all basalt and chestnut soil field locations had above average radionuclide concentrations.

Brown soils, High Mountain soils, Reddish Brown soils and Reddish Yellow Podsol soils in areas containing high concentrations of ^{226}Ra and ^{232}Th radionuclides had no spatial distribution pattern. In areas with Brown soils and Reddish Brown soils, high concentrations of ^{40}K radionuclides had no spatial distribution pattern (Table 4).

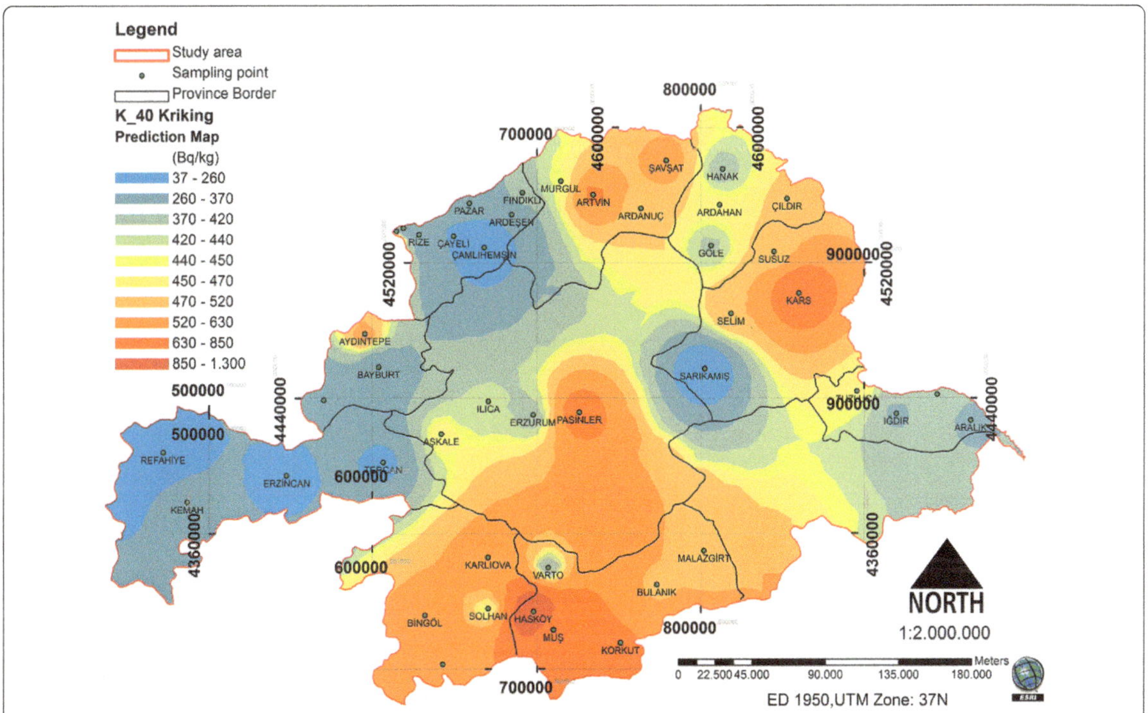

Figure 7 Spatial prediction map for the ordinary kriging interpolation of ^{40}K.

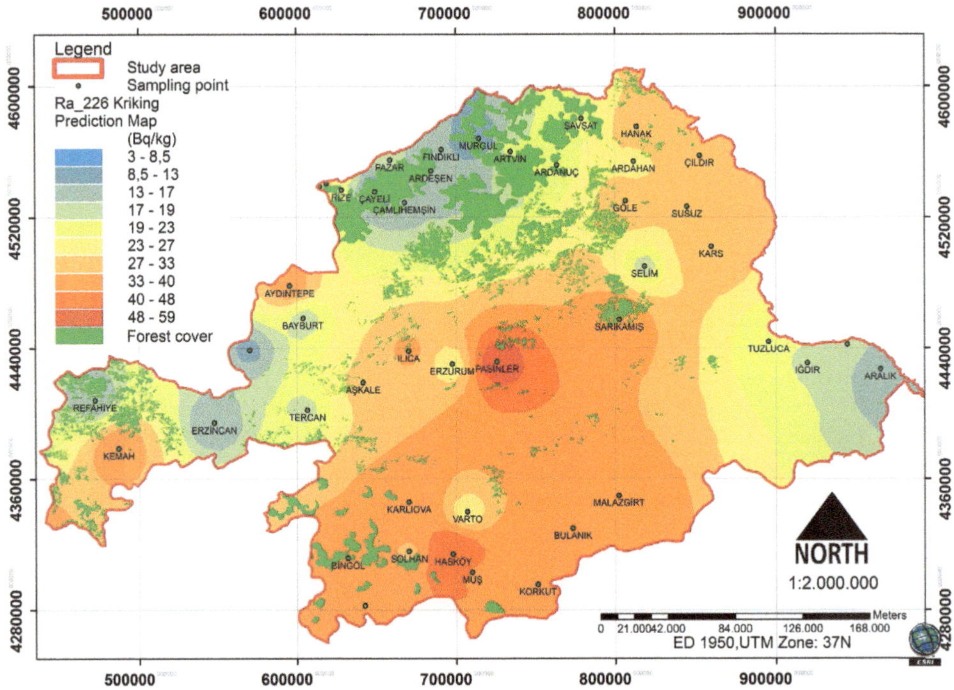

Figure 8 ^{226}Ra and spatial distribution of forest cover.

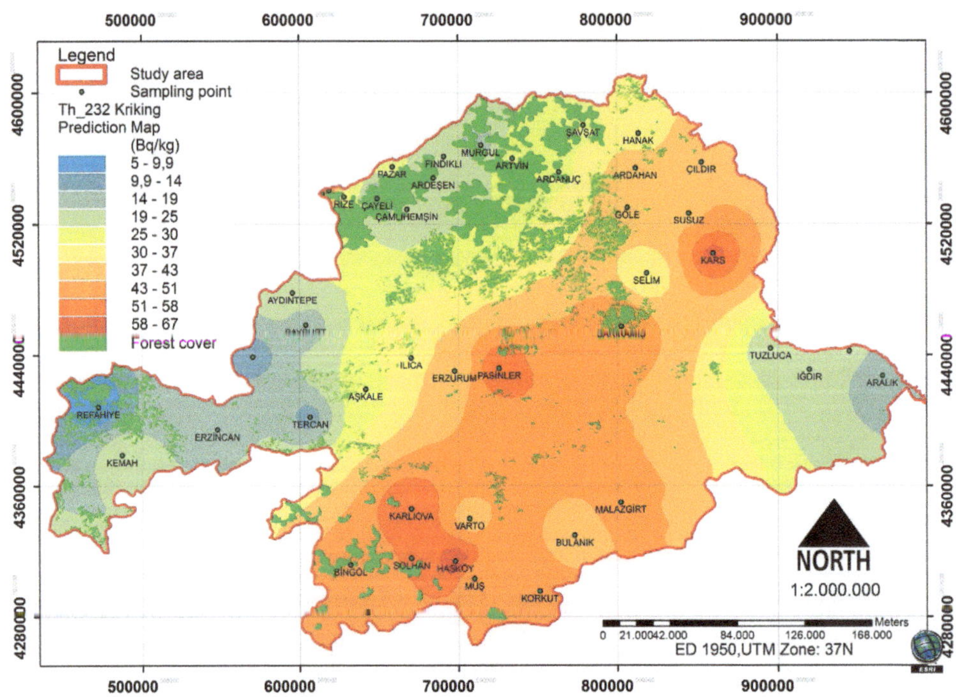

Figure 9 ^{232}Th and spatial distribution of forest cover.

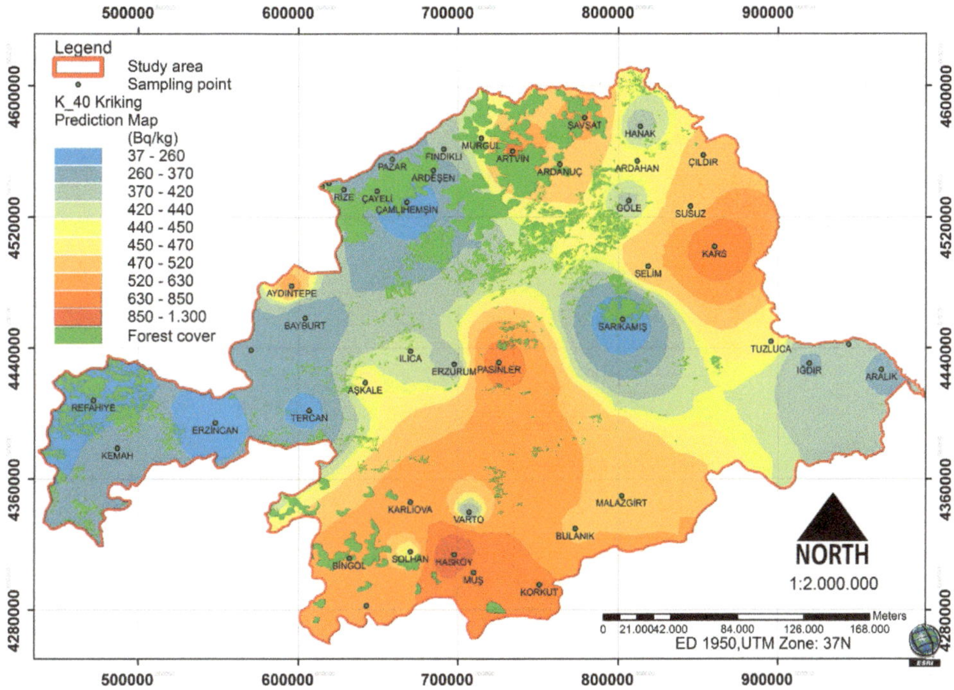

Figure 10 ^{40}K **and spatial distribution of forest cover.**

In summary, changes in the concentrations of radionuclides in the soil depend on the formation of iron oxide and other elements. Some of the acids formed in the soil, through calcium carbonate found in the environment, prevent the retention of the radionuclides. Therefore, radionuclide concentrations in the rocks can be reduced with calcium carbonate; this, in turn, reduces the level of external radiation [28,29]. According to the Anonymous [30], some rocks and a soil type typical of the specific radioactivity values was identified in the follow: For ^{40}K; Granite (1000 Bq/kg), clay stone (700 Bq/kg), Sandstone (350 Bq/kg) Basalt (250 Bq/kg) and limestone (90 Bq/kg). For ^{232}Th; Granite (80 Bq/kg), clay stone (50 Bq/kg), Sandstone (10 Bq/kg), Basalt (10 Bq/kg) and Limestone (7 Bq/kg). Local distribution values can vary greatly according to changing areas [31,32].

Table 3 Correlations test result between radionuclides and forest cover

Parameters	Radionuclides			Forest cover
	^{226}Ra	^{232}Th	^{40}K	
^{226}Ra	1			
^{232}Th	0,865**	1		
^{40}K	0,592	0,718*	1	
Forest cover	−0,008	0,096	0,232	1

**Correlation is significant at the 0.01 level (2-tailed).
*Correlation is significant at the 0.05 level (2-tailed).

Conclusions

Over time, the infiltration of radionuclides has resulted in high radionuclide concentrations in the lower soil layers. The radionuclides in these lower soil layers can move upwards through the roots of plants and be transferred to the plant during the growth process. Since radionuclides can have detrimental health effects on humans, it is important to determine the spatial variation of concentrations of radioactive elements.

This research was conducted to examine to spatial distribution of natural radioactive element (^{226}Ra, ^{232}Th and ^{40}K) concentrations and their relationship with soil groups and forest cover using the Kriging method. According to the statistical analyses, positive correlations were detected between the ^{226}Ra and the ^{232}Th (0.865**), as well as between the ^{40}K and ^{232}Th (0.718*). Negative correlations between forest cover and ^{226}Ra were found, while positive correlations between ^{232}Th and ^{40}K were detected.

The basalt and chestnut soils in the study area were found to have above average concentrations of radionuclides. The Brown soils, High Mountain soils, Reddish Brown soils and Reddish Yellow Podsol soils

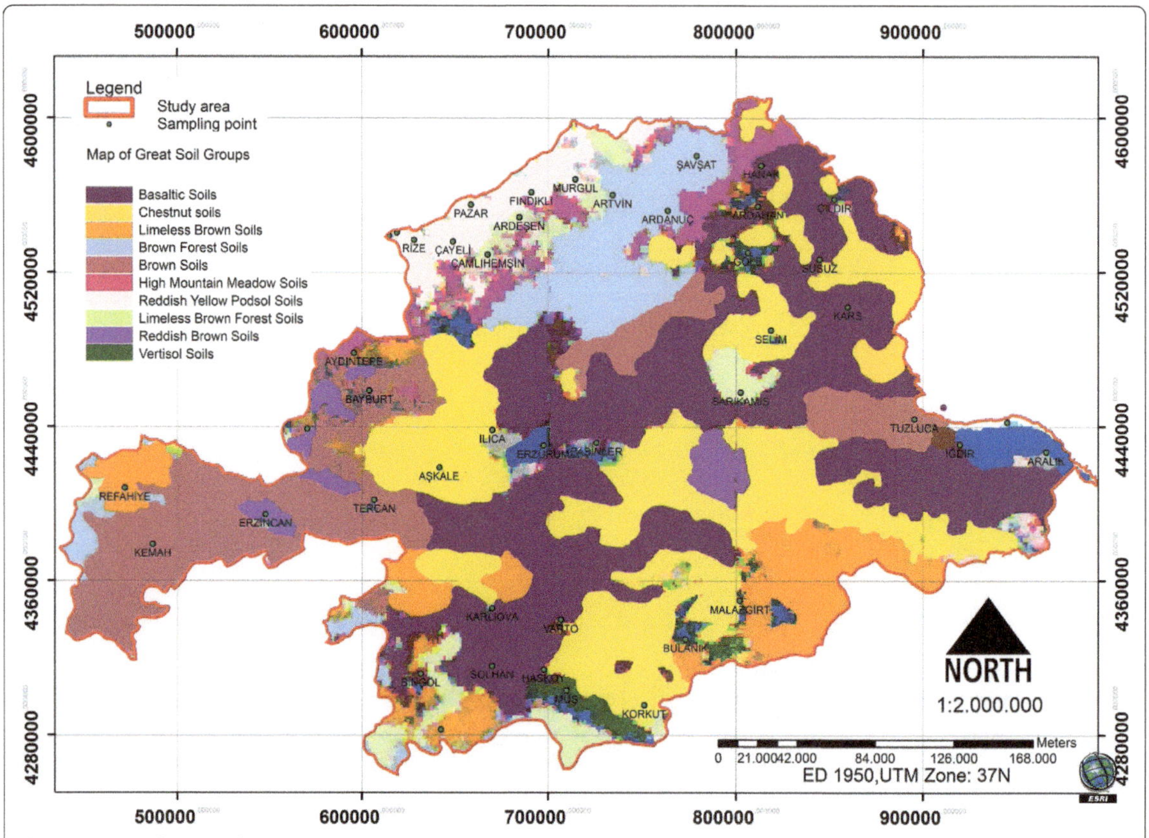

Figure 11 Map of great soil groups.

did not have high concentrations of ^{226}Ra and ^{232}Th. The Brown soils and the Reddish Brown soils also did not have high concentrations of ^{40}K.

Radionuclides are present in different concentrations in the soil, plants and water, which comprise parts of the basic food chain. Excessive exposure to radiation can lead to cancer; it is also the cause of hereditary diseases. Therefore, spatial variations of radioactive element concentrations need to be monitoring for the sustainability of a healthy environment.

Table 4 Spatial changes between radionuclides and great soil groups

Great soil goups	Spatial changes of the radionuclides concentration (Hectare)					
	^{40}K		^{226}Ra		^{232}Th	
	Under optimal concentrations (<400 Bg/kg)	Upper optimal concentrations (>400 Bg/kg)	Under optimal concentrations (<35 Bg/kg)	Upper optimal concentrations (>35 Bg/kg)	Under optimal concentrations (<45 Bg/kg)	Upper optimal concentrations (>45 Bg/kg)
Bazaltic Soils	1187656	1717242	1915127	989771	1876826	1028072
Chesnut Soils	1101871	1129844	1290559	941156	1316923	914792
Limeless Brownish Soils	428955	582383	620178	391160	762213	249125
Limeless Brown Forest Soils	94789	228346	119664	203471	135446	187689
Vertisol Soils	0	76254	0	76254	0	76254
Brown Forest Soils	464221	287303	684116	67408	684116	67408
Brown Soils	1505651	0	1505651	0	1505651	0
High Mountain Soils	262129	159430	421559	0	421559	0
Reddish Yellow Podsol Soils	438377	56680	495057	0	495057	0
Reddish Brown Soils	94684	0	0	94684	0	94684

Competing interests

The author declares that he has no competing interests.

Author's contribution

TD participated in the design of the study and has collected the data and drafted the manuscript used the GIS and makes statistical analysis related data with soil groups and forest area.

Acknowledgment

Authors present their great thanks to Turkey Atomic Energy Agency for data supply.

References

1. Theodorsson P: *Measurements of Weak Radioactivity.* Singapore: World Scientific Pub. Co; 1997.
2. TAEK: **Resource of natural radiation.** http://www.taek.gov.tr/bilgi-kosesi/184-radyasyon-insan-ve-cevre/radyasyonla-birlikte-yasiyoruz/501-dogal-radyasyon-kaynaklari.html Accessed on: 11.03.2014.
3. UNSCEAR: **Report on sources and effects of ionizing radiation to the general assembly, United Nations, Vienna.** 2000, http://www.unscear.org/unscear/en/publications/2000_1.html Accessed on: 25.02.2014.
4. Robertson GP: **Geostatistics in ecology: interpolation with known variance.** *Ecology* 1987, **68:**744–748.
5. Cressie NAC: *Statistics for Spatial Data.* Canada: John Wiley and Sons, Inc; 1993:900.
6. Goovaerts P: *Geostatistics for Natural Resources Evaluation.* New York: Oxford University Press; 1997:483.
7. Ecker MD: *Geostatistics: Past, Present and Future, Encyclopedia of Life Support Systems (EOLSS), Developed under the Auspices of the UNESCO.* Oxford, UK: Eolss Publishers; 2004.
8. Isaaks EH, Srivastava RM: *An Introduction to Applied Geostatistics.* New York: Oxford University Press; 1989.
9. Brown RB, Huddleston JH: **Presentation of statistics data on Map units to the user. In spatial variabilities of soil and landform.** *SSSA Special* 1991, **28:**127–147.
10. Khan HM, Khan K, Atta MA, Jan F: **Measurement of gamma activity of soil samples of Charsadda district of Pakistan.** *J Chem Soc Pakistan* 1994, **16:**183–188.
11. Rühm W, Kammerer L, Hiersche L, Wirth E: **Migration of 137Cs and 134Cs in different forest soil layers.** *J Environ Radioact* 1996, **33:**63–75.
12. Rosén K, Öborn I, Lönsjö H: **Migration of radiocaesium in Swedish soil profiles after the Chernobyl accident, 1987–1995.** *J Environ Radioact* 1999, **46:**45–66.
13. Bergman R: **The distribution of radioactive caesium in boreal forest ecosystems. In Nordic Radioecology, the Transfer of Radionuclides through Nordic Ecosystems to Man.** *Studies in Environmental Science* 1994, **62:**335–379. (ed. H. Dahlgaard) Elsevier, New York, NY.
14. Gorham E: **A comparison of natural and fallout radioactivity in Ontario soils under pine.** *Can J Bot* 1963, **4:**11309–11319. USA.
15. Degering D, Schlenker S, Unterricker S: *Radionuclide Behaviour in Natural Organic Matter (Peat, Cola and Forest Soil Surfaces)*, NRC 5, 5th International Conference on Nuclear and Radiochemistry. Pontresina, Switzerland: Paul Scherrer Institut; 2000:449–452.
16. Sokolik GA, Ivanova TG, Leinova SL, Ovsiannikova SV, Kimlenko IM: **Migration ability of radionuclides in soil-vegetative cover of Belarus after Chernobyl accident.** *Environ Int* 2001, **26:**183–187.
17. UNSCEAR: *Sources and Effects of Ionizing Radiation, Report of the General Assembly With Scientific Annex B.* New York: United Nations Publicaitons; 1993.
18. Hölgye Z, Malý M: **Sources, vertical distribution, and migration rates of ^{239,240}Pu, ^{238}Pu, and ^{137}Cs in grassland soil in three localities of central Bohemia.** *J Environ Radioact* 2000, **47:**135–147.
19. TAEK: Turkey Atomic Energy Agency: *Turkey Atlas of Environmental Radioactivity.* Ankara: 2014. http://www.taek.gov.tr/radyasyon-izleme/turkiye-cevresel-radyasyon-atlasi.html Accessed on: 26.03.2014.
20. OGM: *Forest Cover Map*, General Directorate of Forestry. Ankara: OGM Publications; 2012.
21. ESRİ: **The principels of geostatistical analysis.** 2013, 54. http://maps.unomaha.edu/Peterson/gisII/ESRImanuals/Ch3_Principles.pdf 22.02.2014.
22. Johnston K, Hoef M, Krivoruchko K, Lucas N: *Using ArcGIS Geostatistical Analyst.* New York: ESRI; 2001.
23. Clark I: *Practical Geostatistics.* London: Applied Science Publishers Ltd.; 1979:129.
24. Trangmar BB, Yost RS, Uehara G: **Application of geostatic to spatial studies of soil properties.** *Advances in Argon* 1985, **38:**45–94.
25. Cambardella CA, Moorman TB, Novak JM, Parkin TB, Karlen DL, Turco RF, Konopka AE: **Field-scale variability soil properties in Central Iowa soils.** *Soil Sci Soc Am J* 1994, **58:**1501–1511.
26. Erşahin S: **Alluvial soil in a field, some physical and chemical properties of the spatial variability of the determination.** *SU Journal of the Faculty of Agriculture* 1999, **13:**34–41.
27. Chelmicki V, Mietelski JW, Macharski P, Swicchowicz J: *Natural Factors of Cs-137 Rcdistribution in Soil.* Poland: Institute of Nuclear Physics Cracow, Report No. 1615ID; 1993:19.
28. NCRP: *National Council on Radiation Protection and Measurements*, No.45, Natural Background Radiation in the U.S., Soil Radioactivity. 1975:54.
29. Özger AG: **District of Ceyhan, Yumurtalık and Pozantı Determination of Natural Radioactivity Levels.** In *M.Sc. Thesis.* Çukurova University: Graduate School of Science; 2005.
30. Anonymous: *Federal Ministry for the Environment, Nature Conservation and Nuclear Safety, environmental radioactivity and radiation exposure, Annual Report, Bonn.* ; 1995:43–45.
31. Atakan Y: *Natural radioactivity, natural and human created in the radiation doses*, International Symposium on Medical Geology Participatory Books. 2008:51–63.
32. Vukašinović I, Đorđević A, Rajković M, Todorović D, Pavlović V: **Distribution of natural radionuclides in anthrosol-type soil.** *Turk J Agric* 2010, **34:**539–546.

Biosorption of Hg(II) and Cu(II) by biomass of dried *Sargassum fusiforme* in aquatic solution

Shengmou Huang and Gan Lin*

Abstract

The biosorption of heavy metals Hg(II) and Cu(II) from aquatic solution by biomass of dried *Sargassum fusiforme* was studied in the paper. The *Sargassum fusiforme* was able to absorb appreciable amount of mercury and copper from the aquatic solutions within 60 min of contact time with the metal solution and exhibited high removal of mercury and copper at low equilibrium concentrations. The specific adsorption of both Hg(II) and Cu(II) increased at low concentration of biomass and decreased when biomass concentration exceeded 2.0 g/L. The binding of mercury followed Freundlich model while copper supported Langmuir isotherm for adsorption with their r^2 values of 0.971 and 0.923, respectively. The maximum adsorption per unit masses of *Sargassum fusiforme* (mg/L) at equilibrium (q_{max}) for Hg(II) and Cu(II) were calculated to be 30.86 and 7.69 mg/g, respectively. The biosorption by *Sargassum fusiforme* was best described using a pseudo-second-order kinetic model for copper and mercury ions in solution in the study. The adsorption was pH dependent as the maximum mercury biosorption and copper adsorption was happened at solution pH of 8–10.

Keywords: Biosorption, *Sargassum fusiforme*, Mercury, Copper

Background

The heavy metal is among the most common pollutant found in industrial effluents. The major sources of pollution in the aquatic environment are industries such as paint, pulp and paper, oil refining, electrical, rubber, processing, fertilizer, pharmaceutical and battery manufacturing [1,2]. The major effects of mercury and copper poisoning manifest as neurological and renal disturbances as it can easily pass the blood–brain barrier. Environmental contamination with toxic heavy metals is a significant worldwide problem with their successive accumulation in the food chain and continued persistence in the ecosystem which will hurt human beings. Efforts have been made to remove toxic heavy metal from the wastewater and environment by using conserved technologies such as ion exchange or chemical precipitation, which are sometimes inefficient and expensive, particularly for removal of low concentrated heavy metal ions [3], and also leads to produce toxic sludge that adverse the economical feasibility of the treatment methods.

Indeed, many early studies have shown that nonliving biomass may be even more effective than living cells in sequestering metallic elements. Over the past two decades, much effort has been directed at identifying readily available biomass which, in its nonliving state, is capable of effectively removing heavy metals. It has been demonstrated that biosorption is a potential alternative to traditional treatment processes of metal ions removal. Biosorption is a property of certain types of inactive, dead biomass to bind and concentrate heavy metals from even very dilute aqueous solutions [4]. Biomass exhibits this property, acting just as a chemical substance, as an ion exchange of biological origin. Research on biosorption is revealing that it is sometimes a complex phenomenon where the metallic species could be deposited in the solid biosorbent through different sorption processes of ion exchange, complexation, chelation, microprecipitation, etc.

In these years, the role of seagrass in removal of toxic metal ions from the polluted water have taken more importance as they have a high area-to-volume ratio and therefore provide a large contact area for metal binding [5]. Small bacteria, algae, fungi and yeast have been well recognized for heavy metal removal [6]. Up to date, the role of algae has received increased attention to years

* Correspondence: lingan1978@126.com
School of chemical engineering and food science, Hubei University of Arts and Science, Xiangyang 441053, China

because of it are potential for application of environmental protection as well as recovery of heavy metals. The affinity with various algae species for binding of heavy metals shows different results [7]. Metal ions with greater electro-negativity and smaller ionic radii are preferably absorbed by algae biomass [8]. Metal accumulation capacity of algae biomass is sometimes higher than chemical sorbents therefore algae biomass may serve as an economically feasible to the existing physicochemical methods of metal removal of wastewaters. The major challenge to biosorption studies is to select the most promising biomass from a large pool of available and inexpensive biomaterials. Contributions to *Sargassum fusiforme* in the metal adsorption is of great concern [9].

In the present study, dried biomass of *Sargassum fusiforme* were used and characterized for its Cu(II) and Hg(II) removal potential from synthetic metal solution. The effect of pH, biomass concentration, initial metal concentration and contact time was studied for metal sorption procedure as well as heavy metal equilibrium sorption kinetics was made in lab.

Methods

Biosorbent material

The dry biomass of *Sargassum fusiforme* were purchased from Fuzhou Lantian limited Company, Fujian (China). It was powdered and sieved into less than 1 mm in diameter and dried at 80°C for 12 h with drying oven(01A, Suzhou sinovel oven manufacturing co., LTD). The characteristics of the *Sargassum fusiforme* were determined by F-Sorb type 3400 specific surfaces and pore diameter gauge (Beijing gold spectrum technology co., LTD). The surface BET on the algae was of means with 35-40 m^2/g, total pore volume is of 50-70% and the pore structure is mesoporous material. The FTIR spectrum of the fresh and metal-loaded ones were made by the FTIR920(Tianjin topology instrument co., LTD). The SEM images of the fresh and metal-loaded ones were attained by SU3500 (Hitachi High-Technologies Corporation).

Mercury and copper sorption experiments

Heavy metal solutions were prepared for diluting 200 mg/L of stock solutions, which were made by dissolving copper nitrate and mercury nitrate of analytical grade (Shanghai bo yiu biological technology co., LTD) in double distilled water. Metal sorption studies were carried out to evaluate the capacity of dry biomass of *Sargassum fusiforme* to adsorb metal ions from solutions. In batch ones, 100 mL of synthetic metal solutions having different concentrations (10,20,30,40, and 50 mg/L) of copper or mercury were placed in 250 ml Erlenmeyer flasks with a range of biomass concentrations(0.5,1.0,1.5.2.0,2.5, and 3.0 g/L) as biosorbent. Erlenmeyer flasks were kept under shaking at 120 rpm at 25°C. Samples were taken after 20-120 min and filtered and analyzed for final metal concentration (C_f) using ICP-AES (HK-2000, Huake Beijing tiancheng technology co., LTD) after an acid digestion [10].

To see the effect of pH on Hg(II) and Cu(II) removal, a range of pH (2–10) was adjusted to 0.1 M NaOH or 0.1 M HCl in 100 ml metal solutions containing fixed concentration of metal at 10 mg/L and biomass of 3.0 g/L followed by contact time of 60 min at rotation of 120 rpm. The metal adsorption(q) with *Sargassum fusiforme* and bioremoval efficiency(R) were calculated by the following formulae.

$$q = \left(C_i - C_f\right) * \frac{V}{M} \tag{1}$$

$$R(\%) = \frac{C_i - C_f}{C_i} * 100 \tag{2}$$

Where q = metal adsorption (mg/g); M = dry mass of *Sargassum fusiforme*(g); V = volume of initial metal solution used (L); R = bioremoval efficiency (%); C_i = initial concentration of metal in aquatic solution (mg/L); C_f = final concentration of metal in aquatic solution (mg/L) [11].

Adsorption isotherm

During biosorption, the equilibrium is established between absorbed metal ion on the *Sargassum fusiforme*(q) and unabsorbed metal ions in the solution(C_f). This equilibrium represented by Langmuir and Freundlich adsorption isotherms, are widely used to analyze data for wastewater treatment application [12]. Langmuir equation, which is valid for monolayer sorption onto a surface, with identical sites was given by Eq. 3.

$$q = q_{\max} * b * \frac{C_f}{1 + bC_f} \tag{3}$$

Where q_{max}(mg/g) is the maximum amount of the metal ion per unit weights of algae to form a complete monolayer on the surface bound at high C_f(mg/L), and b is a constant related to the affinity of the binding sites(mg/L), q_{max} represents a practical limiting adsorption capacity when the surface is fully covered with metal ions and assists in the comparison of adsorption performance [13]. The q_{max} and b can be determined from the liner plot of C_f/q versus C_f. The empirical Freundlich equation based on sorption on a heterogeneous surface is given below by Eq. 4.

$$q = k * C_f^{1/n} \tag{4}$$

The k and n parameters are the constants of the Freundlich isotherm. The k and n are indicators of adsorption capacity and adsorption intensity, respectively. The Eq.4 can be linearized in logarithmic forms and Freundlich constants can be determined by the plot. Freundlich isotherm is also more widely used as it provides no information on the monolayer adsorption capacity [14].

Biosorption kinetics

The experimental biosorption kinetic data was modeled using the pseudo-first-order (Eq.5), and pseudo-second-order models (Eq.6). The linear pseudo-first-order model can be represented by the following equation:

$$\log(q_e - q_t) \log q_e - \frac{K_1}{2.303} * t \tag{5}$$

The qe (mg/g) and qt (mg/g) are the amounts of adsorbed metal on the sorbent at the equilibrium time and at any time t, respectively, and $K_1(\mathrm{min}^{-1})$ is the rate constant of the pseudo-first-order adsorption process. The linear pseudo-second-order model can be represented by the following equation:

$$t/q_t = \frac{1}{K_2} * q_e^2 + \frac{t}{q_e} \tag{6}$$

Where K_2 (g*mg^{-1}*min^{-1}) is the equilibrium rate constant of pseudo-second-order [11].

Results and discussion

Effect of pH solution

The pH is one of the important parameters in heavy metal sorption by *Sargassum fusiforme*. Therefore metal sorption studies were carried out at different pH values. Results revealed the maximum biosorption of Hg(II) were at pH 8(70%) and 10(72%) and Cu(II) demonstrated the same result at pH8(90%) and 10(92%) from aquatic solution containing initial 10 mg/L of metal concentration (Figure 1).

It was observed that Hg(II) and Cu(II) adsorption was less than 10% at pH 2. Enhance adsorption of Hg(II) and Cu(II) ions at higher pH was observed which coincides with earlier findings where in most cases the removal efficiency increased steadily with rise in pH [15]. The adsorption of metal ions was lower at low pH because of high concentration of protons in the solution which competed with metal ions in forming a bond between the active sites on the surface of the algae biomass [16]. Selective sorption of specific metals due to distinct pH optima for their sorption may be due to the chemical composition of cell surfaces. A distinct relationship between pH of aquatic metal solutions and involvement of functional group in binding of Hg(II) and Cu(II) onto *Sargassum fusiforme* maxima was observed with the involvement of functional groups such as carboxyl, phosphate and hydroxyl [17].

Metal concentration

Biosorption studies carried out for both Hg(II)and Cu(II) in 100 ml solutions containing metals varying from 10 to 50 mg/L with Hg(II)and Cu(II) by 3.0 g/L of biomass exhibited effective role of initial metal concentration on metal removal. A consistent decrease in metal removal was observed by increasing external metal concentration (Figure 2) where 70-74% removal efficiency was reported on 10 to 20 mg/L Hg(II) solutions followed by decline in solutions to 50 mg/L Hg(II)(Figure 2). Similarly decreases in Cu(II) removal efficiency was observed by increasing external metal concentration on 50 mg/L Cu(II) (Figure 2). Rapid metal adsorption profile of *Sargassum fusiforme* was obtained for both Hg(II) and Cu(II), which is important when the algae are used for biosorption. It

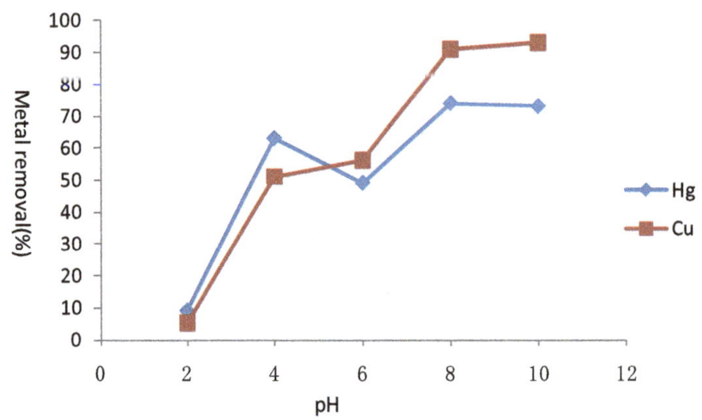

Figure 1 pH dependent sorption of Hg(II) and Cu(II) by *Sargassum fusiforme*(Hg(II):10 mg/L, Cu(II):10 mg/L), standard deviation is less than 5% in triplicates.

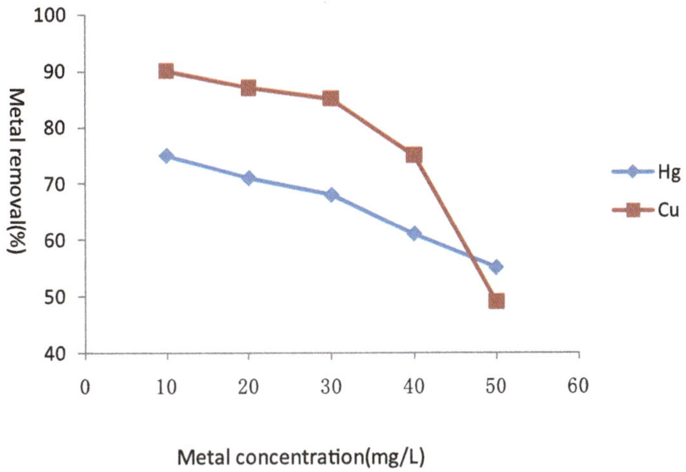

Figure 2 Initial concentration dependent sorption of Hg(II) and Cu(II) by *Sargassum fusiforme*, standard deviation is less than 5% in triplicates.

exhibited rapid biosorption at first 60 min by removing 72% Hg(II) and 90% of Cu(II) from metal solutions. Decreases in metal removal of increasing initial metal concentration was supported by the findings that observed that the removal of metal generally decreases from increasing concentration of metals in the solution [18]. Algae surface has different functional groups of varying the affinity with ionic kinds, therefore decline in metal removal is largely attributed to saturation of adsorption sites [7].

Contact time determination

Rapid metal adsorption profile of *Sargassum fusiforme* was obtained for both Hg(II) and Cu(II), which is important when the material is to be used for biosorption. It exhibited rapid biosorption in first 60 min by removing 71% Hg(II) and 88% of Cu(II) from metal solutions thereafter increase in metal removal was magical. Equilibrium was established between absorbed metal ions after 40 min with maximum removal of 55% and 75% of Hg(II) and Cu(II) (Figure 3).

The *Sargassum fusiforme* biomass showed rapid biosorption at first 60 min. It has been reported that the sorption of heavy metal ions by algae followed mechanism where the metal ion is physically or chemically taken up onto the surface of the algae [19]. In this case, since the algae were dried and biological functions were no longer active, the sorption could only take place on the

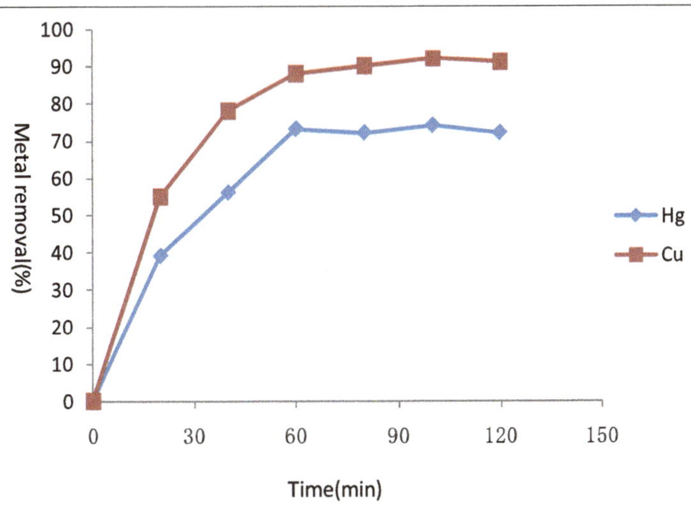

Figure 3 Time dependent removal of Hg(II) and Cu(II) by *Sargassum fusiforme*(Hg(II):10 mg/L, Cu(II):10 mg/L), standard deviation is less than 5% in triplicates.

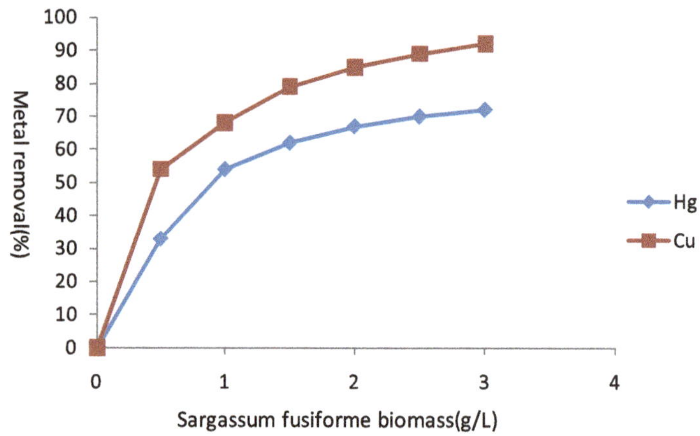

Figure 4 Effect of *Sargassum fusiforme* biomass concentration on Hg(II) and Cu(II) removal(Hg(II):10 mg/L, Cu(II):10 mg/L), standard deviation is less than 5% in triplicates.

cell surface. The increase in Hg(II) and Cu(II) adsorbed by increasing biomass was also expected as a result of increase in available area-to-volume ratio and therefore providing a large contact area for heavy metal binding [20].

Biomass determination

Increase in metal removal efficiency from 10 mg/L manual metal solutions to both Hg(II) and Cu(II) was observed on increasing biomass concentration (Figure 4).

Hg(II) adsorption was increased to 71% by increasing biomass concentration on 0 to 3.0 g/L in 10 mg/L of mercury containing synthetic solutions whereas, same trend was observed in case of Cu(II) with the increase of 90%. The *Sargassum fusiforme* biomass displayed its equilibrium for Hg(II) removal of 3.0 g/L of biomass concentration whereas, a continuous increase in Cu(II) removal of increasing biomass concentration was observed of 3.0 g/L. Metal adsorption studies from solution mass balance revealed a decline in sorption of Hg(II) and Cu(II) respectively by increasing biomass from 0 to 3.0 g/L after 60 min of contact time. The other probable explanations for such a relationship between biomass concentration and adsorption may be limited availability of metal, increased electrostatic interactions between binding sites and reduced mixing at higher biomass concentration [21,22].

The FTIR and SEM analysis

With the determination of functional matrices and group in the heavy metal biosorption of the algae, it is useful for the study of FTIR spectrums. The figures are shown in Figure 5. With the determination of biosorption kinetics and isotherms in the heavy metal biosorption of the algae, the use of SEM images is shown in Figure 6 for the study.

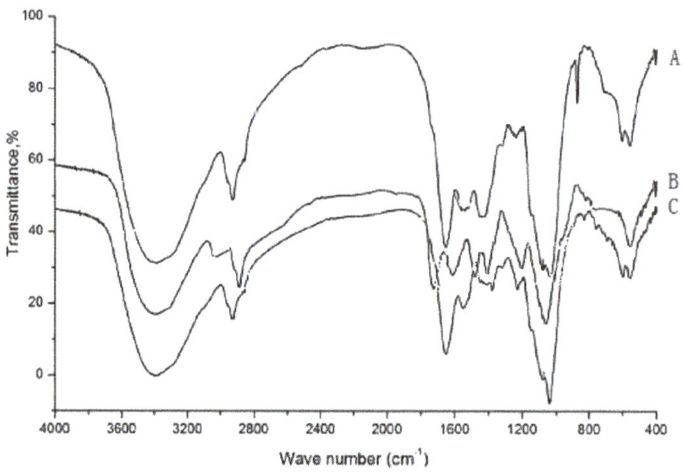

Figure 5 The FTIR spectrum of the adsorbent for fresh and metal loaded ones. A: fresh, **B**: Cu(II) loaded, **C**: Hg(II) loaded.

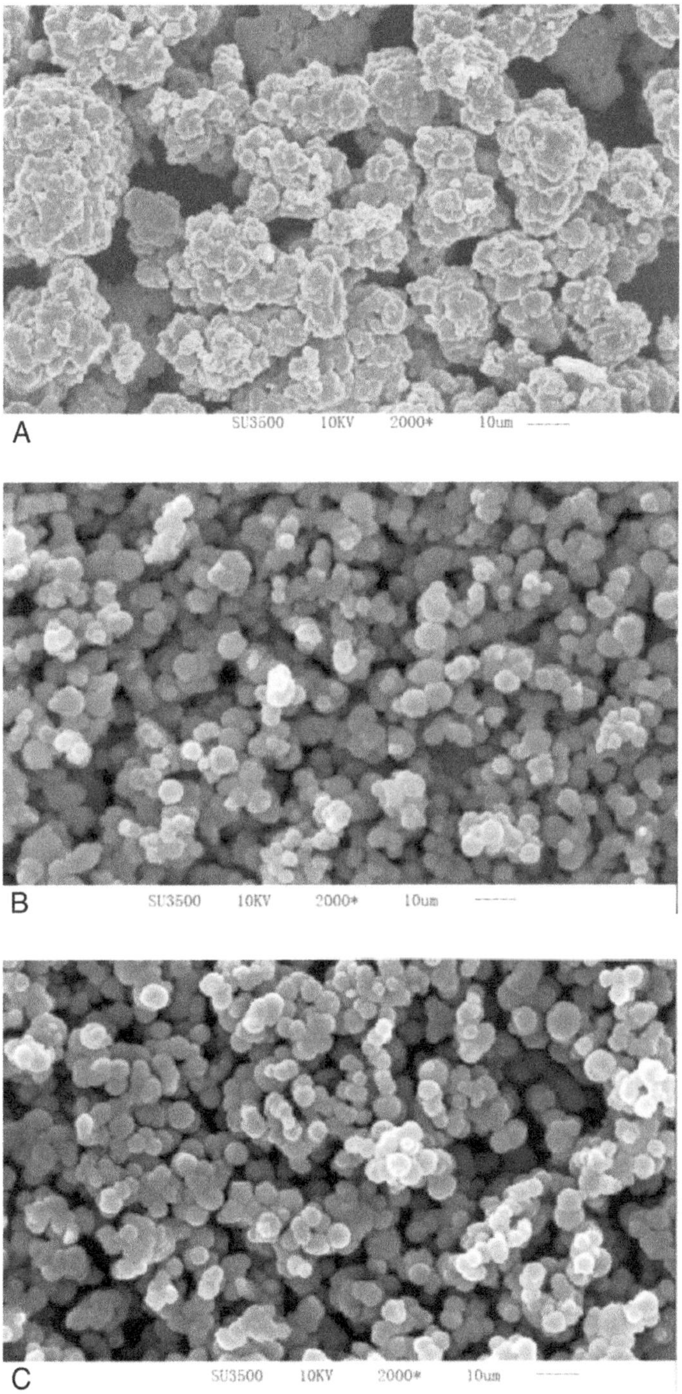

Figure 6 The SEM images of the adsorbent for fresh and metal loaded ones. A: fresh, **B:** Cu(II) loaded, **C:** Hg(II) loaded.

Modeling study

A linear regression of the experimental results from Hg(II) and Cu(II) differed in terms of Hg(II) adsorption fitted better to Freundlich isotherm and Cu(II) to Langmuir isotherms with r^2 values of 0.971 and 0.823 respectively (Table 1). The maximum adsorption per unit masses of

Table 1 Langmuir and Freundlich parameters for the sorption of the test metals by *Sargassum fusiforme*

Metal	Langmuir isotherm			Freundlich isotherm		
	b(L/mg)	r^2	qmax(g/mg)	K(mg/g)	n	r^2
Hg(II)	0.988	0.668	30.86	2.012	3.89	0.971
Cu(II)	1.269	0.923	7.69	0.899	5.41	0.765

Sargassum fusiforme (mg/L), at equilibrium (q_{max}) for Hg (II) and Cu(II) were calculated to be 30.86 and 7.69 mg/g respectively (Table 1).

The sorption isotherm is the relationship between equilibrium concentration on the solution and equilibrium concentration of solute in the sorbent at constant temperature where either Freundlich or Langmuir model can describe the biosorption equilibrium of copper and mercury [23]. An extremely high r^2 value of Freundlich isotherm for Hg(II) sorption indicated that ion exchange interaction takes place between metal ion and the biosorbent, while Cu(II) follows Langmuir isotherm and thus supported physicochemical interactions with each other.

For biomasses of *Sargassum fusiforme,* the kinetics of copper and mercury biosorption were analyzed using pseudo-first-order and pseudo-second-order models. All the constants and regression coefficients are shown in Table 2. In the present study, biosorption by *Sargassum fusiforme* was best described using a pseudo-second-order kinetic models for copper and mercury ions in solution. This adsorption kinetic is typical of the adsorption of divalent metals onto biosorbents.

Conclusions

The goal of the study was to explore and find out the potential use of algae biomass as a low cost sorbent for the removal of heavy metals from aquatic solutions. The heavy metals Hg(II) and Cu(II) from aquatic solution was able to be dealt with dried *Sargassum fusiforme.* The seagrass adsorbed appreciable amount of mercury and copper from the aquatic solutions within 60 min at low equilibrium concentrations. The specific adsorption of both Hg(II) and Cu(II) increased at low concentration while decreased when biomass concentration exceeded 2.0 g/L. The binding of mercury followed Freundlich model but copper supported Langmuir isotherm for adsorption with their r^2 values of 0.971 and 0.923, respectively. The maximum adsorption per unit masses of *Sargassum fusiforme* (mg/L), at equilibrium (q_{max}) for Hg(II) and Cu(II) were calculated to be 30.86 and 7.69 mg/g respectively. The adsorption was pH dependent as the maximum mercury biosorption utilized at pH 8 and 10 and Cu(II) adsorption was at pH 8 and 10. The biosorption by *Sargassum fusiforme* was best described using a pseudo-second-order kinetic model for copper and mercury ions in solution in the study. The present paper emphasizes the *Sargassum fusiforme* is an ideal candidate and can be designed as a practical and economical process for wastewater treatment polluted by heavy metals.

Table 2 First and second order adsorption rate constants for Hg(II) and Cu(II)

Metal	Pseudo-first-order		Pseudo-second-order	
	$K_1(min^{-1})$	r^2	$K_2(g*mg^{-1}*min^{-1})$	r^2
Hg(II)	$5.3*10^{-3}$	0.745	$9.15*10^{-3}$	0.957
Cu(II)	$3.1*10^{-3}$	0.615	$8.84*10^{-3}$	0.963

Competing interests

The authors declare that they have no competing interests.

Authors' contributions

HSM and LG conceived the work, performed the experiments, designed the experiments, analyzed the data, and wrote the manuscript. Both authors read and approved the final manuscript.

Acknowledgments

We greatly thank Chen Guantong from FAU for providing researching materials in this investigation. We are also grateful to Zhang Danfeng for the helpful comments and linguistic revision of the manuscript. This work was supported by grants from the ministry of education from Hubei province, People's Republic of China(project No. Q20122506).

References

1. Rezaee A, Ramavandi B, Ganati F. Biosorption of mercury by biomass of filamentous algae *Spirogyra* species. J Biol Sci. 2006;6(4):695–700.
2. Khodaverdiloo H, Samadi A. Batch equilibrium study on sorption, desorption, and immobilisation of cadmium in some semi-arid zone soils as affected by soil properties. Soil Res. 2011;49:444–54.
3. Lu WB, Shi JJ, Wang CH, Chang JS. Biosorption of lead, copper and cadmium by indigenous isolate *Enterobacter* sp. Processing high heavy metal resistance. J Hazard Mater. 2006;134:80–6.
4. Rezaee A, Ramavandi B, Ganati F. Equilibrium and spectroscopic studies on biosorption of mercury by algae biomass. Pak J Biol Sci. 2006;9(4):777–82.
5. Pandiyan S, Mahendradas D. Application of bacteria to remove Ni(II) Ions from aqueous solution. Eur J Sci Res. 2011;52:345–58.
6. Ekmekyapar F, Aslan A, Bayhan YK, Cakici A. Biosorption of copper (II) by nonliving lichen biomass of *Cladonia rangiformis* hoffm. J Hazard Mater. 2006;B137:293–8.
7. Zouboulis AI, Loukidou MX, Matis KA. Biosorption of toxic metals from aqueous solution by bacterial strains isolated from metal-polluted soils. Process Biochem. 2004;39:909–16.
8. Anjana K, Kaushik A, Kiran B, Nisha R. Biosorption of Cr(VI) by immobilized biomass of two indigenous strains of cyanobacteria isolated from metal contaminated soil. J Hazard Mater. 2007;148:383–6.
9. Naik UC, Srivastava S, Thakur IS. Isolation and characterization of *Bacillus cereus* IST105 from electroplating effluent for detoxification of hexavalent chromium. Environ Sci Pollut Res Int. 2011;19:3005–14.
10. Vijayaraghavan K, Jegan J, Palanivenu K, Velan M. Biosorption of cobalt(II) and nickel(II) by seaweeds: batch and column studies. Sep Purif Technol. 2005;44:53–9.
11. Ok YS, Yang JE, Zhang YS, Kim SJ, Chung DY. Heavy metal adsorption by a formulated zeolite-Portland cement mixture. J Hazard Mater. 2007;147:91–6.
12. Kaewsarn P, Yu Q. Cadmium (II) removal from aqueous solutions by pretreated biomass of marine alga *Padina* sp. Environ Pollut. 2001;112:209–13.
13. Chatterjee SK, Bhattacharjee I, Chandra G. Biosorption of heavy metals from industrial waste water by *Geobacillus thermode* nitrificans. J Hazard Mater. 2010;175:117–25.

14. Lodeiro P, Barriada JL, Herrero R, Sastre deVicente ME. The marine macroalga *Cystoseira baccata* as biosorbent for cadmium (II) and lead (II) removal: kinetic and equilibrium studies. Environ Pollut. 2006;142:264–73.
15. Vilar VJP, Botelho CMS, Boaventura RAR. Lead uptake by algae *Gelidium* and composite material particles in a packed bed column. Chem Eng J. 2008;144:420–30.
16. Costodes VCT, Fauduet H, Porte C, Delacroix A. Removal of Cd(II) and Pb(II) ions from aqueous solutions by adsorption onto sawdust of *Pinus sylvestris*. J Hazard Mater. 2003;105:121–42.
17. Pabst MW, Miller CD, Dimkpa CO, Anderson AJ, McLean JE. Defining the surface adsorption and internalization of copper and cadmium in a soil bacterium *Pseudomonas putida*. Chemosphere. 2010;81:904–10.
18. Sari A, Tuzen M. Biosorption of Pb(II) and Cd(II) from aqueous solution using green alga (*Ulva lactuca*) biomass. J Hazard Mater. 2008;152:302–8.
19. Oliveira SM, Pessenda LC, Gouveia SE, Favaro DI. Heavy metal concentrations in soils from a remote oceanic island, Fernando de Noronha. Braz An Acad Bras Cienc. 2011;83:1193–206.
20. Pardo R, Herguedas M, Barrado E, Vega M. Biosorption of cadmium, copper, lead and zinc by inactive biomass of *Pseudomonas putida*. Anal Bioanal Chem. 2003;376:26–32.
21. Wang XS, Qin Y. Removal of Ni(II), Zn(II) and Cr(VI) from aqueous solution by *Alternanthera philoxeroides* biomass. J Hazard Mater. 2006;138:582–8.
22. Xiong J, He Z, Liu D, Mahmood Q, Yang X. The role of bacteria in the heavy metals removal and growth of *Sedum alfredii* Hance in an aqueous medium. Chemosphere. 2008;70:489–94.
23. Mata YN, Blazquez ML, Ballester A, Gonzalez F, Munoz JA. Characterization of the biosorption of cadmium, lead and copper with the brown alga *Fucus vesiculosus*. J Hazard Mater. 2008;158:316–23.

6

Modelling and evaluation of light railway system's noise using neural predictors

Selçuk Erkaya[1*], Abdurrahman Geymen[2] and Bülent Bostancı[2]

Abstract

Background: Noise is defined as a sound or series of sounds that are considered to be invasive, irritating, objectionable and disruptive to the quality of daily life. Noise is one of the environmental pollutants, and in cities it is usually originated from road traffic, railway traffic, airports, industry etc. The tram is generally considered as environmentally friendly, namely non-polluting and silent. However complaints from residents living along the tramway lines prove that it may sometimes cause annoyance. In this study, a Global Pointing System (GPS) receiver for determining the sampling locations and a frequency based noise measurement system for collecting the noise data are used to analyse the noise level in the city centre. Both environmental (background) and tram noises are measured.

Results: Three types of neural networks are used to predict the noises of the tram and environment. The results of three approaches indicate that the proposed neural network with Radial Basis Function (RBF) has superior performance to predict the noises of the tram and environment.

Conclusions: For making a decision about transportation planning, this network model can help urban planners for evaluating and/or isolating the tram noise in terms of human health.

Keywords: Noise mapping, Neural networks, Radial basis function

Background

The first step of effective noise reduction is to define the main sources of the noise generation. Noise has a clear effect upon person's health in terms of physiological and physical approaches. For example, negative effects on sense of hearing may be considered as a physical effect. These effects may cause temporary or permanent hearing loss. Physiological effects may include increase in blood pressure, cogwheel rigidity, stress, irregular heartbeat, pupil enlargement, insomnia, and tachyon etc. The application of neural networks has been rapidly expanded over the last two decades due to the progress in computer modelling and sensor technologies [1]. In case of system identifications using neural networks, the main purpose is usually to define a dynamically valid model which can be used for system analysis.

Modelling and prediction of noise by using classical approaches is a very complex and nonlinear process, due primarily to involvement of several factors on which noise level depends. To overcome these problems, researchers and acoustical engineers have applied the neural networks (NN) in the field of noise prediction. A literature review concerning the application of neural networks in traffic noise prediction was presented [2]. A back propagation neural network (BPNN) model was used to predict the noise caused by urban traffic. Five characteristics as the number of cars, trucks and motorcycles, the average height of buildings and the road width were used as input to model the equivalent sound pressure level as output [3]. Mathematical logarithmic, statistical linear regression and neural models were presented to predict the maximum A-weighed noise level ($L_{A,max}$) for the Tehran–Karaj express train. Measurements were obtained from sampling locations at distances of 25 m, 45 m and 65 m from the centreline of the track and at a height of 1.5 m [4]. Another study of same research group presented an artificial neural network model to predict hourly A-weighted equivalent sound pressure levels for roads in Tehran at distances less than 4 m from the nearside carriageway edge. Data were obtained from 50 sampling locations near five roads [5]. An experimental study was designed to assess the effect of road traffic noise on human performance [6]. A procedure

* Correspondence: serkaya@erciyes.edu.tr
[1]Engineering Faculty, Mechatronics Engineering Department, Erciyes University, Kayseri 38039, Turkey
Full list of author information is available at the end of the article

for evaluating the noise quality of a cooling system (HVAC system), which frequently works during a day, was studied by using neural network structures [7]. Both experimental and simulation analyses were implemented together. For predicting the sound absorption coefficients of a sandwich structure nonwoven absorber, a general forecasting method was performed using general regression neural network (GRNN) [8]. Artificial neural network model was proposed to estimate the weighted sound insulation index value of wooden windows based on a limited number of windows parameters [9]. BPNN and GRNN models were used to predict the construction noise in Kuwait by considering the 33 construction sites. The GRNN model was superior to the BPNN model in its accuracy of predicting construction noise [10]. A neuro-adaptive active noise control approach with radial basis function neural network (RBFNN) was introduced for both modelling and controlling the system [11]. The feasibility and accuracy of network modelling for road traffic noise prediction was tested during the uninterrupted and interrupted traffic flow conditions [12]. Sixteen locations were identified by neural model comprising the feed forward negative back propagation algorithm. A procedure with neural predictor was proposed to test and evaluate the sound quality of cars with varying running speed [13]. Also, a robust noise analyser with NN was introduced to model and evaluate the joint noise of an industrial robot [14]. A Multi-Layered Perceptron (MLP) neural network model with Levenberg-Marquardt (LM) learning algorithm was developed for urban noise. 289 data from streets in Granada, Spain were obtained. The neural network model included 25 input variables to model the sound pressure level [15]. Noise measurements were made for 16 relevant outdoor points in the central campus area of Yildiz Technical University, Istanbul, Turkey. Artificial neural networks were used to model the variation of noise levels from traffic around the campus area. Six variables in input matrix, that is, sampling location, geographical situation, wind speed and direction, air temperature and relative humidity, and time of day were used to predict the sound pressure level [16].

The goal of this study is to present a neural network based approach to predict the level of environmental and tram line noises. Three types of neural predictor, which are extensively preferred in literature, are used for exact modelling. This paper is organized in the following manner. Section 2 outlines the methods, that is, working area, measurements and neural models. Results and discussion are given in section 3. Conclusions are outlined in section 4 for readers.

Methods

Working area and measurements

Kayseri is a large and industrialized city in Central Anatolia, Turkey. It has got remarkable history and population around 1 Million. The transportation within the city relies mainly on buses, and personal vehicles. A light rail transit system called KAYSERAY was constructed and completed by the end of 2009. According to "Transportation Master Plan in Kayseri", 82,7% of the local transportation was realized by public transportation. When the rail system was put into service in 2009, the rate of the public transportation usage was increased [17]. In order to investigate and evaluate the noise effect of the rail system on people, noise measurements near the city centre, where the traffic was highly intense in terms of the public transportation, was performed. Noise measurements were carried out between 11.1 and 11.6 kilometres of rail system in Kayseri. This area, given in Figure 1, is in the city centre and has got some historic buildings such as inner and outer towers formed by the surrounding walls as well as the old markets. Rail system route passes quite close to the outer tower.

In this study, noise measurements were performed by Bruel-Kjaer (B&K) portable Pulse 3560-L data acquisition, two acoustic sensors with preamplifier and a PC [18]. Also, at the sampling locations, coordinates of locations were measured at ITRF 96 coordinate system by Astech Promark 800 GPS satellite receiver. Two noise measurements were performed at the same point as environmental and tram noises. 48 locations of tram line in the city centre of Kayseri are considered. In case of tram passing, noise measurements were performed within two days at 09:00 hours in the morning and 16:00 hours in the evening. These measurements were carried out five times. The tour interval of tram is nearly 4 minutes. The measuring area is close to tram route right. Due to the environmental conditions, such as reflection from the buildings and castle wall etc., noise values were recorded as cross-section at approximately 5 meter intervals at two points. One of them is at the right side of the tram line and the other is at the left side. Block diagram for experimental and simulation approaches is outlined in Figure 2.

Neural network

Three types of neural network were used to model and evaluate the noise characteristics of tram and environment. Structures of neural models are given in the following subsections.

Radial Basis Function Neural Network (RBFNN)

RBF neural network was firstly introduced to the thematic literature in 1988 [19]. In many engineering and science problems, this type has been widely used owing to the good convergence ability, simple structure and faster learning capability. This network type is a feed-forward network and has three layers. Input layer is the first layer and the input signals (x_i) go from this layer to second layer. Three characteristics, that is, X, Y and Z coordinates of measured points, are considered in input matrix. In

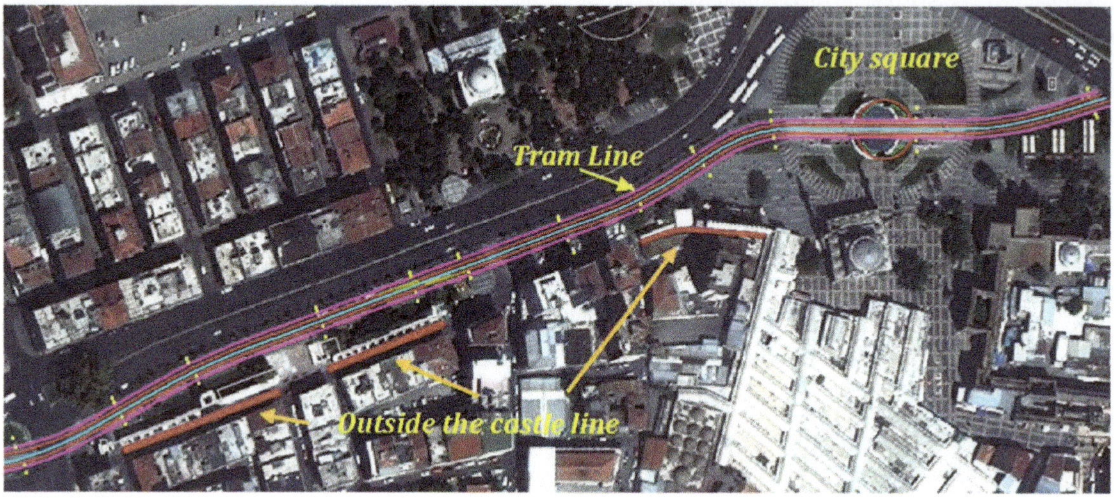

Figure 1 Working area.

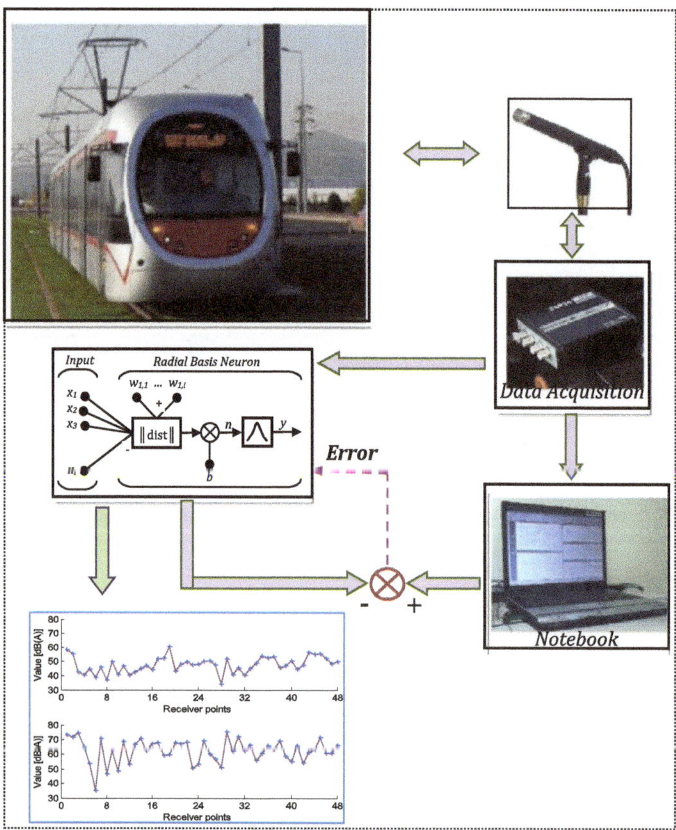

Figure 2 Block diagram of experimental and simulation approaches.

addition, tram type, tram velocity, air velocity and direction can be considered in input matrix for more stable network model. However, these characteristics have nearly zero changing. The sampling points are in the city centre and the traffic intensity is nearly similar in every hour for the daytime. Therefore, these effects were not considered in the current study. Hidden layer composed of RBF neural units is the second layer. The third layer is named as output layer, and the neurons of this layer have got linear transfer functions. Output matrix includes the tram and environmental noises. The neural network toolbox of MATLAB was used for developing the proposed network models [20]. Figure 3 outlines the RBFNN model. Hidden layer has got a non-linear Gaussian function,

$$a_j = \exp\left(-\frac{v_j^2}{2\sigma_j^2}\right) \tag{1}$$

where a_j is defined as output of the jth node in the hidden layer. σ_j is a width of the neuron j, v_j is given as Euclidean norm of the distance between input vector and neuron centre calculated as,

$$v_j(x) = \|x-c_j\| = \sqrt{\sum_{i=1}^{r}(x-c_{j,i})^2} \tag{2}$$

where c_j is defined as a centre of the unit j. The width of a unit is considered as the root mean square distance to the nearest unit j. For the jth unit, the width σ_j is defined as

$$\sigma_j = \left(\frac{1}{\varepsilon}\sum_{h=1}^{\varepsilon}\|c_j-c_h\|^2\right)^{1/2} \tag{3}$$

where $c_1, c_2, \ldots, c_\varepsilon$ outline the nearest unit centres to the unit j. The output value is given as

$$y_k = \sum_{j=1}^{s} d_{jk}a_j \tag{4}$$

where y_k defines the kth subsection of the y in the output layer, d_{jk} is the weight between neuron of jth hidden layer and neuron of kth output layer. The number of hidden units is a crucial factor for determining the predictive properties of the network structure and is automatically calculated until the desired value of error is reached. In order to evaluate the best predictive property, various numbers of RBF units are used in network model. The number and width of RBF units are determined by hidden layer. After processing in hidden layer, the network model has got one weight value connected to the output layer. A linear squares regression algorithm is used to train the weight of output layer [21]. Mean square of the error (MSE) is considered as a performance measuring index of neural model.

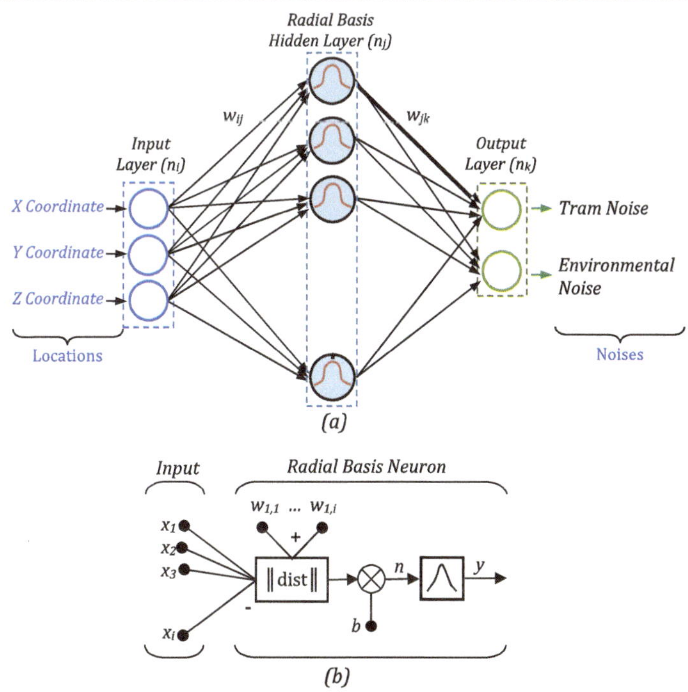

Figure 3 (a) Structure of RBFNN, (b) A neuron model for *i* inputs.

Multi-Layered Perceptron Neural Network (MLPNN)

A MLPNN structure is used as another network model to predict and evaluate the tram and environmental noise characteristics. Each layer has got linear or nonlinear neurons and each individual neuron sums its weighted inputs and gives an output by means of a nonlinear activation function with a bias. In the current study, tangent sigmoid activation function is preferred in the nonlinear neurons,

$$f(x) = \frac{1}{1+e^{-x}} \tag{5}$$

A normalized between 0 and 1 is carried out for the values of training and testing data. In order to minimize the convergence errors between desired and actual outputs of the neuron, neural model weights are updated by Levenberg-Marquardt learning algorithm. The update rule for the network weights according to Gauss–Newton (GN) method, which is a bridge between GN method and gradient descent algorithm, is outlined as:

$$\Delta\omega = -\left[\nabla^2 E(\omega)\right]^{-1} \nabla E(\omega) \tag{6}$$

where $\nabla^2 E(\omega)$ is the Laplacian of the energy function and also referred to as the Hessian matrix. The Hessian term can be given,

$$\nabla^2 E(\omega) = J^T(\omega)\, J(\omega) + S(\omega)$$

where;

$$S(\omega) = \sum_{i=1}^{N} e_i(\omega)\, \nabla^2 e_i(\omega) \tag{7}$$

where $e_i(\omega)$ is the error vector of the neural network for pattern i and $J(\omega)$ is the Jacobian matrix. By using the Taylor expansion, $S(\omega)$ is nearly considered as zero for the GN method. $S(\omega)$ comprises the second derivatives of the network error relative to the network weights. Since the number of computations increases exponentially with the size of the network, this term is very expensive for computing. The combination of the above equations gives the update rule of the GN method as,

$$\Delta\omega = -\left[J^T(\omega)\, J(\omega)\right]^{-1} J^T(\omega)\, e(\omega) \tag{8}$$

By considering the above introduction, the LM modification to the GN method is outlined as,

$$\Delta\omega = -\left[J^T(\omega)\, J(\omega) + \lambda I\right]^{-1} J^T(\omega) e(\omega) \tag{9}$$

If the λ is large, Eq. (9) approximates gradient descent. Otherwise, for a small λ, the algorithm approximates the GN method. If the λ is adaptively adjusted, the LM algorithm can make provision between its two extremes, that is, the gradient descent and the GN algorithm. Therefore, the advantages of gradient descent and the GN algorithms can be combined by LM method.

Generalized Regression Neural Network (GRNN)

A GRNN consists of four layers: input layer, pattern layer, summation layer and output layer. The first layer is input layer and it has got input units. Pattern layer is the second layer and the outputs of this layer go to the third layer (summation layer). The last layer is the output layer. Any iterative training procedure as in back propagation method is not necessary for GRNN [20,22,23]. By considering the training data, this network type can approximate any arbitrary function between input and output vectors. GRNN is a method to estimate the Probability Density Function (PDF) of x and y. PDF can be derived from the data without any preconceptions about its form, the system is perfectly general. If $f(x,y)$ represents the known continuous PDF of a vector random variable, x, and a scalar random variable, y, the conditional mean of y given X is given by

$$E\left[y|X\right] = \int_{-\infty}^{\infty} y f(X,y)dy \Big/ \int_{-\infty}^{\infty} f(X,y)dy \tag{10}$$

If the density $f(x,y)$ is unknown, it must be predicted from a sample of x and y observations. The probability estimator $\hat{f}(X,Y)$ is based upon sample values X^i and Y^i of the random variables (x and y);

$$\hat{f}(X,Y) = \frac{1}{(2p)^{(p+1)/2} s^{(p+1)}} \frac{1}{k} \times \sum_{i=1}^{k} \exp\left[-\frac{(X-X^i)^T(X-X^i)}{2s^2}\right] \exp\left[-\frac{(Y-Y^i)^2}{2s^2}\right] \tag{11}$$

where k is the number of sample observations and p is the x dimension. A physical interpretation of the probability estimate $\hat{f}(X,Y)$ is that it assigns sample probability of width s for each sample X^i and Y^i, and the probability estimate is the sum of those sample probabilities [22]. Defining the scalar function D_i^2,

$$D_i^2 = (X-X^i)^T(X-X^i) \tag{12}$$

and performing the indicated integrations gives,

$$\hat{Y}(X) = \sum_{i=1}^{n} Y^i exp\left(-\frac{D_i^2}{2s^2}\right) \Big/ \sum_{i=1}^{n} exp\left(-\frac{D_i^2}{2s^2}\right) \tag{13}$$

Eq. (13) can be applied to problems comprising the numerical data.

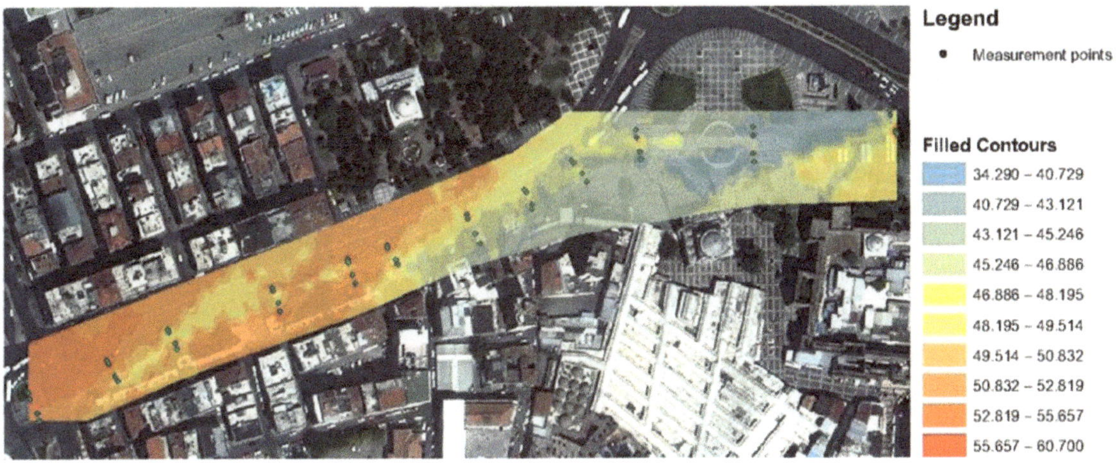

Figure 4 Environmental noise map.

Results and discussion

Neural network predictors for environmental noise, that is, background noise except for tram, and tram noise are presented in the current study. By using the interpolation technique, noise maps of environment and tram are outlined in Figures 4 and 5, respectively,

According to the directive on the assessment and management of the environmental noise accepted in 2010 in Turkey, it is stipulated that the noise level (L_{day}) spread from the rail transport systems around during the day may not exceed the limit value of 65 dBA. However, by evaluating the Figures 4 and 5 together, 22 measurements at the 48 sampling points exceed this limit value.

After the measurements, neural network models for predicting the noise characteristics are constituted. Training and testing stages of the network structures are employed on neural network toolbox of MATLAB. 175 data are used in the training stage of the designed networks. Also, these networks are validated and tested with 52 and 48 data, respectively, in responses to input which have not been used in the training step. The percentage of these data sets is nearly consistence with literature [5,21,23]. After the training and testing stages of networks are completed, the weights are saved and used for predicting and estimating the environmental and tram noises for given an input matrix. Both prediction and experimental results are compared to each other for case of the network stability.

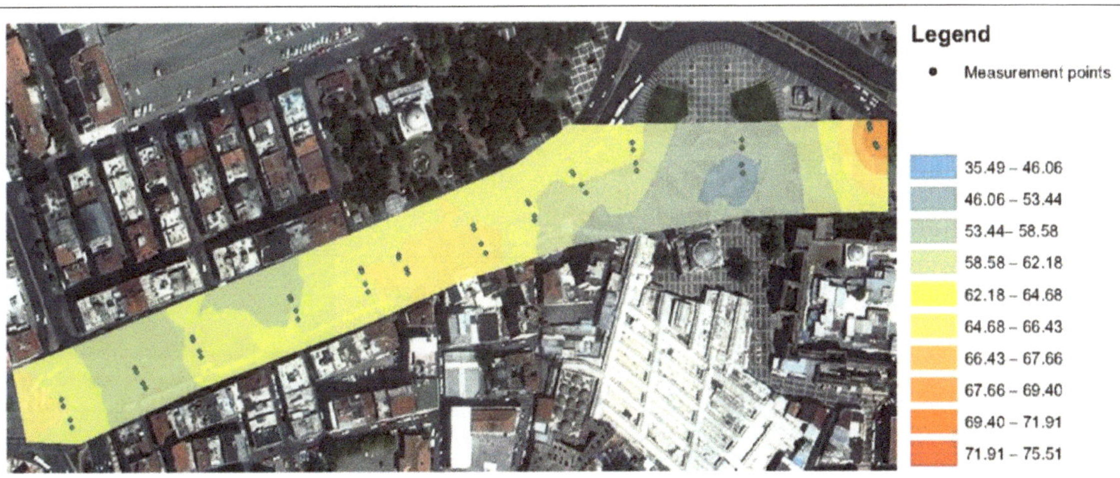

Figure 5 Tram noise map.

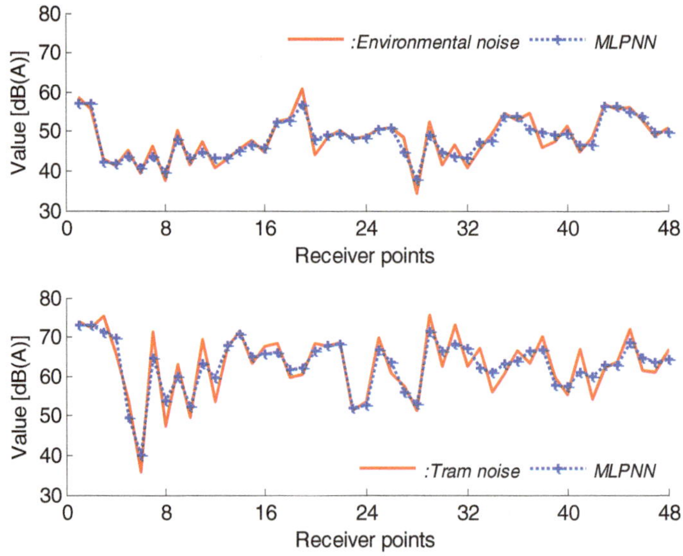

Figure 6 MLPNN results for environmental and tram noises.

Figure 6 gives the results of MLPNN predictor for environmental and tram noises.

By evaluation of Figure 6, it can be concluded that the network outputs nearly follows the measured values. But, this MLPNN predictor is not suitable for modelling the noise characteristics. Because, there is a clear difference between NN outputs and real noise values. These differences can be observed at all points. The second predictor model is based on GRNN. The simulation results for this predictor are given in Figure 7.

As seen from Figure 7, while environmental and tram noises at some points can be predicted correctly, this evaluation for all points is not valid. There is not an exact matching between experimental and neural simulation results. This GRNN predictor is also not suitable for modelling the noise characters. The last predictor model is RBFNN. The simulation result for this predictor is given in Figure 8.

Figure 8 shows that RBFNN model has a great accuracy for predicting and evaluating the environmental and

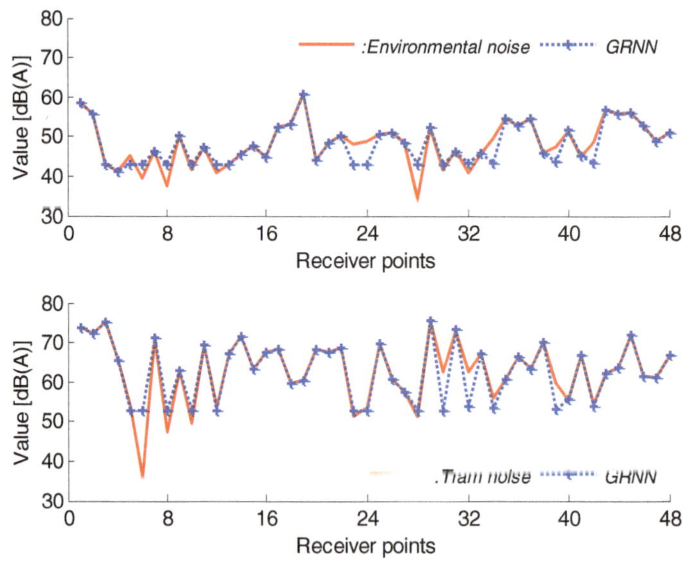

Figure 7 GRNN results for environmental and tram noises.

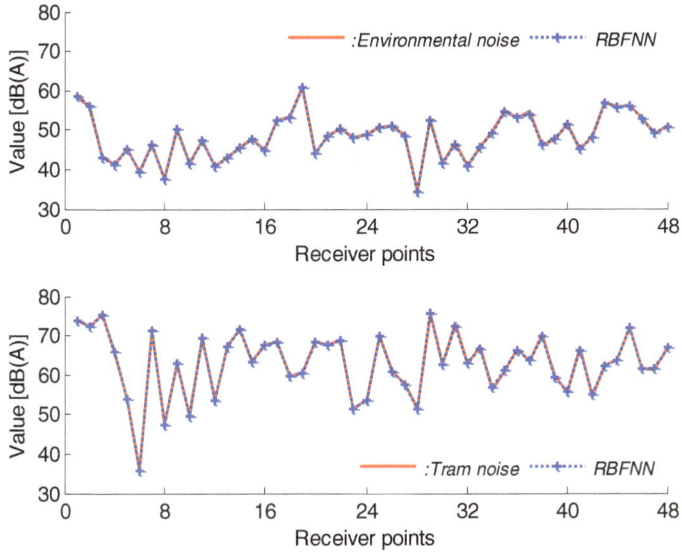

Figure 8 RBFNN results for environmental and tram noises.

tram noise characteristics. The approximation capability of the proposed network type is very suitable for this task. This model can be used to evaluate the intermediate values of the related noises. Training history of RBFNN is outlined in Figure 9.

By considering the differences between measuring and modelled noise values at the same points, convergence errors of the MLPNN, GRNN, RBFNN are outlined in Figure 10. Figure 10(a) and (b) denote the convergence errors for MLPNN predictor for the tram and environmental noises, respectively. Also, these errors for GRNN predictor are outlined in Figure 10(c) and (d) for each noise, respectively. In the case of RBFNN predictor, these errors are given in Figure 10(e) and (f) for the tram and environmental noises, respectively.

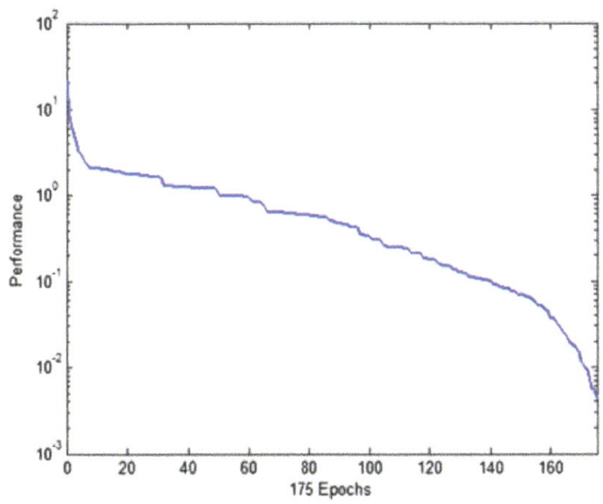

Figure 9 Performance index of neural predictor varying with epoch.

As seen from Figure 10, convergence errors of the RBFNN are smaller than that of the GRNN and MLPNN predictors. This is a good reflection of modelling and predicting capabilities of the proposed RBFNN model. A good convergence was achieved by comparing the measurement results and the results from the RBFNN method. It can be concluded that the prediction of the environmental and tram noises is possible by using the RBFNN. Also, proposed neural model has a great accuracy to predict and estimate the noise characteristics under the received points. When the neglected parameters in input matrix, that is, tram type, measuring hour, tram velocity, air velocity or ground effects etc. have a considerable change, these characteristics should be considered in input matrix for more stable and accurate RBFNN predictor. These arrangements also affect the benefits and/or limits of neural model for noise prediction.

Conclusion

In this study, a neural predictor is proposed to model and evaluate the characteristics of environment and tram noises. At the first stage of this study, the route of Kayseri light railway system, between 11.1 and 11.6 kilometres, is considered to evaluate the environmental and tram noise. 48 sampling points, where the traffic is highly intense in terms of the public transportation, are used for measuring. By considering the directive on the assessment and management of the environmental noise accepted in 2010 in

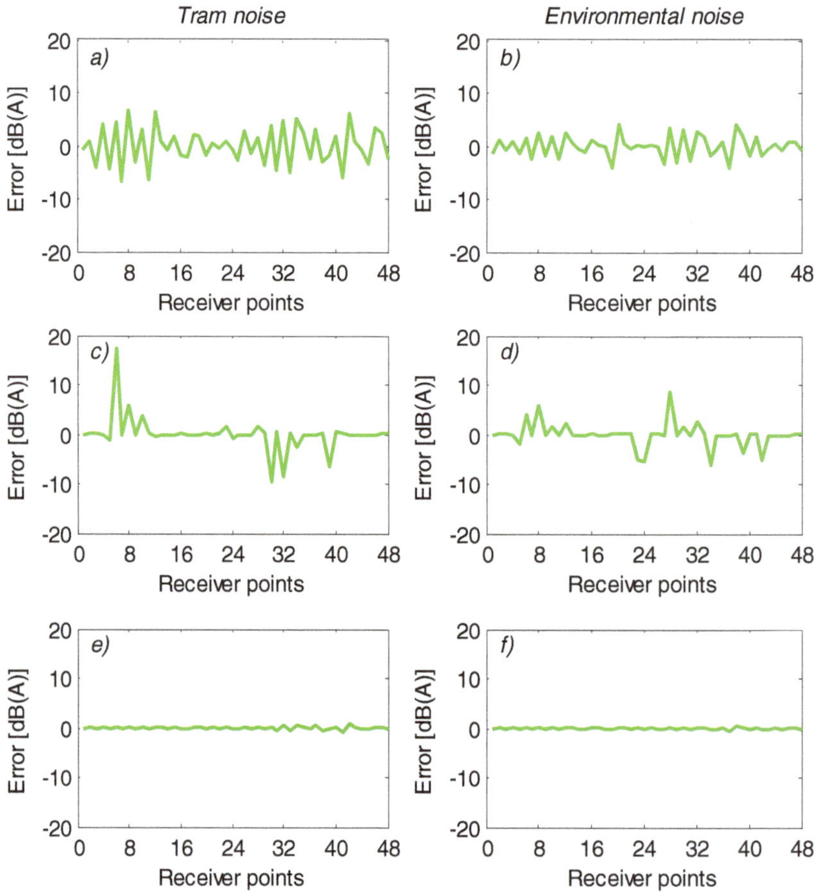

Figure 10 Convergence errors of neural models, a) and b) Error for MLPNN predictor, c) and d) Error for GRNN predictor, e) and f) Error for RBFNN predictor.

Turkey, tram noises at some measured points (22 points) exceed the limit values (65 dBA).

At the second stage of this study, three types of neural networks, that is, multi-layered perceptron, generalized regression and radial basis function neural networks, are used for modelling and predicting the noise values. For training and testing of network structure, noise measurements are carried out to specify the network stability for exact modelling and predicting the noise characteristics. X, Y and Z locations for each point are taken into consideration in input matrix of network. In addition, the output matrix is constituted by environmental and tram noises. The simulation results give that the RBFNN has good convergence and high accuracy ability to predict the noise values at related points. This predictor is robust and stable to model the noise characteristics. On the contrary, other network models, that is, MLPNN and GRNN predictors are not suitable and should not be used to model and predict the noises correctly. The proposed neural predictor may be helpful to urban planners for making a decision about transportation planning. Also, these values can be used to select the correct materials for noise isolation.

Competing interests
The authors declare that they have no competing interests.

Authors' contributions
All authors read and approved the final manuscript.

Acknowledgements
The authors wish to express their thanks to reviewer for their valuable contributions and Kayseri Transport Corporation-Kayseri Metropolitan Municipality.

Author details
[1]Engineering Faculty, Mechatronics Engineering Department, Erciyes University, Kayseri 38039, Turkey. [2]Engineering Faculty, Geomatics Engineering Department, Erciyes University, Kayseri 38039, Turkey.

References

1. Suzuki K. Artificial Neural Networks - Methodological Advances and Biomedical Applications. Rijeka: InTech; 2011.
2. Kumar K, Parida M, Katiyar VK. Road traffic noise prediction with neural networks-a review. Int J Opt Cont Theo Appl. 2012;2(1):29–37.
3. Cammarata G, Cavalieri S, Fichera A. A neural network architecture for noise prediction. Neural Net. 1995;8(6):963–73.
4. Givargis SH, Karimi H. Mathematical, statistical and neural models capable of predicting LA, max for the Tehran-Karaj express train. App Acous. 2009;70:1015–20.
5. Givargis SH, Karimi H. A basic neural traffic noise prediction model for Tehran's roads. J Env Manag. 2010;91:2529–34.
6. Alimohammadi I, Soltani R, Sandrock S, Azkhosh M, Gohari, MR. The effects of road traffic noise on mental performance. Iranian J Env Health Sci Eng. 2013; doi:10.1186/1735-2746-10-18.
7. Erkaya S, Yildirim Ş. Evaluation of Noise Characteristics for a Cooling System Using Neural Network. 11th WSEAS Int Conf Robot Cont Manufac Tech and Multimedia Sys Signal Proces., 8–10 March 2011, Italy, 39–45.
8. Liu J, Bao W, Shi L, Zuo B, Gao W. General regression neural network for prediction of sound absorption coefficients of sandwich structure nonwoven absorbers. App Acous. 2014;76:128–37.
9. Buratti C, Barelli L, Moretti E. Wooden windows: Sound insulation evaluation by means of artificial neural networks. App Acous. 2013;74:740–5.
10. Hamoda MF. Modeling of construction noise for environmental impact assessment. J Const Develop Count. 2008;13:79–89.
11. Tokhi MO, Wood R. Active noise control using radial basis function networks. Cont Eng Prac. 1997;5(9):1311–22.
12. Parbat DK, Nagarnaik PB. Artificial Neural Network Modeling of Road Traffic Noise Descriptors. First Int Conf Emerg Trends in Eng Tech. 2008; doi:10.1109/ICETET.2008.220.
13. Yildirim Ş, Erkaya S, Eski İ, Uzmay İ. Design of neural predictor for noise analysis of passenger car's engines. J Sci Indust Resear. 2008;67(5):340–7.
14. Yildirim Ş, Eski İ. Noise analysis of robot manipulator using neural networks. Robot Comp Integ Manufac. 2010;26:282–90.
15. Genaro N, Torija A, Ramos A, Requena I, Ruiz DP, Zamorano M. Modeling Environmental Noise Using Artificial Neural Networks. Ninth Int Conf Intel Sys Des Appl 2009; doi:10.1109/ISDA.2009.179.
16. Avsar Y, Saral A, Gonullu MT, Arslankaya E, Kurt U. Neural network modelling of outdoor noise levels in a pilot area. Turkish J Eng Env Sci. 2004;28:149–55.
17. Kayseri Transport Corporation, http://www.kayseriulasim.com. Accessed 25 Feb 2015.
18. Brüel & Kjær Sound & Vibration Measurement, http://www.bksv.com. Accessed 25 Feb 2015.
19. Broomhead D, Lowe D. Multivariable functional interpolation and adaptive networks. Complex Sys. 1988;2:321–55.
20. MATLAB (ver 7.0), The MathWorks Inc., 3 Apple Hill Drive, Natick, MA 01760–2098.
21. Erkaya S. Analysis of the vibration characteristics of an experimental mechanical system using neural networks. J Vib Cont. 2012;18:2059–72.
22. Specht DF. A general regression neural network. IEEE Trans Neural Netw. 1991;2(6):568–76.
23. Erkaya S. Prediction of vibration characteristics of a planar mechanism having imperfect joints using neural network. J Mech Sci Tech. 2012;26(5):1419–30.

A parametric study on the decolorization and mineralization of C.I. Reactive Red 141 in water by heterogeneous Fenton-like oxidation over FeZSM-5 zeolite

Ceyda Yaman and Gönül Gündüz*

Abstract

In this study, the heterogeneous Fenton-like degradation of Reactive Red 141 (RR141) in water was investigated over iron containing ZSM-5 zeolite (Si/Al = 42) prepared by ion-exchange (FeZSM-5 (42)). The catalyst was characterized by XRD, SEM, FTIR, TPR, and ICP-AES measurements. The effects of the initial concentrations of the dye and H_2O_2, the initial pH of the solution, catalyst loading, and the reaction temperature were investigated on heterogeneous Fenton-like degradation of RR141. The reduction of the solution initial pH from ca. 7.0 to ca. 3.5 had a positive effect on color removal. A complete color removal was achieved with all the H_2O_2 concentrations in the range of 0.007 - 0.067 M over the FeZSM-5 (42) catalyst after 2 h of reaction. The COD reduction increased from 52% to 81% with an increase in the amount of the catalyst. The COD reduction was affected positively with the increase in temperature from 298 K through 313 K to 323 K and then to 333 K. The initial decolorization rate was described by the equation: $-r_{A0} = 9.4*10^4\ e^{-38.8/RT}\ C_{RR141,0}\ C_{H2O2,0}^{0.184}$ with an H_2O_2 concentration range of 0.007 M – 0.033 M (where R is in kJ/mol).

Keywords: Reactive red 141, Heterogeneous Fenton-like oxidation, Fe-ZSM-5 zeolite catalyst

Background

Sulfonated and unsulfonated azo dyes have a negative aesthetic effect on the wastewater that is highly colored even at a low concentration of dye. On the other hand these dyes are toxic, carcinogenic and mutagenic. It is difficult to remove azo dyes in wastewater produced by textile industries using biological, physical and chemical treatment methods because of the chemical stability of these dyes, the high cost of the processes, and also disposal problems. Therefore, it is necessary to find an effective method for the wastewater treatment of reactive azo dyes. In the last decade, attention has focused on the Advanced Oxidation Processes (AOP) that is based on the generation of highly reactive hydroxyl radicals.

Among them, heterogeneous Fenton's reaction is very promising because it is a cost-effective method with a high reaction yield and regeneration of the catalyst is possible. The removal of the catalyst from the purified water is easy and a narrow range of pH values at which the reaction occurs is not required. On the other hand, leaching of iron ions from the solid catalyst is limited [1-16]. Heterogeneous Fenton-type catalysts have been developed by incorporating transitional metal cations such as iron ions or iron oxides into porous supports such as zeolites and pillared clays [17-21]. In the presence of H_2O_2, hydroxyl radicals ($OH^{\cdot}$) are produced by interaction of H_2O_2 with the iron (II) species present on the porous support. The main reaction mechanism of heterogeneous Fenton process is described as follows [22-26]:

$$X\text{-}Fe^{2+} + H_2O_2 \rightarrow X\text{-}Fe^{3+} + OH^{\cdot} + HO \quad (1)$$

where X presents the surface of the catalyst. Iron (III) can then react through Equations 2–4 with hydrogen

* Correspondence: gonul.gunduz@ege.edu.tr
Chemical Engineering Department, Ege University, 35100 Bornova, İzmir, Turkey

peroxide in order to regenerate iron (II) supporting the Fenton process:

$$X\text{-}Fe^{+3} + H_2O_2 \rightleftarrows X\text{-}FeOOH^{2+} + H^+ \quad (2)$$

$$X\text{-}FeOOH^{2+} \rightarrow HO_2^{\cdot} + X\text{-} Fe^{2+} \quad (3)$$

$$X\text{-}Fe^{3+} + HO_2 \rightarrow X\text{-}Fe^{2+} + O_2 + H^+ \quad (4)$$

The hydroperoxyl radicals ($HO_2^{\cdot}$) generated in Eq.3 are less reactive than the $OH^{\cdot}$ species. In the application of heterogeneous Fenton-like oxidation to dye degradation, the following reactions take place: Firstly, the formed oxidative radicals ($OH^{\cdot}$ and $HO_2^{\cdot}$) react with the activated dye molecules to produce intermediate products and then mineralization products ($H_2O + CO_2$) through Eqs. 5–6:

$$X\text{-}Fe^{3+} + dye \rightarrow X\text{-}Fe^{2+} + {}^{\cdot}dye^+ \quad (5)$$

$$\text{Oxidative radicals} + {}^{\cdot}dye^+ \rightarrow \text{Intermediate products} \rightarrow CO_2 + H_2O \quad (6)$$

Decolorization of the dye is a result of N = N bond destruction with the addition of $OH^{\cdot}$. The mineralization of dye is the total oxidation of the intermediate products to CO_2 and H_2O and it is slower than color removal because of the priority of the $OH^{\cdot}$ attack on the N = N bonds [1].

C.I. Reactive Red 141 (RR141) is a sulfonated, bright red color diazo reactive textile dye and is widely used for the dyeing processes in the textile industry. Procion Red H-E7B and C.I. Reactive Red 141 are the commercial names of the dye. Its empirical formula is $C_{52}H_{22}Na_8O_{26}S_8Cl_2N_{14}$ and is composed of two monochlorotriazine reactive groups. It has a molecular weight of 1774 g/mol and its chemical structure is given in Figure 1. The adsorption spectra of RR141 is characterized by two main bands, one in the visible region (λmax = 543 nm) and the other in the UV region (λmax = 288 nm). In the heterogeneous Fenton-like oxidation of RR141, hydroxyl radical attack on the N = N bonds occurs at 543 nm and this band is responsible for the chromophoric components in the dye.

The degradation of RR141 has been investigated by biodegradation [27-29], by adsorption [22,30,31], by homogeneous Fenton's reaction, by non-catalytic or catalytic photooxidation [32-41], by electrochemical oxidation with conductive-diamond anode [42], and by ultrasound [1]. Few studies have been reported on the heterogeneous Fenton-like degradation of C.I. Reactive Red 141 to date. In one study, iron oxide particles recovered from acid mine drainage were used as an adsorbent or as a catalyst in the oxidation of RR141 through a Fenton-like mechanism to remove the dye from the aqueous solution [22]. However, the main aim of that study was to investigate the dye-adsorption capacity of iron oxide rather than its catalytic effect in the heterogeneous Fenton-like oxidation of dye. Only one experiment has been carried out for dye degradation by heterogeneous Fenton's reaction and a TOC removal of around 3% could only be achieved.

Conventional processes such as adsorption, coagulation/flocculation (CF) etc., may be costly, ineffective and produce a high amount of secondary wastes. CF is still not good enough to be used in industry even when it is combined with microfiltration or ultrafiltration. However, catalytic methods such as heterogeneous Fenton-like oxidation result in permanent chemical degradation of dyes. This process is still simple, non-expensive, a promising, and attractive treatment method for the effective decolorization and degradation of dyes when compared with the conventional processes [25-43].

Many studies are found in literature on the removal of dyes using Fe-ZSM-5 [3,23,24,44], Fe-Y [2,25,45-48], and Fe-clay [26,49-52] catalysts by several advanced oxidation techniques. The catalytic activity and stability of these catalysts depend on the synthesis method in addition to their composition and framework structure. The leakage of iron ions from the support is the other important factor to be considered in dye degradation over an iron containing support: because iron leaching from the catalyst causes a new pollution of the treated water. The studies showed that iron containing ZSM-5 zeolite exhibited better catalytic activity and stability than iron-containing Y zeolites. On the other hand, the activity of iron-containing clay catalysts in the degradation of dyes depends on the careful selection of the preparation method and calcination conditions. However, till now no a detailed parametric study including decolorization kinetics has not been reported on the heterogeneous Fenton-like degradation of dyes on iron containing ZSM-5 zeolites. The objectives of this study are to: (1) investigate the influence of the reaction conditions of the heterogeneous Fenton-like oxidation and optimize them, (2) investigate the decolorization kinetics, and (3) investigate the leakage of iron ions in the reaction for the stability of the catalyst.

Our group previously published a study [53] on the degradation of RR141 using the heterogeneous Fenton-like process over iron containing ZSM-5 zeolites. That work

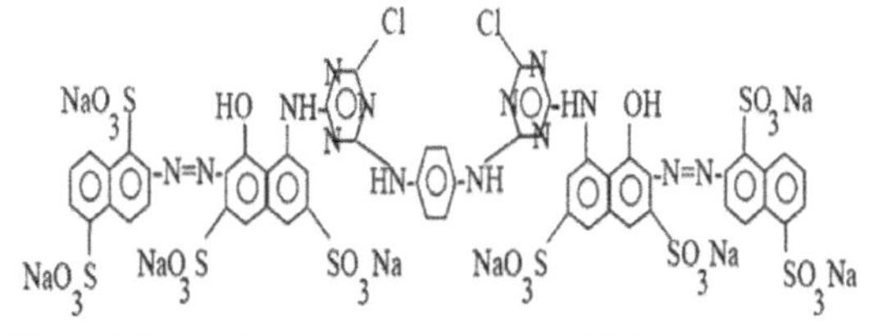

Figure 1 Chemical structure of reactive red 141.

included the preparation of the catalysts by ion-exchange or hydrothermal synthesis and their characterization studies by XRD, SEM, FTIR, ICP-AES, TPR, and nitrogen adsorption. The catalytic activity screening tests of the prepared catalysts were accomplished to determine the catalyst with the highest activity in the degradation of RR141 by heterogeneous Fenton-like oxidation reaction. The highest color removal (97%) was achieved by the catalyst prepared by ion exchange with a silicon/aluminum ratio of 42 zeolite (FeZSM-5(42)). The above mentioned objectives of the presented study was investigated over that iron-containing ZSM-5 zeolite catalyst. The presented study is novel and unique from these points of view.

Methods

Preparation of the catalysts

Ion exchange was used for the preparation of the iron containing the ZSM-5 zeolite catalyst. The method of Schwidder et al. [54] was applied with minor modifications [21] for the ion-exchange. The ZSM-5 zeolite with silicon/alumina = 42 was obtained from Süd-Chemie AG (Germany). An iron exchange of 98.9% could be achieved. The catalyst was coded as FeZSM-5 (42).

Catalyst characterization

The prepared catalyst was characterized by nitrogen adsorption, X-ray diffraction patterns (XRD), scanning electron microscope (SEM), Fourier transform-infrared (FTIR) spectrometer, inductively coupled plasma atomic emission spectrometer (ICP-AES), and by temperature programmed reduction (TPR) measurements. The precise procedures for the characterization of the catalyst are described in Ref [53].

Heterogeneous Fenton-like oxidation of RR141

C.I. Reactive Red 141 (Procion Red H-E7B) was purchased from Dystar (Germany) with a dye content of >85% and was used as received without further purification. The heterogeneous Fenton-like degradation of RR141 was carried out under isothermal conditions in a temperature controlled shaded glass batch reactor with a volume of 470 mL equipped with a mechanical stirrer at ca. 280 rpm (Heidolph, Germany) and a pH electrode (Mettler Toledo). Figure 2 presents the picture of the experimental set-up. In a typical run, 0.15 dm^3 of aqueous dye solution (0.1 g-dye/dm^3-soln = 5.64×10^{-5} M) was placed into the reactor and the temperature was adjusted to 333 K. When the temperature reached to 333 K, the pH of the dye solution was measured and 0.15 g of catalyst (1 g-cat/dm^3 –soln.) was introduced into the solution under continuous stirring. After the adsorption equilibrium was established (roughly in 10–15 min) the solution was analyzed to determine the dye removal by adsorption. Then a solution of 35% H_2O_2 (Merck, Germany) (40 mmol/0.15 dm^3 solution, namely 0.267 M) was added to the dye solution. After the addition of H_2O_2, the pH of the solution was again measured. This was recorded as the starting time of the reaction. The samples taken periodically were centrifuged for 0.5 h to remove the catalyst and kept at 273 K to stop the reaction before the analysis with the UV spectrophotometer (Jasco 7800 UV/vis).

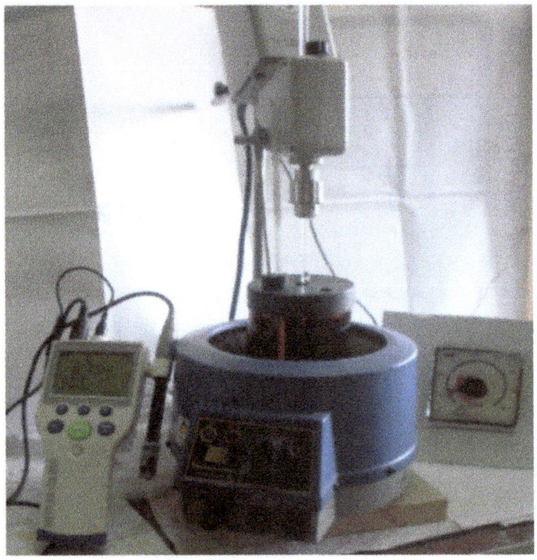

Figure 2 Experimental set-up.

The decrease of the intensity of the band at 543 nm was used as a measure of decolorization degree. The reduction in the chemical oxygen demand (COD) of the dye solution was determined using a Lovibond (Germany) Checkit Direct COD Vario device for each run after a reaction time of 2 h.

The blank run with the above conditions, but without H_2O_2 showed that dye removal by adsorption was not greater than 3% and 21% in 15 min and 120 min of reaction, respectively. A color removal of 11% could be achieved in the presence of H_2O_2 only in 2 hour of reaction.

Each experiment was conducted in duplicate and the standard deviation of the average of the independent runs for color removal changed in the range of ±0.51 to ±1.29.

Results and discussion

Catalyst characterization studies

The X-ray diffraction patterns of the FeZSM-5 catalyst sample showed the typical diffractograms of the MFI structure ($2\theta = 7–9^0$ and $23–25^0$). The incorporation of iron in the MFI lattice did not damage the zeolite structure [53].

The SEM images of the catalyst sample depicted that the crystallites in the FeZSM-5 (42) sample were a spherical shape (Figure 3).

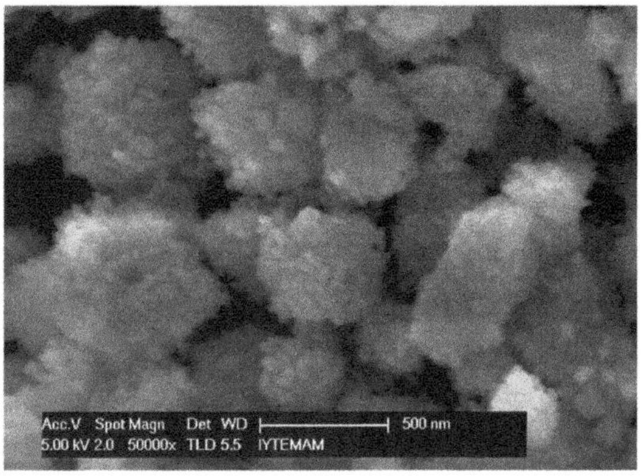

Figure 3 SEM image of the catalyst.

Iron content and Si/Al ratio of the catalyst were determined with the ICP-AES method and found to be 4.98 wt % and 42.8, respectively. The BET surface area, total pore volume, average pore diameter and micropore area of the catalyst were found to be 469 m^2/g, 0.321 cm^3/g, 0.73 nm (using the Horvath-Kawazoe method), and 236 m^2/g, respectively.

The FTIR spectra of the catalyst showed bands at 450, 550, 800, 1100, 1225, and 1650 cm^{-1} which were assigned to different vibrations of the tetrahedral and framework structure of the ZSM-5 zeolite [53].

The temperature-programmed reduction with hydrogen (H_2-TPR) of the catalyst showed that a major hydrogen consumption peak was obtained at 397 K which reflected the reduction of out of framework iron oxides [53].

Influence of the initial pH of solution on the degradation of dye

The effect of solution pH on the degradation of dye was investigated at an initial dye pH of ca. 7 and at a pH of 3.5 which was regulated by the addition of 0.1 N sulphuric acid to the dye solution.

Figure 4 shows the effect of the solution pH on the color and COD removals for RR141 degradation with the catalyst. The reduction of pH to around 3.5 positively affected

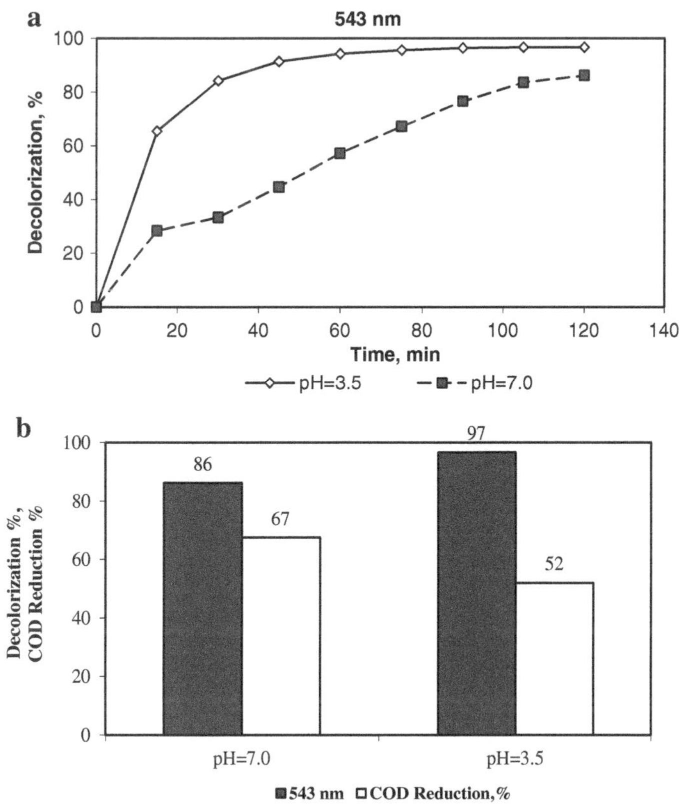

Figure 4 The influence of the initial pH of the solution on the degradation of RR141. (Initial dye concentration = 0.1 g/dm^3, catalyst loading 1 g-cat/dm^3-soln, H_2O_2 concentration = 0.267 M, and temperature = 333 K). **a)** Decolorization as a function of time, **b)** Decolorization, %, and COD removal, %, after a reaction duration of 2 h.

the color removal. The acidic environment increased the decolorization degree of the dye from 86% to 97% after a reaction duration of 2 h. The pKa of the sodium sulfonate groups of the dyes is very low (<1), therefore, the RR141 is expected to exist as anionic groups ($-SO_3^-$) at a pH > 1.0. On the other hand, the interaction between the anionic groups of dye and surface acid sites of the Fe-ZSM-5 zeolite catalysts becomes stronger at a low pH. The observed increase in decolorization at a low pH can be attributed to a greater adsorption of dye on the catalyst surface and consequently it results in a higher decolorization of the dye [40]. However, a decrease in COD removal from 67% to 52% was observed with the regulation of the solution pH to a ca. 3.5. This may be due to the formation of intermediates such as monoazo, naphthalene, and naphthol disulfonic acid intermediates whose degradation is hindered at acidic pH [20,29].

The amount of iron loss from the catalyst into the solution was determined by measuring the iron concentration in the solution after a reaction duration of 2 h, with an atomic absorption spectrophotometer (Varian 10 plus). The leaching of iron cations from the zeolite into the solution depended strongly on the pH [4]. As expected, with the regulation of pH from 7 to about 3.5 the iron leaching increased from 0.3×10^{-3} g/dm^3 to 0.9×10^{-3} g/dm^3. It means that iron loss changed from 0.59% to 1.77%. As seen, the iron leaching was considerably low (being below the EU directives of < 2×10^{-3} g/dm^3).

Influence of the hydrogen peroxide concentration on the degradation of dye

The effect of the H_2O_2 concentration on the degradation of RR141, while maintaining constant all the other operating parameters (catalyst loading: 1 g-cat/dm^3–soln., initial pH ~ 3.5, initial concentration of dye = 0.1 g-dye/dm^3-soln., temperature = 333 K) was investigated and is given in Figure 5. The increase in H_2O_2 concentration from 0.007 M to 0.017 M and to 0.033 M positively affected the initial rate of color removal (Figure 5a.). This result is expected because of the increase of the OH· radicals produced with the increasing amount of H_2O_2, Eq.1. Nevertheless the increase in H_2O_2 concentration from 0.033 M to 0.067 M and to 0.267 M slowed the initial decolorization of RR141. A complete color removal was

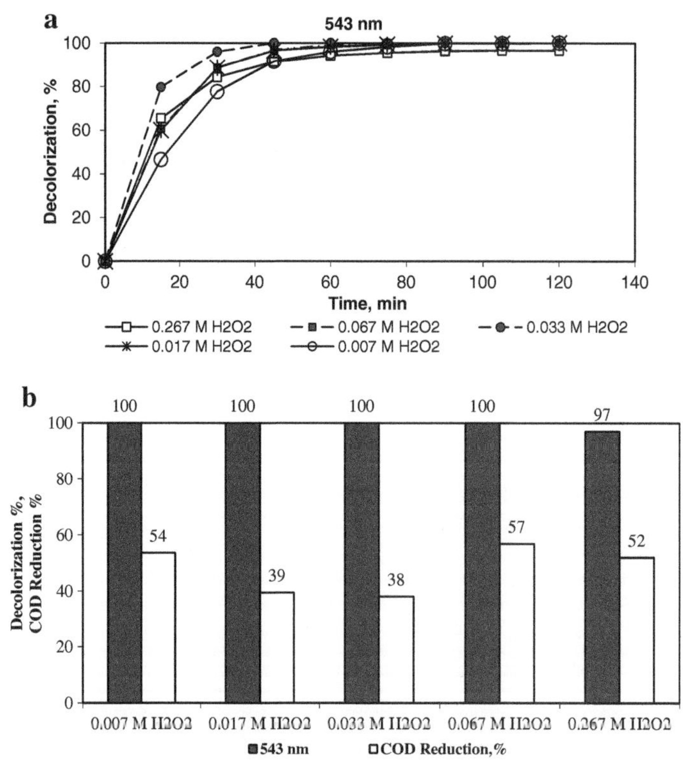

Figure 5 The influence of the initial H_2O_2 amount on the degradation of RR141. (Initial dye concentration = 0.1 g/dm^3, catalyst loading 1 g-cat/dm^3-soln, initial pH ~ 3.5, and temperature = 333 K). **a)** Decolorization as a function of time, **b)** Decolorization, %, and COD removal, %, after a reaction duration of 2 h.

achieved with all the initial concentrations of H_2O_2 studied, except with 0.267 M (97%) after 2 h of oxidation. The slight decrease in the initial decolorization of RR141 with an increasing H_2O_2 can be attributed to the reaction between the H_2O_2 and generated hydroxyl radicals to produce less reactive hydroperoxyl radicals ($HO_2^{\cdot}$):

$$H_2O_2 + OH \rightarrow HO_2^{\cdot} + H_2O \quad (7)$$

The dominant response from the two opposite effects given in Equations 1 and 7 directs the reaction. Similar results have been reported by Neamtu et al. [2] and Ramirez et al. [4], in the Fenton-like oxidation of Procion Marine H-EXL and Orange II, respectively.

Figure 5b presents the percentages of decolorization and COD removal in the degradation of RR141 after a reaction time of 2 h. COD reduction reached 57% in the presence of 0.067 M of H_2O_2, while it was 54% at a dose of 0.007 M H_2O_2 and decreased to 38% with the increase in H_2O_2 concentration from 0.007 M to 0.033 M. A COD removal of 52% was obtained at a dose of 0.267 M H_2O_2. The COD removal is significantly lower than the color removal at all doses of H_2O_2. This result signifies the priority of the $OH^{\cdot}$ attack on the N = N bonds and the slower destruction of the aromatic/olefinic carbons in the dye [1]. For cost considerations, the optimum H_2O_2 concentration can be selected as 0.007 M.

In literature, the COD (chemical oxygen demand), TOC (Total Organic Carbon), and DOC (dissolved organic carbon) removals were measured in the degradation of RR141 by several advanced oxidation techniques. For instance a TOC removal of about 3% was achieved in the heterogeneous Fenton-like oxidation of RR141 over iron oxides particles recovered from acid mine drainage [22].

A 17%-23% TOC removal was achieved in the degradation of RR141 by the ferrioxalate-Fenton/UV-A and TiO_2/UV-A processes [32].

A 100% DOC removal was obtained for RR141 after a 90 min treatment under homogeneous Fenton assisted solar light [34].

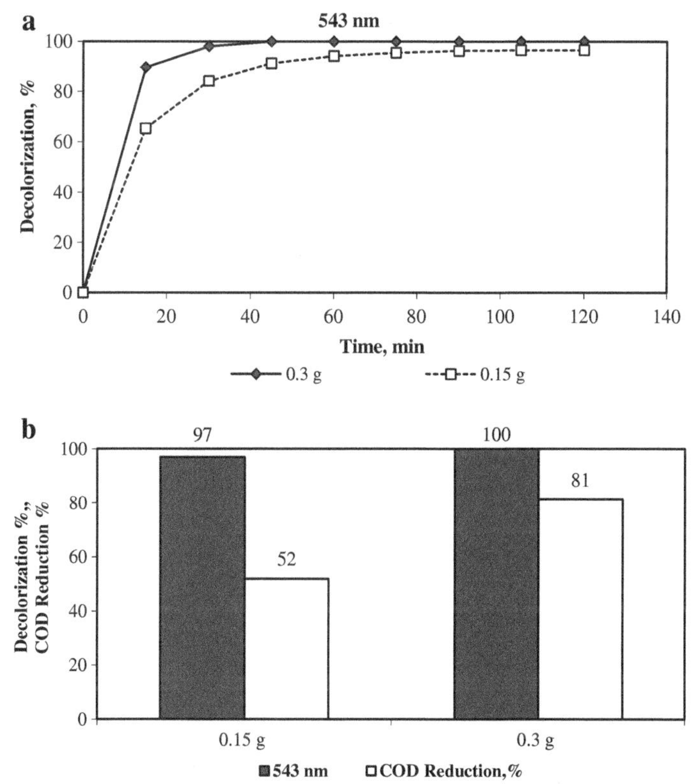

Figure 6 The influence of the catalyst amount on the degradation RR141. (Initial dye concentration = 0.1 g/dm^3, initial pH = 3.5, H_2O_2 concentration = 0.267 M, and temperature = 333 K). **a)** Decolorization as a function of time, **b)** Decolorization, %, and COD removal, %, after a reaction duration of 2 h.

A decrease of 64% in COD was reached in the degradation of RR141 within 5 hours using the UV/H_2O_2 advanced oxidation process [37].

COD was reduced from 120 mg/L to 23 mg/L (81%) in the solar nano-photocatalytic degradation of RR141 using TiO_2 [38].

A 37% removal of TOC was achieved in the photocatalytic degradation of RR141 for the Zn_2SnO_4 photocatalyst after 270 min of sunlight irradiation [39].

A TOC reduction of 29% was achieved in the degradation of RR141 with a TiO_2 coated pebble bed photocatalytic reactor having a solar collector [40].

A COD removal of 100% was obtained in the electrolyse of an aqueous solution of RR141 with a conductive-diamond anode [42].

The influence of the catalyst amount on the degradation of dye

The effect of the catalyst amount was investigated on the Fenton-like degradation of RR141 using catalyst amounts of 0.15 g and 0.3 g for 0.150 dm^3 dye solution under the following reaction conditions: an initial RR141 concentration of 0.1 g/dm^3, a temperature of 333 K, an initial pH = 3.5, an initial H_2O_2 concentration = 0.267 M. The results are shown in Figure 6. Doubling the amount of catalyst slightly increased the color removal from 97% to 100% after 2 hours of reaction. The COD reduction increased from 52% to 81% with an increase in the amount of the catalyst. This remarkable increase in COD removal may be attributed to the production of more hydroxyl radicals in the degradation reaction of RR141. Because increasing the catalyst amount provides more active catalytic sites of Fe^{2+}/Fe^{3+} species to enhance degradation. A similar trend where the catalyst amount influences the degradation of dye was reported in literature, as well [2,4,20].

Influence of the temperature on the degradation of dye

Experiments were conducted to investigate the effect of temperature on the degradation of an aqueous dye solution at four different temperatures, 298, 313, 323, and 333 K under the following conditions: an RR141 initial concentration of 0.1 g/dm^3, a catalyst amount of 0.15 g/ 0.150 dm^3 dye solution, an initial pH of 3.5, and an H_2O_2 amount of 0.033 M (at which the initial decolorization rate was the highest). The results are presented in Figure 7. It

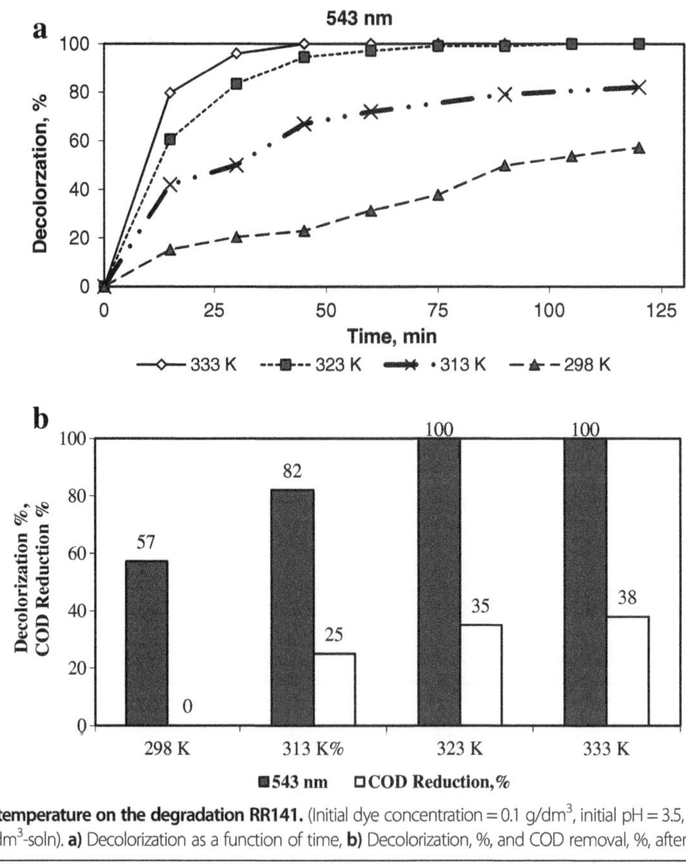

Figure 7 The influence of temperature on the degradation RR141. (Initial dye concentration = 0.1 g/dm^3, initial pH = 3.5, H_2O_2 concentration = 0.033 M, and catalyst loading 1 g-cat/dm^3-soln). **a)** Decolorization as a function of time, **b)** Decolorization, %, and COD removal, %, after a reaction duration of 2 h.

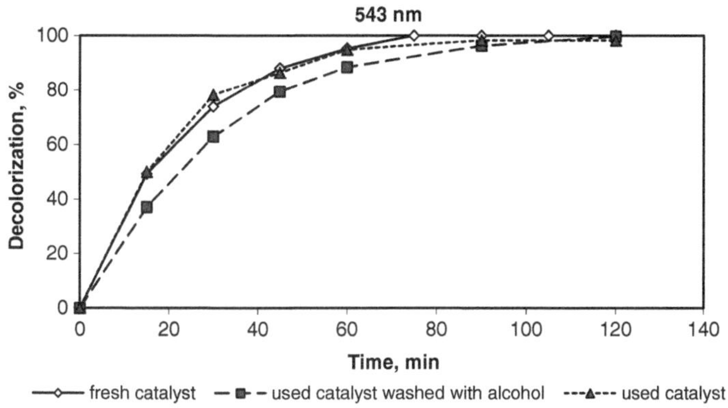

Figure 8 Stability of the catalyst in the oxidation of RR141. (Initial dye concentration = 0.1 g/dm^3, initial pH = 3.5, H_2O_2 concentration = 0.033 M, catalyst loading 1 g-cat/dm^3-soln, and temperature = 333 K).

was clearly seen that the color removal rate increased with the increase in temperature from 298 K through 313 K to 323 K and then to 333 K. These results agree with the fact that the Fenton reaction was accelerated with the increasing temperature, describing an Arrhenius behavior [33]. Because both the collision frequency of the molecules at the surface of the catalyst and the fraction of molecules that possess energy in excess of the activation were increased. Temperature has a significant role at enhancing the extent of the decolorization of dye with the generated OH$^{\cdot}$, since it is a thermodynamic state function that enhances the feasibility of a chemical process [26]. The lowest degradation degree was measured at a temperature of 298 K. Furthermore, while the color removal increased with the increase in temperature no COD reduction was observed at 298 K, however the COD reduction was enhanced with the temperature being 25%, 35%, and 38% at temperatures higher than 298 K, respectively. Regarding the time required to achieve, for instance 40% of RR141 degradation, it was found that this time significantly decreased when the temperature was increased, with t = 78.0, 14.5, 10.0, and 7.5 min at 298, 313, 323, and 333 K, respectively.

In literature, similar results have been reported in the catalytic wet peroxide oxidation (CWPO) of Orange II over an Fe-saponite catalysts [4], in the CWPO of phenol over pillared clays containing iron [55] and in the wet oxidation of 2.4.6-trichlorophenol in water using an Fe^{3+}, Co^{2+}, Ni^{2+} supported MCM-41 catalysts [18].

Stability of the catalyst

For the stability studies, the runs were carried out using an 0.15 dm^3 of 0.1 g/dm^3 RR141 aqueous solution with an addition of 0.033 M H_2O_2 at 333 K, and at a pH of 3.5. To recover the catalyst, after 2 h of oxidation the final effluent was filtrated and dried or washed with ethanol and then water. These catalysts were labeled as used catalyst and used catalyst washed with alcohol, respectively. The latter one was calcined by heating to 423 K and holding there for 15 min then heating to 873 K and keeping at this temperature for 2 h to remove the adsorbed organic species from the active sites [4,56]

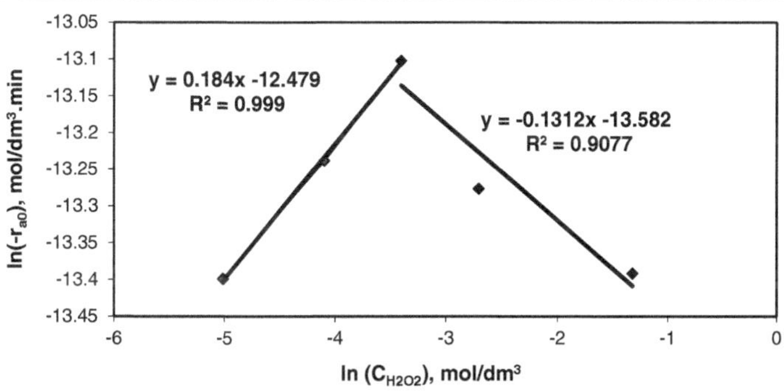

Figure 9 The variation of the initial rate with respect to the initial concentration of H_2O_2.

Table 1 Reaction rate constants at different temperatures

Temperature (T), K	$-r_{A0}$ (mol/dm^3.min)	k (dm^3/mol)^{0,184} min^{-1}	C_{RR141} (mol/dm^3)	$C^{0,184}_{H2O2}$ (mol/dm^3)$^{0.184}$
333	2.041*10^{-6}	0.0677	5.64*10^{-5}	0.535
323	1.708*10^{-6}	0.0567	5.64*10^{-5}	0.535
313	1.122*10^{-6}	0.0328	5.64*10^{-5}	0.535
298	4.171*10^{-6}	0.0138	5.64*10^{-5}	0.535

and their performances reached in terms of RR141 decolorization are presented in Figure 8. The same color removal results were obtained after 2 h oxidation of RR141 over fresh, used and used catalyst washed with alcohol. A slight decay in the initial decolorization rate was obtained only on the used catalyst washed with ethanol. The loss of activity can be attributed to the poisoning of the active catalytic sites due to the adsorbed organic species or oxidation of Fe^{2+} to Fe^{3+}.

In literature, similar results were reported in the studies on the CWPO of Orange II over Fe-saponite catalysts [4] and on CWPO of propionic acid over a FeZSM-5 catalyst [57].

Decolorization kinetics of the Fenton-like oxidation of RR141

In the Fenton-like oxidation of RR141, the reaction mixture was stirred vigorously at around 280 rpm. The external diffusion effects were calculated using Hougen's criterion and it was found that $(C_b-C_s)/C_b \approx 0.04$, so it was assumed that $C_b \approx C_s$. The internal diffusion resistance was negligible due to the small size of the catalyst particles (500 nm). To calculate the internal diffusion effects, the generalized Thiele modulus based on the reaction rate was determined and found to be 0.339×10^{-6} and hence the effectiveness factor was assumed to be unity [58].

The decolorization kinetics was determined at an initial pH of 3.5 using the initial decolorization rates and a first order dependency was obtained on the dye concentration with $R^2 = 1$. This result was in good agreement with those reported in literature for decolorization kinetics of RR141 degraded by several advanced oxidation techniques [1,32,34,37,38,40,59]. However, the photo-catalytic degradation of RR141 on Zn_2SnO_4 followed the zero order kinetics under sunlight [41].

The order with respect to H_2O_2 concentration was determined by plotting the initial rate, $-\ln(-r_{A0})$, against the initial H_2O_2 concentration, $\ln(C_{H2O2,0})$. Figure 9, presents the variation of the initial rate with respect to the initial concentration of H_2O_2 for 0.1 g/dm^3 dye concentration at 333 K.

As it is seen in Figure 9, there is a break at the H_2O_2 concentration of 0.033 M. Namely, order of reaction depends on the amount of H_2O_2 (shifting-order reaction). The order of reaction is 0.184 with respect to H_2O_2 in the range of 0.007 M-0.033 M H_2O_2 and −0.131 with respect to H_2O_2 greater than 0.033 M H_2O_2. The initial rate is expressed by equations (8) and (9) based on the amount of H_2O_2.

$$-r_{A0} = k\, C_{RR141,0} C_{H2O2,0}{}^{0.184} \qquad (0.007\text{-}0.033\ \text{M}) \qquad (8)$$

$$-r_{A0} = k\, C_{RR141,0} C_{H2O2,0}{}^{-0.131} \qquad (> 0.033) \qquad (9)$$

In these equations, $-r_{A0}$ has the units of mol/dm^3 min, and $C_{RR141,0}$ and $C_{H2O2,0}$ are in units of mol/dm^3, and k is the reaction rate constant. As seen from Equation 7,

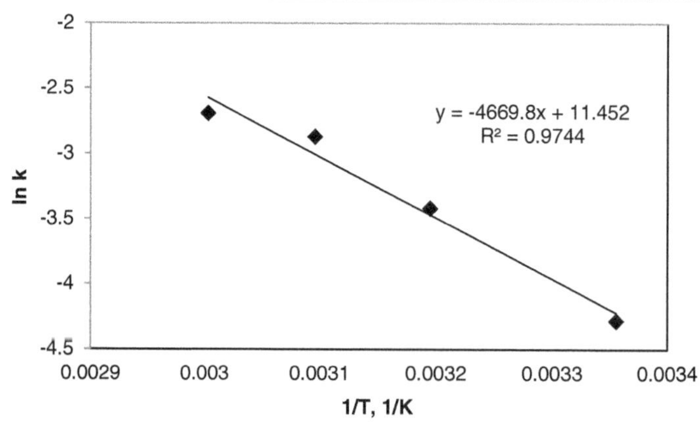

Figure 10 lnk versus 1/T dependency for the decolorization of RR141.

at high H_2O_2 concentrations it reacts with $OH^{\cdot}$ radicals to generate less reactive perhydroxyl radicals, $HO_2^{\cdot}$, causing a decrease in the color removal rate. Table 1 shows the reaction rate constant, k, calculated at different temperatures (298, 313, 323, and 333 K) by using the initial rate equation (8).

Figure 10 presents the Arrhenius plot of lnk vs. 1/T obtained by using the data in Table 1. From the slope of the Arrhenius plot ($R^2 = 0.97$) in Figure 10, –E/R, where R is the universal gas constant (8.314 J/mol K), and the activation energy, E, was calculated to be 38.8 kJ/mol. Finally, the initial decolorization rate of RR141 can be expressed by the following equation for the range of 0.007 M - 0.033 M H_2O_2;

$$-r_{A0} = 9.4 * 10^4 e^{-38.8/RT} C_{RR141,0} C_{H2O2,0}{}^{0.184} \tag{10}$$

In literature, the activation energy for the heterogeneous Fenton-like reaction of RR141 has not been declared. This study is a useful reference in the decolorization kinetics of RR141 for the design of RR141 removal reactors. In the homogeneous photo-Fenton reaction of RR141, activation energy was estimated to be 1.26 kJ/mol [34]. The lack of mass transfer resistances facilitates the homogeneous catalytic reactions with low activation energies. Decomposition of RR141 with the ferrioxalate-Fenton/UV-A process was fitted to the empirical Langmuir-Hinshelwood kinetic model [32]. An activation energy of 35.9 kJ/mol was reported for the rapid decolorization of azo dye methyl orange in an aqueous solution by nanoscale zerovalent iron particles [60]. This value is very close to the activation energy (38.8 kJ/mol) obtained in this study for the heterogeneous Fenton-like oxidation of Reactive Red 141. Moreover, in literature, the activation energy of the homogeneous catalytic Fenton oxidation of Reactive Brillant Blue X-BR azo dye was given to be 25.21 kJ/mol [61].

Conclusions

The heterogeneous Fenton-like degradation of Reactive Red 141 (RR141) in water was investigated over iron containing ZSM-5 zeolite (Si/Al = 42) prepared by ion-exchange. The catalyst seems to have a promising efficiency in RR141 degradation. A complete color removal could be achieved with the catalyst at a pH of 3.5 in an H_2O_2 concentration range of 0.007 M-0.067 M after two hours of reaction. The increase in H_2O_2 concentration up to 0.033 M increased the initial decolorization due to the increase of the $OH^{\cdot}$ radicals formed. However, at H_2O_2 concentrations higher than 0.033 M the initial decolorization rate of RR141 was decelerated. The highest COD removal was obtained to be 81% with a complete color removal at an H_2O_2 concentration of 0.267 M and at 333 K with a catalyst amount of 0.3 g for 0.15 dm^3 a dye solution of 0.1 g/dm^3. An increase in temperature positively affected the decolorization of dye as well as the COD removal. The initial decolorization rate was described as $-r_{A0} = 9.4{*}10^4\ e^{-38.8/RT}\ C_{RR141,0}\ C_{H2O2,0}^{0.184}$ in the H_2O_2 concentration range of 0.007 M – 0.033 M. Iron leaching remained below the EU directives. The small iron leaching makes it possible for the catalyst to have long term stability without generating iron hydroxide sludge.

It can be concluded that this study offers a significant potential for the application of heterogeneous Fenton-like oxidation over iron containing a ZSM-5 zeolite for the degradation of RR141 aqueous solutions. It will be a good alternative to the oxidation methods currently used in the degradation of RR141.

Competing interests

The authors declare that they have no competing interests.

Authors' contributions

CY carried out the experiments under the guidance of GG, participated in the interpretation of the data, helped to draft the manuscript. GG participated in the design of the study, conceived of the study and drafted the manuscript. Both authors read and approved the final manuscript.

Acknowledgement

The authors acknowledge the financial support from TÜBİTAK (The Scientific and Technological Research Council of Turkey) under Project number of 108 M175 and from the Ege University Scientific Research Fund under project number of 08MÜH023.

References

1. Tezcanlı-Guyer G, Ince NH. Degradation and toxicity reduction of textile dyestuff by ultrasound. Ultrason Sonochem. 2003;10:235–40.
2. Neamtu M, Zaharia C, Catrinescu C, Yediler A, Macoveanu M, Kettrup M. Fe-exchanged Y zeolite as catalyst for wet peroxide oxidation of reactive azo dye Procion Marine H-EXL. Appl Catal B Environ. 2004;48:287–94.
3. Stolyarova IV, Kovban IB, Prikhod'ko RV, Kushko AO, Sychev MV, Goncharuk VV. FeZSM-5 zeolites in oxidative degradation of dyes and the nature of their active centers. Russ J Appl Chem. 2007;80(5):746–53.
4. Ramirez JH, Costa CA, Madeira LM, Mata G, Vicente MA, Rojas-Cervantes ML, et al. Fenton-like oxidation of Orange II solutions using heterogeneous catalysts based on saponite clay. Appl Catal B Environ. 2007;71:44–56.
5. Wailling C. Fenton's reagent revisited. Acc Chem Res. 1975;8:125–31.
6. Neamtu M, Yediler A, Siminiceanu I, Kettrup A. Oxidation of commercial reactive azo dye aqueous solutions by the photo-Fenton and Fenton-like processes. J Photoch Photobio A Chem. 2003;161:87–93.
7. Bertanza G, Collivignarelli C, Pedrazzani R. The role of chemical oxidation in combined chemical-physical and biological processes: experiences of industrial wastewater treatment. Water Sci Technol. 2001;44:109–16.
8. Solozhenko EG, Soboleva NM, Goncharuk VV. Decolourization of azo dye solutions by Fenton's oxidation. Water Res. 1995;29:2206–10.
9. Kang SF, Chang HM. Coagulation of textile secondary effluents with Fenton's reagent. Water Sci Technol. 1997;36:215–22.
10. Gemeay AH, Mansour IA, El-Sharkawy RG, Zaki AB. Kinetics and mechanism of the heterogeneous catalyzed oxidative degradation of indigo carmine. J Mol Catal A Chem. 2003;193:109–20.
11. Ishtchenko VV, Huddersman KD, Vitkovskaya RF. Part 1. Production of a modified PAN fibrous catalyst and its optimisation towards the decomposition of hydrogen peroxide. Appl Catal A Gen. 2003;242:123–37.
12. Letaief S, Casal B, Aranda P, Martín-Luengo MA, Ruiz-Hitzky E. Fe-containing pillared clays as catalysts for phenol hydroxylation. Appl Clay Sci. 2003;22:263–77.
13. Tachiev G, Roth JA, Bowers AR. Kinetics of hydrogen peroxide decomposition with complexed and "free" iron catalyst. Int J Chem Kinet. 2000;32:24–35.

14. Martínez F, Calleja G, Melero JA, Molina R. Heterogeneous photo-Fenton degradation of phenolic aqueous solutions over iron-containing SBA-15 catalyst. Appl Catal B Environ. 2005;60:181–90.
15. Bahmani P, Kalantary RR, Esrafilli A, Gholami M, Jafari AJ. Evaluation of Fenton oxidation process coupled with biological treatment for the removal of reactive black 5 from aqueous solution. J Environ Health Sci Eng. 2013;11(13):1–9.
16. Zazouli MA, Yousefi Z, Eslami A, Ardebilian B. Municipal solid waste landfill leachate treatment by Fenton, photı-Fenton and Fenton-like processes: effect of some variables. Iran J Environ Health Sci Eng. 2012;9(3):1–9.
17. Phu NH, Hoa TTK, Van Tan N, Thang HV, P H, Le K. Characterization and activity of Fe-ZSM-5 catalysts for the total oxidation of phenol in aqueous solutions. Appl Catal B Environ. 2001;34:267–75.
18. Chaliha S, Bhattocharyya KG. Wet oxidative method for removal of 2,4,6-trichlorophenol in water using Fe(III), Co(II), Ni(II) supported MCM-41 catalysts. J Hazard Mater. 2008;150:728–36.
19. Dükkancı M, Gündüz G, Yılmaz S, Yaman YC, Prihod'ko RV, Stolyarova IV. Characterization and catalytic activity of CuFeZSM-5 catalysts for oxidative degradation of Rhodamine 6G in aqueous solutions. Appl Catal B Environ. 2010;95:270–8.
20. Dükkancı M, Gündüz G, Yılmaz S, Prihod'ko RV. Heterogeneous Fenton-like degradation of Rhodamine 6G in water using CuFeZSM-5 zeolite catalyst prepared by hydrothermal synthesis. J Hazard Mater. 2010;181:343–50.
21. Bolova E, Gündüz G, Dükkancı M, Yılmaz S, Yaman YC. Fe Containing ZSM-5 Zeolite as Catalyst for Wet Peroxide Oxidation of Orange II. Int J Chem React Eng. 2011;9:S1.
22. Flores RG, Andersen SLF, Maia LKK, Jose HJ, Moreira RFPM. Recovery of iron oxides from acid mine drainage and their application as adsorbent or catalyst. J Environ Manage. 2012;111:53–60.
23. Chen A, Ma X, Sun H. Decolorization of KN-R catalyzed by Fe containing Y and ZSM-5 zeolites. J Hazard Mater. 2008;156:568–75.
24. Prihod'ko R, Stolyarova I, Gündüz G, Taran O, Yashnik S, Parmon V, et al. Fe exchanged zeolites as materials for catalytic wet peroxide oxidation. Degradation of Rodamine G dye. Appl Catal B Environ. 2011;104:201–10.
25. Rache M, Garcia AR, Zea HR, Silva AMT, Madeira LM, Ramirez JH. Azo-dye orange II degradation by the heterogeneous Fenton-like process using a zeolite Y-Fe catalyst- Kinetics with a model based on the Fermi's equation. Appl Catal B Environ. 2014;146:192–200.
26. Azmi NHM, Ayodele OB, Vadivelu VM, Asıf M, Hameed BH. Fe-modified local clay as effcetive and reusable heterogeneous photo-Fenton catalyst for the decolorization of Acid Green 25. J Taiwan Inst Chem Eng. 2014;45:1459–67.
27. O'Neil C, Lopez A, Esteves S, Hawkes FR, Hawkes DL, Wilcox S. Azo-dye degradation in an anaerobic-aerobic teratment system operating on simulated textile effluent. Appl Microbial Biotechnol. 2010;53:249–54.
28. Bell J, Buckley CA. Treatment of a textile dye in the anaerobic baffled reactor. Water SA. 2003;29(2):34.
29. Telke A, Kalyani D, Jadhav J, Govindwar S. Kinetics and mechanism of Reactive Red 141 degradation by a banterial ısolate Rhizobium radiobacter MTCC 8161. Acta Chim Slov. 2008;55:320–9.
30. Netpradit S, Thiravetyan P, Towprayoon S. Adsorption of three azo dyes by metal hydroxide sludge: effect of temperature, pH and electrolytes. J Colloid Interf Sci. 2004;270:255–61.
31. Dolphen R, Sakkyawong N, Thiravetyan P, Nakbanpote W. Adsorption of Reactive Red 141 from wastewater onto modified chitin. J Hazard Mater. 2007;145:250–5.
32. Arslan İ, Balcıoğlu IA, Bahnemann DW. Advanced chemical oxidation of reactive dyes in simulated dye house effluents by ferrioxalate-Fenton/UV-A and TiO_2/UV-A processes. Dyes Pigments. 2000;47:207–18.
33. Torrades F, Garcia-Montano J, Garcia-Hortal JA, Nunez L, Domenech X, Peral J. Decolorisation and mineralization of homo and hetero-bireactive dyes under Fenton and photo Fenton conditions. Color Technol. 2004;120:188–94.
34. Nunez L, Garcia-Hortal JA, Torrades F. Study of kinetic parameters related to decolourization and mineralization of reactive dyes from textile dyeing using Fenton and photo-Fenton processes. Dyes Pigments. 2007;75:647–52.
35. Garcia-Montano J, Perez-Estrada L, Oller I, Maldonado MI, Torrades F. Pilot plant scale reactive dyes degradation by solar photo-Fenton and biological processes. J Photoch Photobio A Chem. 2008;195:205–14.
36. Gültekin I, İnce NH. Degradation of Reactive Azo Dyes by UV/H_2O_2: impact of radical scavengers. J Environ Sci Heal A. 2004;39(4):1069–81.
37. Racyte J, Rimeika M. UV/H_2O_2-Advanced Oxidation processes possibilities for textile reactive dyes decolorization. Lithuania: The 7th Int. Conference Faculty of Environmental Eng., Vilnius Gediminas Technical Univ., May 22–28; 2008. p. 684–9.
38. Jeni J, Kanmani S. Solar Nanophoto catalytic decolorisation of reactive dyes using titanium dioxide. Iran J Environ Health Sci Eng. 2011;1(8):15–24.
39. Foletto EL, Battiston S, Simoes JM, Bassaco MM, Pereira LSF, Moraes Flores EM, et al. Synthesis of $ZnAl_2O_4$ nanoparticles by different routes and the effcet of its pore size on the photocatalytic process. Micropor Mesopor Mat. 2012;163:29–33.
40. Rao NN, Chaturvedi V, Li PG. Novel pebblebed photocatalytic reactor for solar treatment of textile wastewater. Chem Eng J. 2012;184:90–7.
41. Foletto EL, Simoes JM, Mazutti MA, Jahn SL, Muller EI, Pereira LSF, et al. Application of Zn_2SnO_4 photo catalyst prepared by microwave-assisted hydrothermal route in the degradation of organic pollutant under sunlight. Ceram Int. 2013;39:4569–74.
42. Aquino JM, Rodrigo MA, Rocha-Filho RC, Saerz C, Carizares F. Influence of the supporting electrolyte on the electroyses of dyes with conductive-diamond anodes. Chem Eng J. 2012;184:221–7.
43. Harrelkas F, Azizi A, Yaacoubi A, Benhammou A, Pons MN. Treatment of textile dye effluents using coagulation-flocculation coupled with membrane proxesses or adsorption on powdered activated carbon. Desalination. 2009;235:330.
44. Kasiri MB, Aleboyeh H, Aleboyeh A. Degradation of Acid Blue 74 using Fe-ZSM-5 zeolite as a heterogeneous photo-Fenton catalyst. Appl Catal B Environ. 2008;84:9–15.
45. Hassan H, Hameed BH. Oxidative decolorization of Acid Red 1 solutions by Fe-zeolite Y type catalyst. Desalination. 2011;276:45–52.
46. Jamalludin NA, Abdullah AZ. Low frequency sonocatalytic degradation of azo dye in water using Fe-doped zeolite Y catalyst. Ultrason Sonochem. 2014;21:743–53.
47. Aleksik M, Koprivanae N, Bozic AL, Kusic H. The potential of Fe-exchanged Y zeolite as a heterogeneous Fenton-type catalyst for oxidative degradation of Reactive Dye in water. Chem Biochem Eng Q. 2010;24:309–19.
48. Alwash AH, Abdullah AZ, Ismail N. Zeolite Y encapsulated with Fe/TiO_2 for ultrasound-assisted degradation of amaranth dye in water. J Hazard Mater. 2012;233–234:184–93.
49. Xu HY, He XL, Wu Z, Shan LW, Zhang WD. Iron-loaded natural clay as heterogeneous catalyst for Fenton-like discolorization of dyeing wastwater. Bull Kor Chem Soc. 2009;30:2249–52.
50. Hassan H, Hameed BH. Fe-clay as effective heterogeneous Fenton catalyst for the decolorization of Reactive Blue 4. Chem Eng J. 2011;171:912–8.
51. Hassan H, Hameed BH. Fenton-like oxidation of Acid Red 1 solutions using heterogeneous catalyst based on ball clay. Int J Environ Sci Dev. 2011;2(3):1–3.
52. Bankovic P, Nikolic AM, Mojovic Z, Jovicic NJ, Zunic M, Dondur V, et al. Al, Fe-pillared clays in catalytic decolorization of aqueous tartrazine solutions. Appl Clay Sci. 2012;58:73–8.
53. Yaman YC, Gündüz G, Dükkancı M. Degradation of C.I. Reactive Red 141 by heterogeneous Fenton-like process over iron containing ZSM-5 zolites. Color Technol. 2013;29:69–75.
54. Schwidder M, Kumar MS, Klementiev K, Pahl MM, Brückner A, Grünert W. Selective reduction of NO with Fe-ZSM-5 catalysts of low Fe content: I. Relations between active site structure and catalytic performance. J Catal. 2005;231:314–30.
55. Guelou E, Barrault J, Fournier J, Tatibouet J-M. Active iron species in catalytic wet peroxide oxidation of phenol over pillared clays containing iron. Appl Catal B Environ. 2003;44:1–8.
56. Catrinescu C, Teodosiu C, Macoveanu M, Miehe-Brende J, Dred RL. Catalytic wet peroxide oxidation of phenol over Fe-exchanged pillared beidellite. Water Res. 2003;37:1154–60.
57. Centi R, Parathoner S, Torre T, Verduna MG. Catalytic wet oxidation with H_2O_2 of carboxylic acids on homogeneous and heterogeneous Fenton-type catalysts. Catal Today. 2000;55:61–9.
58. Smith JM. Chemical Engineering Kinetics, McGrow Hill. 3rd ed. 1981. p. 405–84.
59. Neamtu M, Siminiceanu I, Yediler A, Kettrup A. Kinetics of decolorization and mineralization of reactive azo dyes in aqueous solution by the UV/H_2O_2 oxidation. Dyes Pigments. 2002;53:93–9.

60. Fan J, Guo Y, Wang J, Fan M. Rapid decolorization of azo dye Methyl Orange in aqueous solution by nanoscale zerovalent iron particles. J Hazard Mater. 2009;166:904–10.
61. Xu H, Zhang D, Xu W. Monitoring of decolorization kinetics of Reactive Brilliant Blue X-BR by aniline spectrophotometric method in Fenton oxidation process. J Hazard Mater. 2008;158:445–53.

In-situ Pb^{2+} remediation using nano iron particles

Mohammad Reza Fadaei Tehrani[1*], Abolfazl Shamsai[1] and Manoochehr Vossughi[2]

Abstract

Originally, application of nano zero valent iron (nZVI) particles for the removal of lead (Pb^{2+}) in porous media was studied. At first, stabilized nZVI (S-nZVI) was prepared and characterized, then used in batch and continuous systems. Based on the batch experiments, corresponding reaction kinetics well fitted with the pseudo-first-order adsorption model, and reaction rate ranged from 0.01 to 0.04 g/mg/min depend on solution pH and the molar ratio between Fe and Pb. In batch tests, optimal condition with more than 90% removal efficiency at 60 min was observed at a pH range of 4 to 6 and Fe/Pb ratio more than 2.5. Continuous experiments exposed that Pb^{2+} remediation was as well influenced by seepage velocity, grain size, and type of porous media. The maximum Pb^{2+} removal efficiency in batch and bench-scale systems were 97% and 81%, correspondingly. The results have shown the ability of S-nZVI to use in permeable reactive barriers, as an efficient adsorbent for Pb^{2+}, because of its excellent stability, high reducing power, and a large surface area.

Keywords: nZVI, *in-situ*, Remediation, Lead, Bench-scale

Background

During the last two decades, presence of heavy metal ions in the environment, especially in water sources, was becoming a major concern due to their non-biodegradability, toxicity, wide-spread presence, and tendency to accumulate in living organisms [1]. Lead, a main concern metal pollutant, is widely used in battery manufacturing, electroplating industry, painting and printing processes, plumbing and the combustion of automobile petrol [2]. The U.S. Environmental Protection Agency (U.S.EPA) has set a permissible limit of 0.015 mg/L in drinking water and has placed it on top of the priority list of toxic pollutants [3]. Lead pollution can cause nervous system damage, renal kidney disease, mental retardation, cancer, and anemia in humans [2]. Chemical reduction, ion exchange, chemical precipitation, mineral adsorption, membrane separation, and bio-sorption are the most frequently used treatment technologies for Pb^{2+} removal [4] which are *ex-situ* techniques. Most of these methods are only suitable for the removal of Pb^{2+} in low concentrations and often require extensive processing as well as being too expensive.

Recently, *in-situ* techniques such as permeable reactive barriers (PRB) have become promising alternatives to *ex-situ* methods owing to their lower operating costs [5]. Nano zero valent iron particles could be used as reducing agents in PRBs for removing the wide range of pollutions that promises to be significantly more effective than granular iron, the reaction rates are 25 to 30 times faster, and the sorption capacity is much higher compared with granular iron [2].

The high reactivity of nZVI is the consequence of greater total surface area, higher density of reactive sites on the particle surface, and/or more intrinsic reactivity of the surface sites [6]. Iron nano particles have been extensively studied to remediate pollutants such as chlorinated compounds and metal ions [7], nitrate [8], carbon tetrachloride, benzoquinone [9], metalloids such as arsenic [10], and organic compounds [11]. However, there are many uncertainties regarding to the features of nZVI-based remediation technologies, which have made it difficult to engineer applications for optimal performance or to assess the risk to human or ecological health. In this study, application of surface modified nZVI (S-nZVI) for Pb^{2+} remediation in porous media was experimented that consists of following steps: (1) synthesis, stabilization, and characterization of S-nZVI; (2) determination of kinetics of Pb^{2+} removal by nZVI and the key factors affecting the reaction; (3) investigation of the effects of flow characteristics on the removal rate; (4) bench-scale modeling of lead remediation under natural conditions.

* Correspondence: fadaei@mehr.sharif.edu
[1]Department of Civil Engineering, Sharif University of Technology, Tehran, Iran
Full list of author information is available at the end of the article

Methods

Materials

Lead nitrate ($Pb(NO_3)_2$), used as the source of Pb^{2+} in all experiments, and other chemical reagents, including $FeCl_3.6H_2O$, $NaBH_4$, and $NiCl_2.6H_2O$, were supplied by Merck, Germany. The concentration of lead, divalent and total, was determined using an atomic absorption spectrometer (Varian SpectrAA 220, Germany).

NZVI preparation

The iron nano particles were prepared on-site to prevent more oxidation of nZVI surface. To synthesize the nZVI particles, 0.15 M $NaBH_4$ solution was added slowly with the rate of 1 to 2 mL/min into 0.1 M $FeCl_3.6H_2O$ aqueous solution at ambient temperature and vigorously stirred at 400 rpm [12]. During this reaction, ferric ions were reduced into black particles by sodium borohydride as the reductant, according to the following reaction [13]:

$$4Fe^{3+}{}_{(aq)} + 3BH_4 + 9H_2O \rightarrow 4Fe^{o}{}_{(s)}\downarrow + 3H_2BO_3 + 12H^{+}{}_{(aq)} + 6H_{2(g)}\uparrow \quad (1)$$

The black precipitates were filtered by vacuum filtration through 0.45 μm filter papers and then washed with DI water and ethanol three times.

NZVI stabilization

Previous researches have indicated that nZVI particles aggregate quickly, after decreasing surface area for reaction and limiting mobility. To control nano particle agglomeration, various particle stabilizing strategies have been reported that surface modification with surfactant is one of the most important approaches [14]. Surfactants, such as starch, could be coated on existing nZVI particles in a post-synthesis process; or synthesizing nZVI in the presence of polymer in a pre-synthesis process. The post-synthesis stabilization approach has been shown to decrease reactivity whereas the pre-synthesis approach has improved reactivity and significantly increased surface area [15]. In the present study, nZVI was stabilized by starch in a pre-synthesis process, according to He and Zhao method [16], which is termed here as S-nZVI.

Batch experiments

The batch experiments were conducted to find the finest condition for columns tests. In addition, useful information could be obtained about the effect of some key parameters. As listed in Table 1, the effects of several main variables were investigated in batch tests, one parameter changed while others were kept constant. Batch experiments were carried out in sealed flasks at 20°C. Predefined S-nZVI and 125 mL buffered Pb^{2+} solution with initial concentration of 200 mg/L and pH 4.0 were added to each flask, and the suspension was stirred. Aliquots of the samples were taken at certain time intervals and analyzed immediately following paper filtration. All experiments were conducted in duplicate and the results were averaged.

Continuous experiments

Continuous experiments were performed in two configurations:

1 - Transparent column with 55 mm diameter and 650 mm length filled with glass beads (Figure 1);
2 - bench-scale apparatus consisted of two PVC columns with 300 mm diameter and 1250 mm height filled with packed sand (Figure 2).

Prior to each run, in the first system, glass beads were soaked in hydrogen peroxide solution for 10 hr, washed with de-ionized water, and finally baked at 105°C for 24 hr [17]. For the continuous system, sands were prepared by baking at 500°C for 24 hr to eliminate adsorbed organic matter. In this set of experiments, the pH of the solution was adjusted to 4 ± 0.2 using 0.1 N HCl.

The effects of some flow parameters were investigated by transparent column model, including seepage velocity and S-nZVI loading. Seepage velocity tests, consisted of 5, 10, 20, and 40 m/d, were conducted by distilled water with initial Pb^{2+} concentrations of 200 mg/L, and 5 g S-nZVI injection. S-nZVI loading tests were experimented by initial Pb^{2+} concentrations of 200 mg/L, seepage velocity of 10 m/d, and frequent 5, 10, and 15 g S-nZVI injection.

Table 1 Experimental design in present study* all experiments were conducted in ambient temperature 15–20°C

Experimental set			Variable parameter						Controlled conditions
Batch		1-1	Controlled pH	2.0	4.0	6.0	8.0		S-nZVI: 0.5 g/L, C_o: 200 mg/L
		1-2	Initial Pb^{2+} (mg/L)	100	200	400	800		S-nZVI: 0.5 g/L, pH: 4.0
		1-3	S-nZVI con.(g/L)	0.1	0.2	0.5	1.0	2.0	C_o: 200 mg/L, pH: 4.0
continuous experiments	Transparent column	2-1	Seepage velocity (m/d)	5	10	20	40		C_o = 200 mg/L, pH: 4, Seepage velocity: 10 m/d
		2-2	S-nZVI loading (g)	1	2	5	10		nZVI: 5 g, pH: 4, C_o = 200 mg/L
	Bench-scale	3-1	Seepage velocity (m/d)	10	20	40			nZVI: 15 g, pH: 4, C_o = 200 mg/L

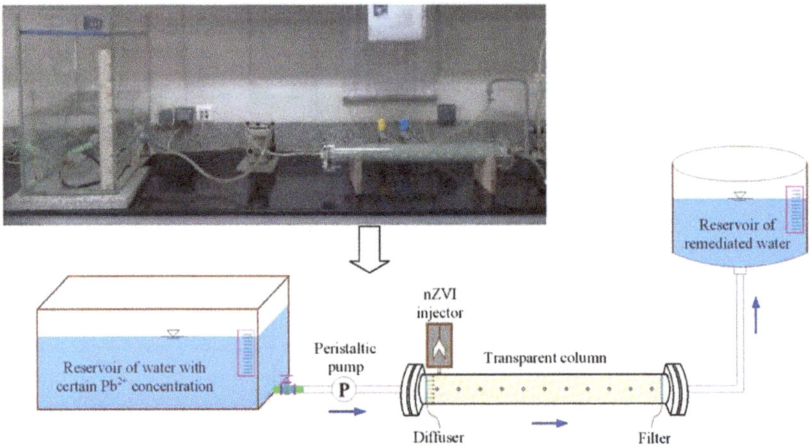

Figure 1 Picture and schematic of transparent column model filled with glass beads.

The bench-scale experiments were planned based on the results of the batch and transparent column tests. The S-nZVI injected into the bottom center of the column forms a permeable reactive zone which reduced inlet pb^{2+}. This configuration is applicable to study the effects of groundwater ionic strength, porous media type, seepage velocity, initial concentration of pb^{2+} and nano particle loading, at the same time. Three treatments, consisted of 5, 10, and 15 g initial S-nZVI loading, were carried out in the bench-scale model. Other conditions were kept as seepage velocity 10 m/d, pH 4, and were used wastewater with initial Pb^{2+} concentration of 200 mg/L.

Results and discussion

Characteristics of S-nZVI

To characterize the stabilized iron nano particles, X-ray powder diffraction (XRD), scanning electron microscopy (SEM), and dynamic light scattering (DLS) were recorded as the results shown in Figure 3. The starched nZVI particles displayed much less agglomeration than those prepared without a stabilizer while S-nZVI remained suspended in water for several hours, non-starched particles agglomerated and precipitated within minutes. XRD results, obtained by a D8 Advanced Bruker diffractometer, indicated the presence of Fe° (peaked at $2\theta = 42$, 67, 82), and Fe_2O_3 ($2\theta = 35$, 53). SEM analyses, by a S4160 FE-SEM device, denoted that the S-nZVI were present as discrete particles as opposed to dendritic flocs for non-starched particles. DLS was performed using a S-red Badge model ZEN1600. The mean particle size was estimated to be 78 nm with a standard deviation of 14 nm, which translated to a surface area of at least 25 m^2/g.

Batch experiments

a. Effect of solution pH

Generally, pH of solution is an important factor for heavy metal ions removal by nZVI. It is widely accepted that low pH has a negative effect on metal adsorption by nZVI [18]. When pH is lower than zero point charge (pH_{zpc}), the positive charge surface of nZVI will repulse

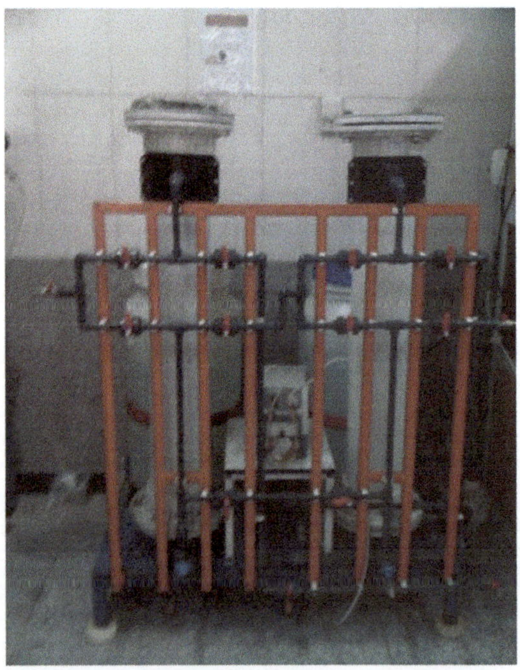

Figure 2 Picture of bench-scale model.

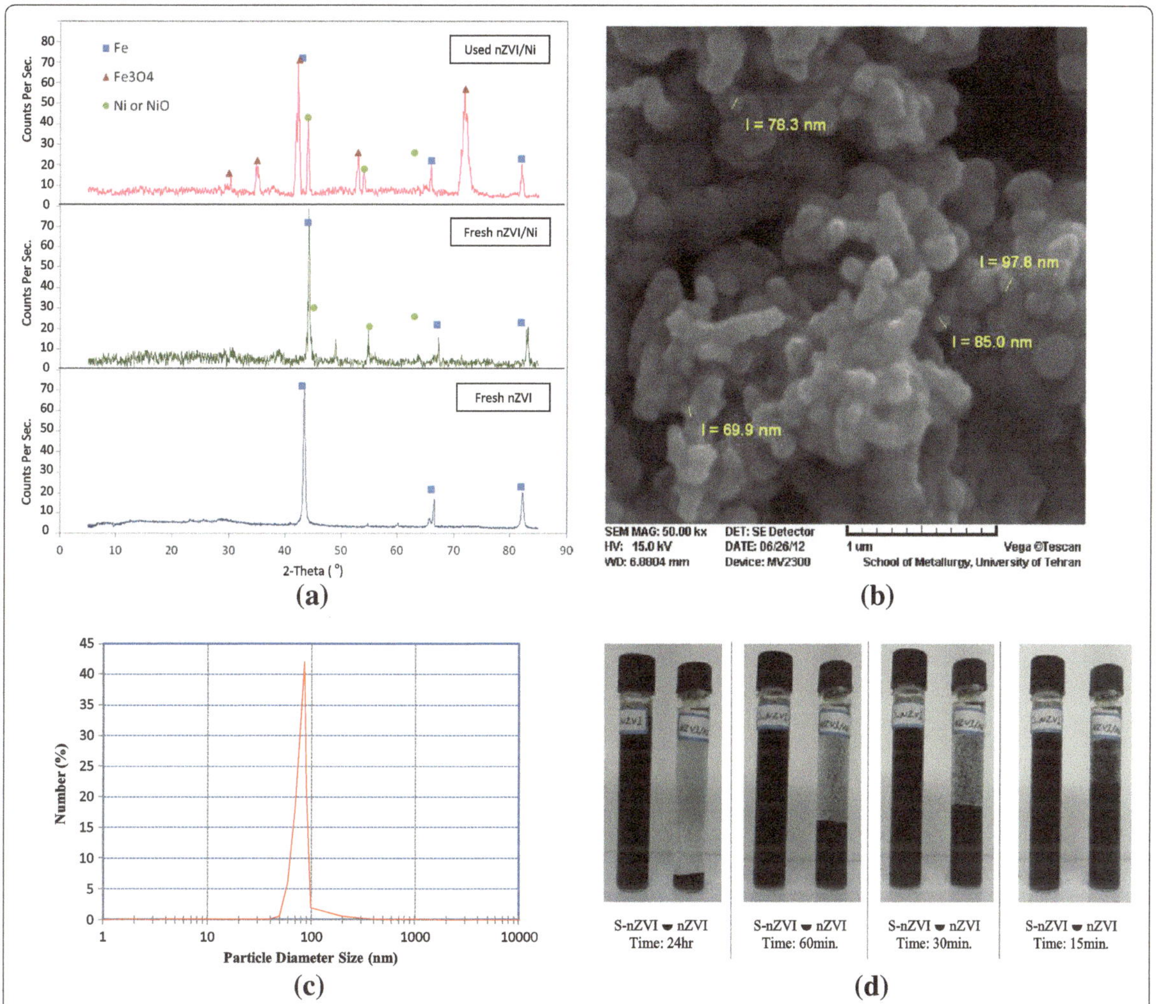

Figure 3 Characteristic of synthesized nZVI, (a) XRD diagram, (b) SEM image, (c) DLS results, (d) stabilization status.

metal cations, and results lower removal efficiency [19]. On the other hand, it is found out from equation 2 that H^+ is strongly produced along the Pb^{2+} reduction reaction that point to an alkaline environment is preferred by the Pb^{2+} removal in aqueous solution [20].

$$2Fe^o + 3Pb^{2+} + 4H_2O \rightarrow 2FeOH + 3Pb^o + 2H^+ \quad (2)$$

Figure 4a presents the results of batch experiments in which S-nZVI are exposed to Pb^{2+} buffered solution with different pH values. At pH <4.0 or >6.0 after 60 min, less than 60% of Pb^{2+} was degraded, while more than 80% removal efficiency was obtained after 60 min at pH 5 ± 1. The results suggest that rapid reduction of Pb^{2+} into Pb^o occurs while pH < 6, and adsorption was optimized by adjusting the pH > 4. Thus, it can be concluded that pH around 5 favors for Pb^{2+} removal by nZVI.

b. Effect of initial Pb^{2+} concentration

As shown in Figure 4b, the effect of initial concentration of Pb^{2+} on removal efficiency was investigated in the range of 100 to 800 mg/L. The equilibrium time became longer and the final removal efficiency of Pb^{2+} decreased as the initial Pb^{2+} concentration increased; So, the percentage of Pb^{2+} removed within 60 min at an initial concentration of 100 mg/L was nearly 85%, and it was only 58% at an initial concentration of 800 mg/L. Furthermore, as revealed in Figure 5b, the plot well fitted to the pseudo first order adsorption model, where

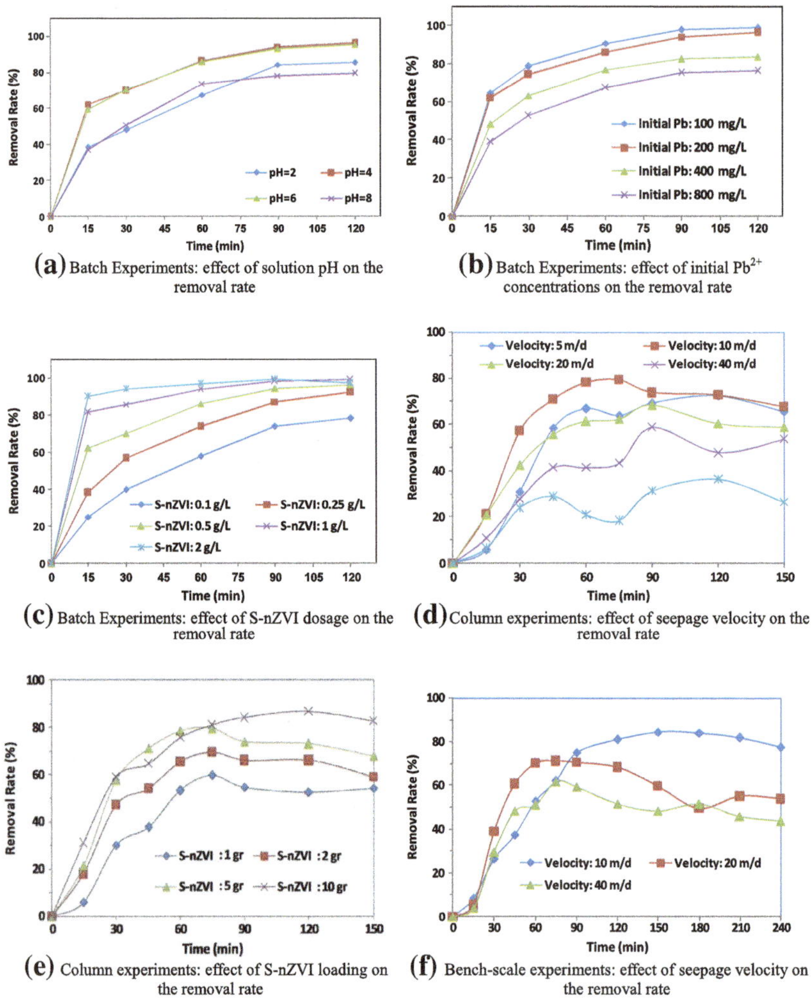

(a) Batch Experiments: effect of solution pH on the removal rate

(b) Batch Experiments: effect of initial Pb^{2+} concentrations on the removal rate

(c) Batch Experiments: effect of S-nZVI dosage on the removal rate

(d) Column experiments: effect of seepage velocity on the removal rate

(e) Column experiments: effect of S-nZVI loading on the removal rate

(f) Bench-scale experiments: effect of seepage velocity on the removal rate

Figure 4 Results of Pb^{2+} removal by experiments in batch, column and bench-scale models.

the observed rate constant decreased significantly as the initial Pb^{2+} concentration increased. Generally, when nZVI concentration was constant, the lower efficiency and slower rate of Pb^{2+} removal were found at higher initial concentrations of Pb^{2+}.These results suggest that the capacity of the S–nZVI for lead removal is about 430 mg Pb/g S-nZVI.

c. Effect of S-nZVI concentration

As shown in Figure 4c, the Pb^{2+} removal efficiency improved as the S-nZVI concentration increased. The removal efficiency of Pb^{2+} was about 50% using S-nZVI at 0.1 g/L for 60 min, but was nearly 95% when the S-nZVI concentration was higher than 1 g/L. In the same conditions, K_{obs} raised as the S-nZVI concentration increased. These phenomena can be attributed to the increase in available active sites resulting from the increase in S-nZVI concentration, where the lead reduction occurred. Additionally, lead ions removal sharply enhanced by increasing contact time for the first 60 min, and then gradually approached equilibrium after approximately 120 min.

d. Kinetics of the Pb^{2+} reduction

The adsorption kinetics of Pb^{2+} ions was studied to determine the required time to achieve equilibrium adsorption of lead ions on the adsorbents. It was reported that nZVI can remove metal ions from aqueous solutions by various mechanisms, including electrostatic adsorption, complex formation, reduction, and

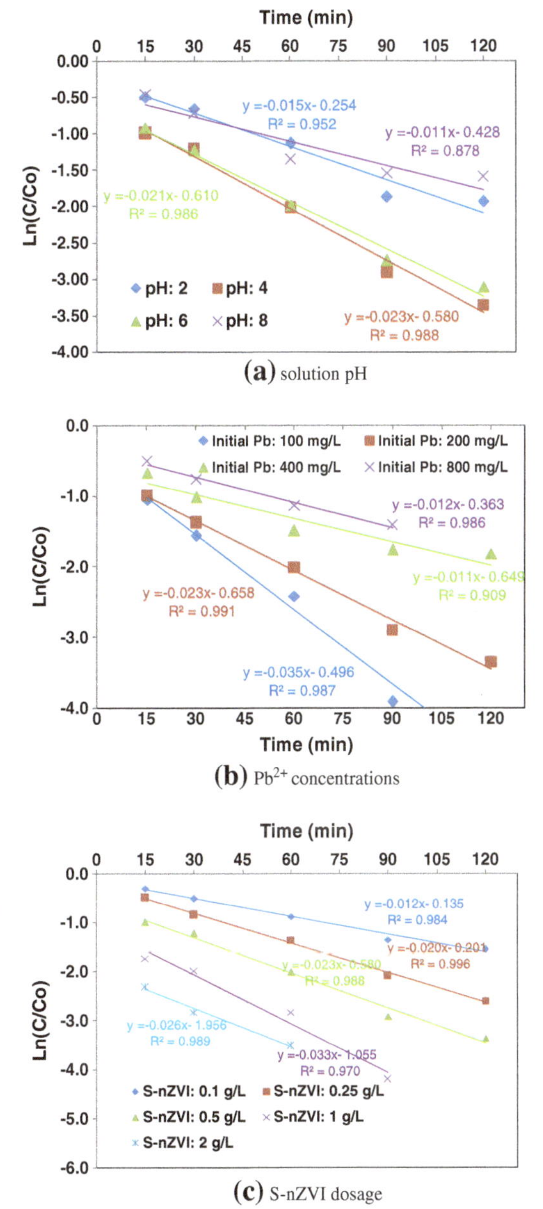

Figure 5 Pseudo first-order adsorption kinetic plots (corresponding to Figure 4a, b and c, respectively).

precipitation [21]. It seems that when nZVI was used, the nano particles captured aqueous lead ions easily and rapidly because of their large surface areas and high reactivity.

In this research, the kinetics was investigated experimentally under different values of initial Pb^{2+} concentration, solution pH, and S-nZVI dosage by using pseudo first-order reaction model that can be represented as following:

$$\ln(C/C_o) = -K_{obs}t \tag{3}$$

where C_o and C are the concentration of Pb^{2+} (mg/g) at initial and time t (min), respectively. K_{obs} (min^{-1}) is the equilibrium rate constant for first order adsorption. Therefore, by plotting $ln(C/C_o)$ against t, the values of K_{obs} can be found from the slope of the revealed plots.

Several studies have investigated the kinetic of Pb^{2+} removal by nZVI. Among a number of kinetic models, such as pseudo zero-order, pseudo first-order and pseudo second-order kinetic models, the pseudo first-order kinetic model was the most suitable which approves the best fit with the experimental data of Pb^{2+} removal compared to the rest of models [2]. As seen in Figure 5, the experimental data were well fitted to the pseudo first-order adsorption model with the high correlation coefficients. The parameters obtained by linear regression analysis were offered in Table 2. The results indicated a decrease in K_{obs} values from 0.04 to 0.01 g/mg/min, when initial Pb^{2+} concentration increased from 100 to 800 mg/L. The rate constant K_{obs} also increased by increasing S-nZVI dosage, and by approaching to a solution pH of 5.

e. Adsorption isotherms

Experimental data were modeled using the well known adsorption models described by the Freundlich and Langmuir equations to study the ability of Pb^{2+} ions to adsorb on S-nZVI [22].

Based on the results of our experimental data fitting on these isotherms, in Table 3, nZVI has the good ability to reduce Pb^{2+} to Pb^o which can then be absorbed by the nZVI easily. Furthermore, data fitting by using the

Table 2 Pseudo first-order adsorption kinetics constants for Pb^{2+} removal by S-nZVI

Parameters	pH:2.0	4.0	6.0	8.0	
K_{obs} (1/min)	−0.015	−0.024	−0.022	−0.011	
R^2	1.0	0.999	0.998	0.991	
Fixed conditions: Initial Pb^{2+} 200 mg/L, S-nZVI 0.5 g/L					
Parameter	**Initial Pb^{2+}: 100 mg/L**	**200**	**400**	**800**	
K_{obs} (1/min)	−0.035	−0.023	−0.011	−0.012	
R^2	0.999	0.999	0.999	0.997	
Fixed conditions: S-nZVI 0.5 g/L, pH 4.0,					
Parameter	**S-nZVI:0.1 g/L**	**0.25**	**0.5**	**1.0**	**2.0**
K_{obs} (1/min)	−0.012	−0.020	−0.024	−0.033	−0.026
R^2	0.999	0.981	0.999	1.0	1.0
Fixed conditions: Initial Pb^{2+} 200 mg/L, pH 4.0,					

Table 3 Freundlich and Langmuir adsorption isotherms constants for Pb^{2+} removal by S-nZVI

Parameters	pH:2.0		4.0	6.0	8.0	
Freundlich	1/n	−0.51	−0.18	−0.21	−0.65	
	K_n	1996	571	629	3662	
Langmuir	q_{max}	0.14	0.24	0.23	0.12	
	K_l	0.05	0.21	0.16	0.04	
Fixed conditions: Initial Pb^{2+} 200 mg/L, S-nZVI 0.2 g/L						
Parameter		**Initial Pb^{2+}: 100 mg/L**	**200**	**400**	**800**	
Freundlich	1/n	−0.11	−0.17	−0.45	−0.67	
	K_n	208	564	4615	43143	
Langmuir	q_{max}	0.13	0.24	0.33	0.50	
	K_l	0.71	0.20	0.03	0.01	
Fixed conditions: S-nZVI 0.2 g/L, pH 4.0,						
Parameter		**S-nZVI:0.1 g/L**	**0.25**	**0.5**	**1.0**	**2.0**
Freundlich	1/n	−0.85	−0.39	−0.18	−0.05	−0.03
	K_n	43228	2335	571	204	38
Langmuir	q_{max}	0.42	0.29	0.24	0.16	0.09
	K_l	0.02	0.06	0.21	1.43	2.83
Fixed conditions: Initial Pb^{2+} 200 mg/L, pH 4.0,						

Langmuir model give a better fit than by using the Freundlich model. This can be seen from the fitting data obtained that the correlation coefficient is higher for the Langmuir adsorption isotherm (~0.92) compared to that of the Freundlich model (~0.84).

Continuous experiments

Transparent column

a. Effect of seepage velocity

The results of seepage velocity tests are shown in Figure 4c. It was observed that a seepage velocity of 10 m/d yielded the maximum removal rate. Furthermore, any variation, increasing or decreasing of this velocity, had a negative effect on the Pb^{2+} removal. Higher seepage velocities enhanced the mobility of nano particles through porous media and reduced the contact time and as a result, reduced the remediation efficiency.

b. Effect of S-nZVI loading

As shown in Figure 4e, when S-nZVI loading rose from 1 to 10 g, the Pb^{2+} removal efficiency within 60 min increased from about 50% to 80%. It is found out that when further amount of S-nZVI was injected, the Pb^{2+} removal has been improved.

Bench-scale model

The results of bench-scale experiments, illustrated in Figure 4f, indicated that the removal efficiency through sand materials were higher than glass beads. In addition, increasing seepage velocity had a decreasing effect on the Pb^{2+} remediation. Through bench-scale experiments, the best Pb^{2+} remediation efficiency was achieved, i.e. about 81%. In pH of 4, initial concentration of 200 mg/L, and 15 g S-nZVI injection, finally 31 L of treated water with Pb^{2+} concentration less than 20 mg/L was acquired. Therefore, it could be proposed that the capacity of S-nZVI for *in-situ* lead removal is about 300 mg Pb^{2+}/g S-nZVI.

Conclusions

Findings of this study indicated that starched nZVI has a good feasibility for *in-situ* lead remediation in contaminated water. Batch experiments proved that pH of solution was an important parameter while kinetics coefficients were directly related to pH with correlation coefficients $R^2 > 0.90$. In addition, increasing of S-nZVI dosage or decreasing Pb^{2+} initial concentration, both lead to enhancement in removal efficiency. It means that if mass-ratio between nZVI and Pb is kept constant, i.e. about 2.5, the removal rate would be invariable.

Transparent column experiments revealed that Pb^{2+} remediation also was mostly influenced by seepage velocity, grain size, and type of porous media. Bench-scale results confirmed the batch and transparent column outcomes. As a final point, because of the fast reaction kinetics and high Pb^{2+} removal capacity, S-nZVI has the fine potential to become an effective remedial agent in PRB for *in-situ* immobilization of lead in polluted groundwater resources.

Abbreviations
nZVI: nano Zero Valent Iron particles; S-nZVI: Stabilized nano Zero Valent Iron particles; U.S.EPA: U.S. Environmental Protection Agency; PRB: Permeable Reactive Barriers; XRD: X-Ray powder Diffraction; SEM: Scanning Electron Microscopy; DLS: Dynamic light scattering.

Competing interests
The authors declare that they have no competing interests.

Authors' contributions
MR Fadaei Tehrani designed and developed the physical models, carried out the experiments and performed the analysis of results. As well as prepared the draft of manuscript. A Shamsai participated in the design of the study and performed the statistical analysis. M Vosughi conceived of the study, and participated in its design and coordination and helped to draft the manuscript. All authors read and approved the final manuscript. Furthermore, MR Fadaei Tehrani is the PHD candidate for Water Engineering doing his thesis under the supervisions of A Shamsaei and M Vosoughi in Civil Engineering Faculty of Sharif University of Technology.

Acknowledgments
This work was supported by the Institute of Biotechnology and Environment (IBE) in Sharif University of Technology, Tehran, Iran.

Author details
[1]Department of Civil Engineering, Sharif University of Technology, Tehran, Iran. [2]Institute of Biotechnology and Environment (IBE), Department of Chemical Engineering, Sharif University of Technology, Tehran, Iran.

References
1. Xu D, Tan X, Chen C, Wang X. Removal of Pb(II) from aqueous solution by oxidized multiwalled carbon nanotubes. Journal of Hazardous Materials. 2008;154(1–3):407–16.
2. Zhang X, Lin S, Lu X-Q, Chen Z-l. Removal of Pb(II) from water using synthesized kaolin supported nanoscale zero-valent iron. Chemical Engineering Journal. 2010;163(3):243–8.
3. U.S.EPA: Drinking Water Contaminants, http://water.epa.gov/drink/contaminants/index.cfm (accessed June 1, 2014). 2014.
4. Machida M, Mochimaru T, Tatsumoto H. Lead(II) adsorption onto the graphene layer of carbonaceous materials in aqueous solution. Carbon. 2006;44(13):2681–8.
5. Li L, Benson CH, Lawson EM. Modeling porosity reductions caused by mineral fouling in continuous-wall permeable reactive barriers. Journal of Contaminant Hydrology. 2006;83(1–2):89–121.
6. Cundy AB, Hopkinson L, Whitby RLD. Use of iron-based technologies in contaminated land and groundwater remediation: A review. Science of The Total Environment. 2008;400(1–3):42–51.
7. Rangsivek R, Jekel MR. Removal of dissolved metals by zero-valent iron (ZVI): Kinetics, equilibria, processes and implications for stormwater runoff treatment. Water Research. 2005;39(17):4153–63.
8. Yang GCC, Lee H-L. Chemical reduction of nitrate by nanosized iron: kinetics and pathways. Water Research. 2005;39(5):884–94.
9. Zhang X, Deng B, Guo J, Wang Y, Lan Y. Ligand-assisted degradation of carbon tetrachloride by microscale zero-valent iron. Journal of Environmental Management. 2011;92(4):1328–33.
10. Kim K-R, Lee B-T, Kim K-W. Arsenic stabilization in mine tailings using nano-sized magnetite and zero valent iron with the enhancement of mobility by surface coating. Journal of Geochemical Exploration. 2012;113:124–9.
11. Fagerlund F, Illangasekare TH, Phenrat T, Kim HJ, Lowry GV. PCE dissolution and simultaneous dechlorination by nanoscale zero-valent iron particles in a DNAPL source zone. Journal of Contaminant Hydrology. 2012;131(1–4):9–28.
12. Peng S, Wang C, Xie J, Sun S. Synthesis and stabilization of monodisperse Fe nanoparticles. Journal of the American Chemical Society. 2006;128(33):10676–7.
13. Lee C, Jee YK, Won IL, Nelson KL, Yoon J, Sedlak DL. Bactericidal effect of zero-valent iron nanoparticles on Escherichia coli. Environmental Science and Technology. 2008;42(13):4927–33.
14. Chris M, Kocur DMOA, Carroll Brent E. Impact of nZVI stability on mobility in porous media. Journal of Contaminant Hydrology. 2013;145:17–25.
15. Nataphan Sakulchaicharoen DMOC, Jose EH. Enhanced stability and dechlorination activity of pre-synthesis stabilized nanoscale FePd particles. Journal of contaminant hydrology. 2010;118:117–21.
16. He F, Zhao D. Preparation and characterization of a new class of starch-stabilized bimetallic nanoparticles for degradation of chlorinated hydrocarbons in water. Environ Sci Technol. 2005;39:3314–20.
17. Kanel SR, Neppolian B, Choi H, Yang JW. Heterogeneous catalytic oxidation of phenanthrene by hydrogen peroxide in soil slurry: Kinetics, mechanism, and implication. Soil and Sediment Contamination. 2003;12(1):101–17.
18. Yalei Zhang YS, Xuefei Z, Chaomeng D, Keller AA. A new insight on the core–shell structure of zerovalent ironnanoparticles and its application for Pb(II) sequestration. Journal of Hazardous Materials. 2013;263:685–93.
19. X.Q. Li WXZ. Sequestration of metal cations with zero valent iron nano particles- a study with high resolution X-ray photoelectron spectroscopy (HR-XPS). J Phys Chem. 2007;111:6939–46.
20. Ponder SM, Darab JG, Mallouk TE. Remediation of Cr(VI) and Pb(II) aqueous solutions using nanoscale zero-valent iron. Environ Sci Technol. 2000;34:2564–9.
21. Yunfei Xi MM, Ravendra N. Reduction and adsorption of Pb2+ in aqueous solution by nano-zero-valent iron-A SEM, TEM and XPS study. Materials Research Bulletin. 2010;45:1361–7.
22. Freundlich HMF. Adsorption in solids. *Zeitschrif t fuer Physikalisch-Chemie.* Stoechiometrie Verwandtschaftslehre. 1906;57:385–470.

9

4-chlorophenol removal from water using graphite and graphene oxides as photocatalysts

Karina Bustos-Ramírez[1,2,3], Carlos Eduardo Barrera-Díaz[1], Miguel De Icaza-Herrera[3], Ana Laura Martínez-Hernández[2,3], Reyna Natividad-Rangel[1] and Carlos Velasco-Santos[2,3*]

Abstract

Graphite and graphene oxides have been studied amply in the last decade, due to their diverse properties and possible applications. Recently, their functionality as photocatalytic materials in water splitting was reported. Research in these materials is increasing due to their band gap values around 1.8-4 eV, and therefore, these are comparable with other photocatalysts currently used in heterogeneous photocatalytic processes. Thus, this research reports the photocatalytic effectiveness of graphite oxide (GO) and graphene oxide (GEO) in the degradation of 4-chlorophenol (4-CP) in water. Under the conditions defined for this research, 92 and 97% of 4-CP were degraded with GO and GEO respectively, also 97% of total organic carbon was removed. In addition, by-products of 4-CP that produce a yellow solution obtained only using photolysis are eliminated by photocatalyst process with GO and GEO. The degradation of 4-CP was monitored by UV-Vis spectroscopy, High Performance Liquid Chromatography (HPLC) and Chemical Oxygen Demand (COD). Thus, photocatalytic activity to remove 4-CP from water employing GO and GEO without doping is successfully showed, and therefore, a new gate in research for these materials is opened.

Keywords: 4-chlorophenol, Photocatalyst, Graphite oxide, Graphene oxide, Water pollution

Background

With increasing global air and water pollutions, photocatalysis has attracted considerable attention because this method provides a promising pathway to attenuate environmental pollution problems, mainly due to the capacity of photocatalyst to degrade organic contaminants [1].

Chlorophenols represent an important group of organic water pollutants due to their toxicity and low biodegradability. They are considered priority pollutants and are employed in numerous industrial processes; in particular, 4-CP is involved in the synthesis of many pesticides, pharmaceuticals and dyes [2-5].

Most polluting organic compounds, including 4-CP, are difficult to degrade, so, it is important to develop more effective methods to promote their degradation [6]. Different biological, physical and chemical methods have been applied for chlorophenol degradation [7,8]. Other established alternative methods, such as Advanced Oxidation Processes (AOP) [9], have been reported to be effective for the degradation of soluble organic contaminants from water, providing almost total degradation. Several technologies are included under AOP such as photo-Fenton, ozonation, photocatalysis, etc. [10,11].

Thus, the remediation of wastewater with chlorophenols using photocatalysis has been widely studied, but not in the case of 4-CP; however, the complexity of degradation processes with heterogeneous catalysts and the high sensitivity of the reaction to experimental conditions represent two main disadvantages, that make it difficult to compare different related systems. Several studies have evaluated the effects of different substituent groups in the aromatic ring in phenolic compounds, as well as the influence of metal ions and/or oxidant compounds, on the adsorption equilibrium and kinetic parameters of degradation during UV irradiation of a suspension in a photocatalytic process with a semiconductor.

The photocatalytic activity is governed by the catalyst, which is a semiconductor (e.g., TiO_2 (the most used), ZnO and Fe_2O_3) [12]. These compounds have two primary characteristics: the first, their band edge energy; semiconductors

* Correspondence: cylaura@gmail.com
[2]División de Estudios de Posgrado e Investigación, Instituto Tecnológico de Querétaro, Av. Tecnológico s/n Esq. M. Escobedo, Col. Centro Histórico, 76000 Querétaro, México
[3]Centro de Física Aplicada y Tecnología Avanzada, Universidad Nacional Autónoma de México, Boulevard Juriquilla 3001, 76230 Querétaro, México
Full list of author information is available at the end of the article

with more negative band edge energy than the reduction potential of water (or protons), and that remain stable when are in contact with water can be considered as appropriate catalyst materials [13]; the second characteristic is the particle size, of primary importance in heterogeneous photocatalysis because it is directly related to the efficiency of the catalyst through the definition of its specific surface area [12].

An increasing amount of works has been addressed in searching alternative materials to TiO_2. Anyway, the information gathered indicates that exist a valid alternative to the use of modified-TiO_2 for photocatalytic process, although the intrinsic electronic and physico-chemical properties of some compounds reported in the literature suggest more investigation. In the degradation of 4-CP, the TiO_2 has been applied in the following cases: 1) Photocatalytic degradation method using 1% silver loaded TiO_2 (Ag-TiO_2), the degradation/transformation of 4-CP is extremely high compared to neat TiO_2, this latter requires longer exposure time to obtain the same degree of degradation than the compound Ag-TiO_2 [14]; 2) Cobalt-modified TiO_2 (Co-TiO_2) is able to bring about the photocatalytic degradation of pollutants such as 4-chlorophenol, the best photoactivity was observed for an amount of cobalt between 0.2% and 0.5% Co/TiO_2 w/w [15]; 3) the mesoporous anatase is able to degrade 100% 4-CP, while Degussa P-25 degraded 57% in time of 180 min, the enhanced photocatalytic activity of the mesoporous titania samples when compared to Degussa P-25 was related to smaller crystallite size, presence of pure anatase phase, higher average pore diameter, and surface area [16]; these are some published works, but in the case of research applying graphite oxide and graphene oxide without doping to degrade photocatalytically 4-CP, it is non-existent until this time.

In the development of new photocatalysts, the graphite oxide (GO), a polymer-like semiconductor made of only carbon, oxygen and hydrogen, has a large exposed area and can be extensively dispersed in water on the molecular scale. These structural features, both due to their chemical and physical aspects, suggest the favourable role of graphite oxide as a photocatalyst. Therefore, graphene oxide (GEO) derivatives of GO can also be good photocatalysts. The difference between them is the number of stacked layers. Both materials (GO and GEO) have photocatalytic activity, as it was reported recently and showed by water splitting and hydrogen production [12,17,18].

Also, nanostructured semiconductor materials are anticipated as new photocatalysts to open up new opportunities and employ the renewable energy sources, such as: Iodine-doped TiO_2 nanoparticles, titanium oxynitride porous thin films, TiO_2/SnO_2 nanofibers, square Bi_2WO_6 nanoplates, and Si nanowires. All these materials have been explored and exhibited interesting photoactivities. These materials with optical gap of 2.7 eV have been recognized as a very promising metal free photocatalyst, and its photocatalytic activity is confirmed to be even higher than the commercial nitrogen-doped TiO_2. But like the TiO_2, the rapid recombination of electrons and holes is one of the main reasons for the low photocatalytic efficiency of these kinds of photocatalysts [19-21]. But in the case of GO and GEO, the anti-recombination is a given characteristic in current works of research related to the topic of photocatalysts. This effect can be attributed to their nanometric thickness, surface area and the presence of oxygenated groups. Also, both carbon structures can be doped with different materials or atoms to improve their performance as photocatalysts [22]. Additionally, reduced graphene oxide (RGO) modified with different compounds has been used successfully as a photocatalytic material in the remediation treatment of heavy metals and organic compounds [23-26]. Also, a recent work has studied about the photocatalytic effectivity of graphene oxide in the removal of 4-CP by computational method [27]. However, the photocatalytic activities of unmodified GO and GEO have not been studied experimentally, for the removal of organic compounds in water. Thus, it is important to verify the photocatalytic activity of these unmodified carbon materials for the removal of organic compounds in water. GEO has attracted great interest because of its easy availability in bulk quantities, readiness for functionalization by chemical reaction, good dispersion in water and high biocompatibility [26]. Thus, in this research is showed for the first time the capacity of graphene and graphite oxides to remove 4-CP from aqueous solutions under UV-light. Both undoped oxides (GEO and GO) present sufficient activity to remove the organic pollutant from water.

Materials and methods

Materials

Graphite (Electron Microscopy Sciences, No. 70230), distilled water (J.T. Baker), 4-chlorophenol (≥99% Sigma Aldrich), Sulfuric acid (H_2SO_4, Baker, 98%), potassium permanganate ($KMnO_4$, Merck), hydrogen peroxide (H_2O_2, Baker, 30%) and distilled water (H_2O) were used as received. Graphite oxide (GO) and graphene oxide (GEO) were synthesized from graphite by a methodology reported in a previous work [28], and described briefly below.

Synthesis of graphite and graphene oxides

First, H_2SO_4 (46 mL) was added into the reaction flask maintained at 0°C (±2°C) (ice bath), then graphite (2 g) and $KMnO_4$ (6 g) were added slowly. After an increase in temperature to 35°C (±2°C), the mixture was stirred by a magnetic stirring bar and mixed for 2 h. Later, the excess water was incorporated to the mixture and H_2O_2 (10 ml) was added until there was no gas production.

Then, filtration was performed with distilled water in a glass filter, and the obtained brown GO was dried in an oven (Barnstead Thermoline, Model 3478) at 65°C for 12 h. After that, a solution containing 100 mg of dried GO in 10 mL of H_2O was prepared. This solution was sonicated for 3 h at room temperature with the assistance of an ultrasonic bath (Branson 1510R-MTH) at 55 degassing units, in order to obtain graphene oxide sheets (GEO).

Adsorption test

Adsorption test consisted on placing an aqueous solution of 4-CP with a concentration of 30 ppm and neutral pH into a tubular glass reactor, adding graphite oxide or graphene oxide (0.8 g/L in both cases) with magnetic stirring (1000 rpm) and then, the reactor was covered with aluminium foil to prevent contact with external light. The reaction time was 100 minutes and aliquots were taken at 20, 40, 60, 80 and 100 minutes.

Photolysis test

For these experiments, 30 mL of 4-CP solution (30 ppm) at neutral pH were placed in the same reactor used for the adsorption test and induced with UV irradiation from a lamp (Pencil UV lamp, 254 nm, 5.5 W). Light source was located in the centre of the vessel along with a magnetic stirrer (1000 rpm). The reactor temperature was maintained at 24°C +/- 2°C and the reactor was covered with aluminium foil to prevent contact with external light. The reaction time was 100 minutes and aliquots were taken after 20, 40, 60, 80 and 100 minutes.

Photocatalyst test

The photocatalytic efficiencies of the GO and GEO were determined in the same tubular glass reactor used for the photolysis test with the same continuous stirring (1000 rpm). The total reaction volume was 30 ml. The tests were performed using 0.8 g/L of graphite and graphene oxides, with 30 ppm of 4-CP at neutral pH. The reactor temperature was maintained at 24°C +/- 2°C and aluminium foil was placed around the reactor. A UV lamp (Pencil UV lamp, 254 nm, 5.5 W) was placed in the centre of the reactor to provide UV light radiation. The reaction time was 100 minutes and aliquots were taken after 20, 40, 60, 80 and 100 minutes.

Chemical Oxygen Demand (COD)

Method 8000/reactor digestion method in the high range (0–1500 mg/L), programmed in the HACH DR5000 spectrophotometer was used to determine the COD in the initial and final solutions of 4-CP.

Characterization

Fourier transform infrared spectroscopy (FT-IR) of GO and GEO samples was performed using a Bruker-Vector 33 with a scanning range of 4000-500 cm^{-1} with resolution of 1 cm^{-1}.

Raman spectroscopy of the carbon samples was carried on a Micro-Raman (Dilor, Lab Ram), with measurements at 488 nm incident laser light with a spectral resolution of 1 cm^{-1}.

UV-vis spectroscopy was carried out on a HACH DR5000 spectrophotometer at wavelengths of 200–1100 nm to determine the absorption bands characteristic of the 4-CP solution and monitor the progress of 4-CP removal from the solution by adsorption, photolysis and the photocatalytic processes.

HPLC (High Performance Liquid Chromatography) was performed with a mobile phase of H_2O_2 with 5 mmol H_2SO_4 and methanol (80:20), a flow rate of 1 mL/min and an Ascentis Express C_{18} 3 cm × 4.6 mm (2.7 μm) SUPELCO column for the determination of intermediate compounds.

Mineralization of 4-CP was followed by measuring the chemical oxygen demand (COD) in a typical reaction. An aliquot was taken at the end of the reaction and the COD was measured by a colorimetric method on the HACH DR5000 spectrophotometer.

Results and discussion

FT-IR spectroscopy

The effect of chemical modification due to reaction of graphite with acids is observed in the FT-IR spectra (Figure 1). Pure graphite is inactive as is observed in spectrum (a), whereas GO and GEO spectra (b and c respectively) show several distinctive signals such as: 1732 cm^{-1}, ν(C = O) at carboxyl groups; 1620 cm^{-1}, ν(C = C); and 1065 cm^{-1}, ν(C-O), giving evidence for the presence of oxygen-containing groups, caused by the chemical reaction and reported in previous work [28].

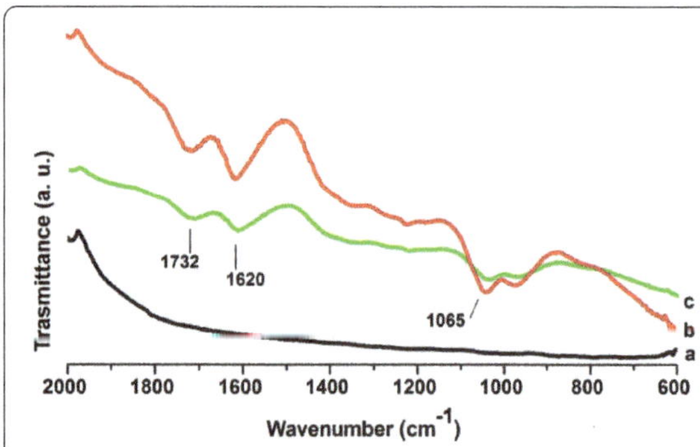

Figure 1 FT-IR spectra of graphite (a), (b), (c).

Raman spectroscopy

Raman spectroscopy shows the characteristic bands assigned to the carbon materials, indicating the modification in the hybridization and defects produced at the surface of materials synthetized by chemical reaction. Figure 2, shows distinctive signals: a strong band close to 1580 cm^{-1} (G band), a line around 1350 cm^{-1} (D band) and 2D band in the region of 2700 cm^{-1}, characteristic for GO and GEO, these bands have been reported by different authors and also in a previous work of this research group [28].

UV-vis spectroscopy

Figure 3 shows the UV-vis spectrum of 4-CP; two characteristic bands of this compound as aqueous solution are observed at 280 and 225 nm [3,29].

The UV-vis spectra in Figure 4 correspond to GO and GEO and show the maximum absorption peaks at 227 and 305 nm that each material exhibits, the bands are attributed to the π-π* electronic transitions of the aromatic C-C bonds and the n-π* transition of the C = O bond, respectively [25]. These spectra are also used to obtain the band gap values for both oxides. Tauc's method is applied, and the calculated values are around 2–4.7 eV for graphite oxide and 1.8–4 eV for graphene oxide; these values are comparable with other semiconductors used as photocatalysts; in addition, these results are very similar to those reported in previous work [13].

Adsorption test

To confirm the degradation of 4-CP due to photocatalysis, samples of graphite and graphene oxides are tested as adsorbents of this pollutant. Figure 5 shows 4-CP removal using GO (A-GO) as adsorbent. In this process, it is observed that the absorption intensity of the band at 280 nm produced by the solution after adsorption with GO is more intense in comparison with the band of only 4-CP (sample 0), indicating that under these conditions GO adsorbs molecules of 4-CP; however, the solution shows a light yellow colour, indicating that the adsorption process may produce some by-products, since it cannot degrade the benzene ring of the 4-CP. The interaction between the two compounds in water may lead to derivatives and by-products of 4-CP, corroborated by the yellow colour of the solution and the increment in absorption of the corresponding band at 225 nm for the benzene ring. Thus, this effect indicates that 4-CP is being adsorbing via link in the GO by C–Cl linkages, with 29% of the 4-CP ultimately removed (calculated by calibration curves used in each experiment). In the case of GEO in the adsorption test (A-GEO), Figure 6 shows the spectra of the carbon samples, where the band at 280 nm decreases; although, in the same way, it can be seen that the band is not eliminated, this could indicate that the functional groups present in the graphene oxide adsorb the complete molecule in a different way than GO. GEO is more efficient in adsorption and it can be considered that no intermediate groups are generated. In the case of GO, the oxygen-containing functional groups between layers do not interact with the 4-CP. However, in 2 dimensions GEO

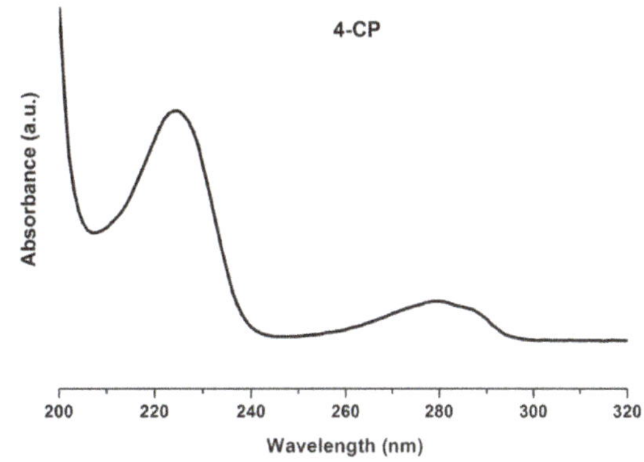

Figure 3 UV-Vis spectrum of 4-chlorophenol (4-CP).

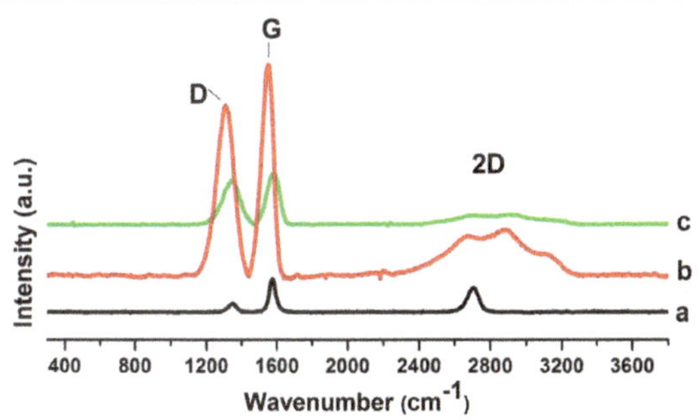

Figure 2 Raman spectra of: graphite (a), graphite oxide (b), graphene oxide (c).

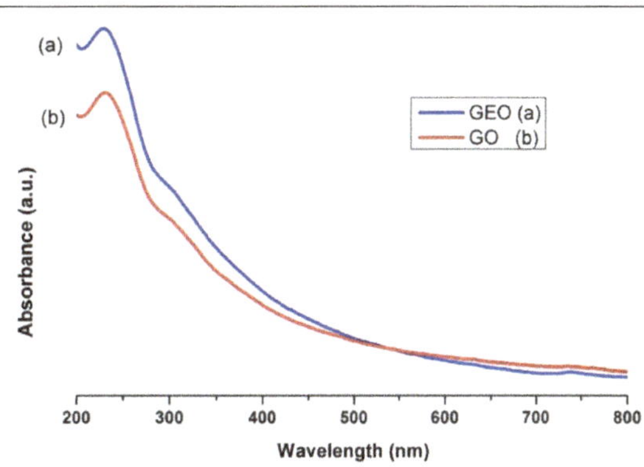

Figure 4 UV-Vis spectra of graphene oxide-GEO (a) and Graphite Oxide-GO (b).

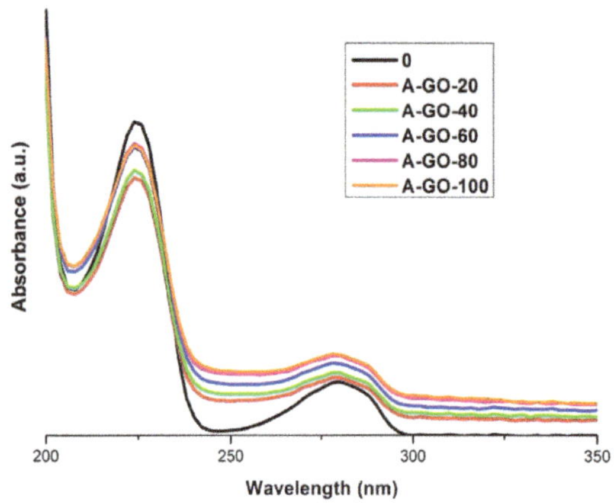

Figure 5 UV-Vis spectra of adsorption test for 4-CP solution using GO as adsorbent. Taking aliquots at 0, 20, 40, 60, 80 and 100 minutes of reaction.

produces better adsorption. The band at 225 nm in the GEO absorption spectra decreases more than in the GO spectra. GEO has a higher capacity as an adsorbent material, with 36% of the removed pollutant (4-CP). These adsorption results are useful when comparing the performance of GO and GEO as photocatalytic materials. Those tests are presented in the next sections.

Photolysis test

Photo dissociation of the C-Cl bond in 4-CP has been reported using UV laser excitation [30]. The photochemical reaction is the first stage in the C-Cl bond cleavage of 4-CP, with subsequent decomposition of the intermediate ion or radical [31]. It is important to consider the band at 280 nm, which defines the generation of intermediate compounds, in the progression of 4-chlorophenol degradation.

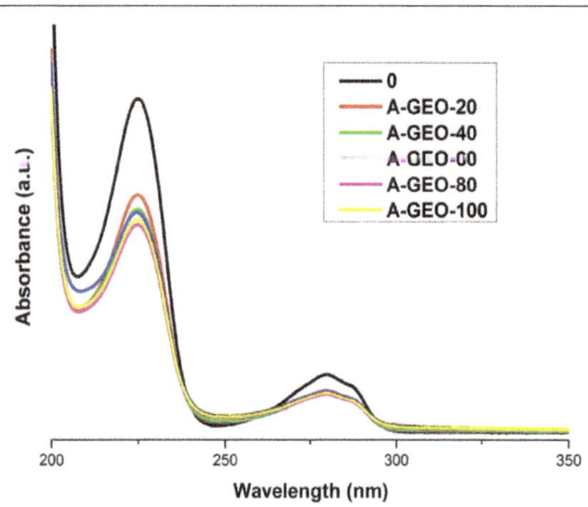

Figure 6 UV-Vis spectra of adsorption test for 4-CP solution using GEO as adsorbent. Taking aliquots at 0, 20, 40, 60, 80 and 100 minutes of reaction.

Figure 7 shows UV-vis spectra obtained from the photolysis test, which corroborate the interaction between the UV light and the water. It is observed, that the characteristic bands in the UV-vis spectrum of 4-CP are affected, and degradation is evident. This indicates that the wavelength emitted by the used lamp is capable of activate OH groups in the solution, causing oxidation due to air trapped in the reactor where the reaction takes place and breaking the C-Cl bonds present in 4-CP. Also, as presumed, the generation of intermediate compounds is apparent, because in the spectrum obtained we can see that the band at 280 nm has a significant shift and increased absorption. It is important to remember, that the by-products in many cases are more toxic, so that the photolysis process alone is not a sufficient method to completely degrade 4-CP.

Photocatalytic activity

Figures 8 and 9 show the UV-vis spectroscopy obtained during the photocatalytic tests using GO (P-GO) and GEO (P-GEO) as photocatalysts, respectively. The degradation of the absorption bands of 4-CP are clearly observed. Comparing the absorption spectra of the two photocatalysts, it can be observed that the degradation of 4-CP is very similar, but after 20 minutes of photocatalysis reaction, the band at 225 nm diminish more considerably with GEO (Figure 9) than with GO (Figure 8). This effect, observed in both spectra, implies that in the GEO the energy caused by UV light at 254 nm is able to quickly activate the movement of electrons, generating OH radicals in the carbon surface, allowing better contaminant degradation. However, in GO, this effect is less significant. It is suggested, that the size (carbon dimension) and disposition of functional groups play an important role in 4-CP degradation. Also, the spectra of Figures 8 and 9 show that the band at 280 nm disappears from all the samples. This

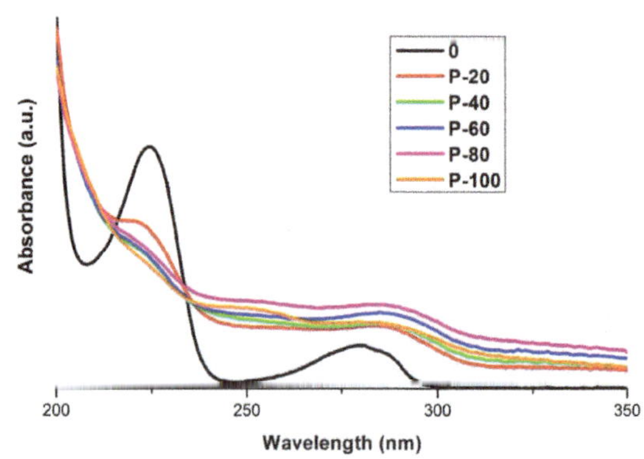

Figure 7 UV-Vis spectra of photolysis test for 4-CP solution. Taking aliquots at 0, 20, 40, 60, 80 and 100 minutes of reaction.

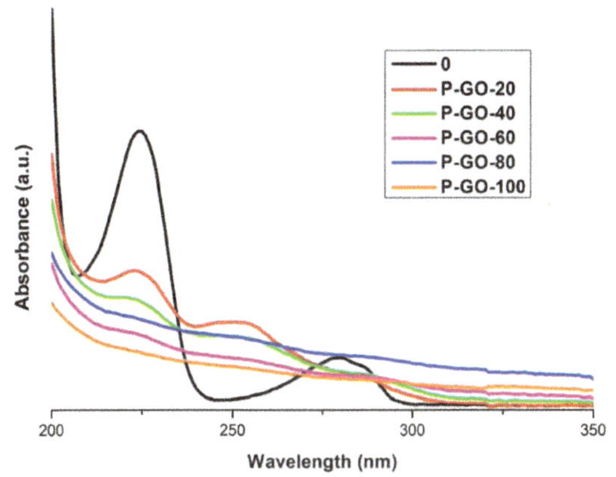

Figure 8 UV-Vis spectra of photocatalytic test for 4-CP solution using GO as photocatalyst. Taking aliquots at 0, 20, 40, 60, 80 and 100 minutes of reaction.

effect is attributed to a minimal generation of intermediate compounds, a good photocatalytic response and the degradation of the pollutant by both materials (GEO, GO). In addition, these results showed that degradation obtained via photocatalysis using GEO is faster than that achieved with GO.

As it was mentioned before, a common characteristic of the presence of by-products generated by chlorophenols, as result of degradation process, is the yellow colouration of the solution, which indicates that intermediates are generated; however, if the final solution is transparent, it indicates that by-products generated are not excessive. Compounds such as hydroquinone and benzoquinone give a yellow colour to the final solution of a treated chlorophenol. Figure 10 shows the final solutions obtained by photolysis (Figure 10a) and photocatalysis

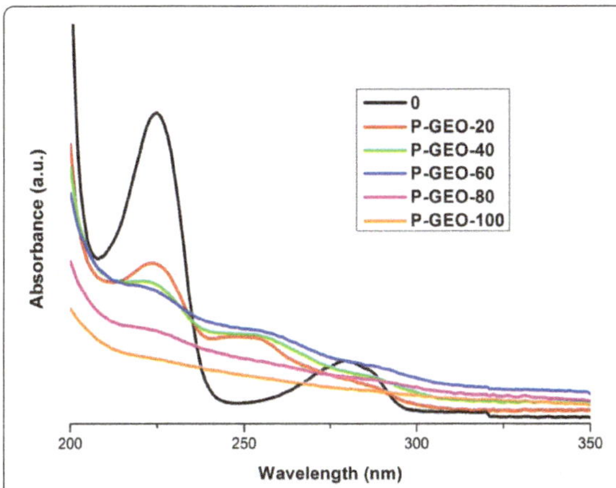

Figure 9 UV-Vis spectra of photolysis test for 4-CP solution using GEO as photocatalyst. Taking aliquots at 0, 20, 40, 60, 80 and 100 minutes of reaction.

with GO (Figure 10b) and GEO (Figure 10c), respectively, it is observed that the yellow colour is prominent after photolysis, but the solution is only slightly yellow after photocatalysis performed with GO and practically colourless in photocatalysis with GEO, indicating that the best process for removing 4-CP is photocatalysis with GEO.

On the other hand, in Figure 11 is observed over 50% of 4-CP degradation at 20 minutes by the sample of GEO; with photocatalysis using GO, the percentage of 4-CP removed is very similar, indicating that both photocatalysis tests have superior removal compared to the photolysis process. Photolysis at 100 minutes reaches 50% of 4-CP degradation in 100 minutes, while GO and GEO achieve 78% and 81% of removal in the photocatalysis test, respectively. The characteristic bands (225 nm and 280 nm) disappear independently in the spectra of GO and GEO in the photocatalyst tests, it is standard to calculate the removal percentage with the band at 225 nm, which is the distinguishing band for this quantification [29-32]. Also in the Figure 11, it can be observed that the degradation process is faster in photocatalysis with GEO than using the other two processes. This can be attributed to structural features of the GEO that have already been mentioned in this paper, as well as in other researches [13,17,18,20,33]; thus, it is presumed that the oxygen-containing functional groups present in the GEO sheets function as oxidizing radicals in the process and accelerate the degradation of 4-CP, influenced by the nanometric size of GEO and carbon material in 2 dimension. The enhanced photocatalytic activity for GEO could be attributed to the ability to capture and transport electrons, and to promote charge separation. It is known that the higher separation efficiency of electron–hole pairs will enhance photocatalytic activity and results in a large number of holes participating in the photocatalytic process [34]. On the other hand, it is important to note that electron-hole recombination could be lower in GEO compared to GO. However, again, the advantages of corrugated sheets of GEO favour the available surface area; this is the great advantage of this graphitic material as a photocatalyst compared to conventional photocatalysts.

Degradation of 4-CP, using TiO_2 as photocatalysts activated in UV zone supported in different materials such as: activated carbon, silica, zeolite have been reported [35,36]. Also graphene has been used as supported of other materials to produce photocatalytic effect in other researches [37]. However, carbon materials without doping, or specifically graphene oxide materials as photocatalysts have not been reported to degrade 4-CP. Other materials activated in UV zone used as photocatalysts in the degradation of 4-CP are enlisted in the Table 1 in comparison with the carbon materials (GO and GEO) analysed in this research. It is observed that GO and

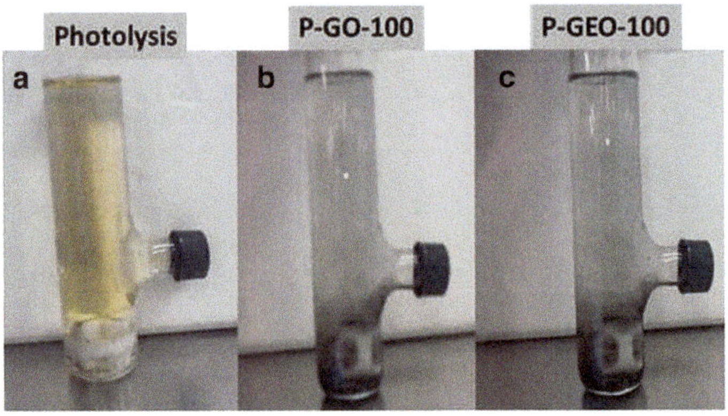

Figure 10 Pictures of the final solutions from the Photolysis. **(a)**, Photocatalytic process with graphite oxide (P-GO) **(b)** and Photocatalytic process with graphene oxide (P-GEO) **(c)**. Differences in colour between yellow and colourless is observed, indicating the generation of by-products (yellow solution).

GEO are efficient materials for the degradation of this organic molecule in comparison with other photocatalysts, either compounds or hybrid materials.

Intermediate degradation of 4-chlorophenol analysed by HPLC

Table 2 shows the concentrations of by-products generated in the reactions of photolysis and photocatalysis as determined by HPLC. In the photocatalytic degradation with both catalysts and with photolysis, aromatic intermediates and carboxylic acids are detected. Three aromatic intermediates are generated during 4-CP degradation, namely benzoquinone, 4-chlorocatechol and hydroquinone. It is known that these three aromatic compounds are commonly the intermediates generated in the TiO_2 photocatalytic degradation of 4-chlorophenol [14,31]. The HPLC analysis was performed on the final sample from each reaction, after 100 min of photolysis or photocatalysis with GO and GEO. Considering the initial 4-CP concentration of 30 ppm, all three processes gave successful degradation. The concentration of benzoquinone in the three cases is the same, 4.8 ppm. The concentration of 4-chlorocatechol is very low, since it is determined to be less than 1 ppm in the final solution in the case of photocatalysis and above 1 ppm in photolysis, although the difference of 0.3 ppm reflects the more effectiveness of the photocatalytic process employed. In the Table 3 it can be observed that the intermediate hydroquinone is present in the samples treated with photolysis and GO as photocatalyst; however, the sample treated with GEO as a photocatalyst does not contain this intermediate. These results indicate that the degradation of 4-CP is more effective with photocatalysis, and GEO is more effective in the degradation process.

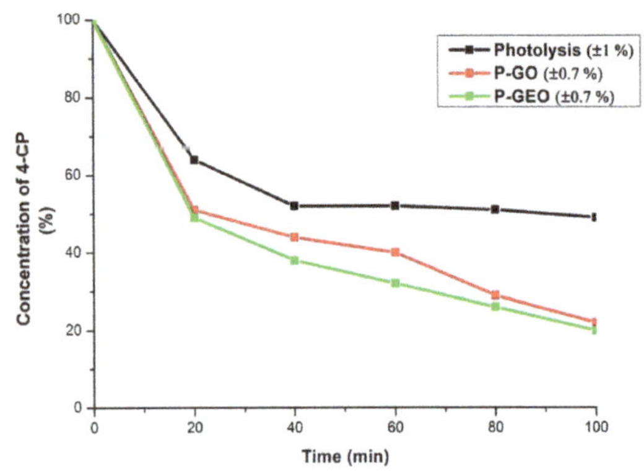

Figure 11 Degradation percentage (%) of concentration of 4-CP solution in the photolysis. Photocatalytic process with graphite oxide (P-GO), and Photocatalytic process with graphene oxide (P-GEO), at 100 min of reaction time. Values of percentage error are included in parentheses.

Table 1 Materials used as photocatalyst to removal 4-CP at different reaction times

Catalysts	Removal of 4-CP (%)	Reaction time (min)	Reference
Ag–TiO2	98	60	[14]
TP2.5 (P-modified TiO2)	78	270	[32]
TiO2-325 mesh	97	180	[35]
MgO TiO2	100	120	[38]
An(P25):Ru(P25)	80	120	[39]
Mesoporuos titania	77-100	180	[16]
ZnO	75	75	[40]
TiO2 synthesized	84	75	[40]
ZnO-TiO2	93	75	[40]
Graphite oxide (GO)	92	100	*This research*
Graphene oxide (GEO)	97	100	*This research*

Table 2 Concentration in ppm of aromatic intermediate compounds generated during the degradation of a 4-CP solution in photolysis and photocatalysis

HPLC	Aromatics compounds (ppm)		
	Benzoquinone	4-chlorocatechol	4-chlorophenol
Photolysis	4.8	1.1	0.7
P-GO	4.8	0.8	0.4
P-GEO	4.8	0.8	0.2

Also, in Table 3, the carboxylic acids generated in the 4-CP degradation process are showed. The highest concentration obtained is oxalic acid, at 5.1 ppm after photolysis; however, in the photocatalytic reactions with GO and GEO the concentration of oxalic acid is 3.8 and 3.3 ppm, respectively. Moreover, in the production of succinic acid the lowest concentration is present in the solution from the photocatalytic process with GEO. The by-products generated in our experimental processes are very similar with those found in other reports, although the amounts or concentrations of these compounds are not reported previously [29,38].

Mineralization of 4-chlorophenol evaluated by COD

The COD test is used to measure the total quantity of oxygen-consuming substances during the complete chemical breakdown of organic substances in water. Figure 12 illustrates the mineralization of 4-CP percentages achieved by photolysis, and photocatalysis with P-GO and P-GEO. It is possible to observe that, the photolysis process eliminates 60% of organic matter, but the photocatalytic processes remove more than 90% (92% and 97% for P-GO and P-GEO, respectively). In addition it is worthy of indicate that the by-products generated in the photocatalytic reaction processes are practically eliminated, in contrast with the photolysis process, because the intermediate compounds are present at the same time in the reactions. Thus, the fact that the photolysis process alone is not enough to degrade 4-CP and the intermediate compounds is corroborated.

Table 3 Concentration in ppm of intermediate compounds (carboxylic acids) generated during the degradation of a 4-CP solution by photolysis and photocatalysis

HPLC	Carboxylic acids (ppm)			
	Oxalic acid	Formic acid	Succinic acid	Hydroquinone
Photolysis	5.1	2.4	3.3	2.7
P-GO	3.8	0.5	2.4	1
P-GEO	3.3	0.5	1.5	0

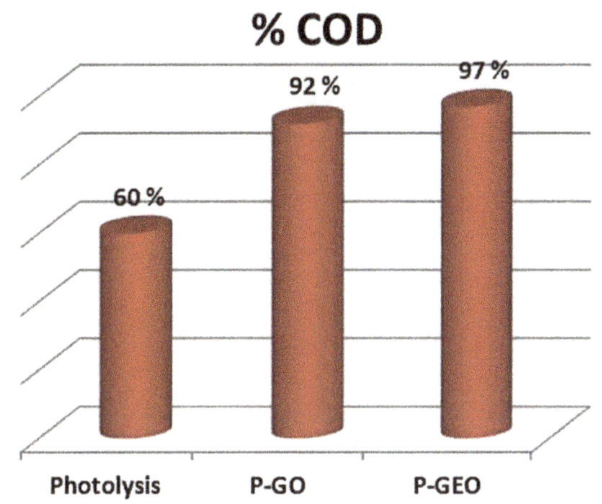

Figure 12 Degradation percentage (%) of organic matter (COD). Determined at the end of the photolysis and photocatalysis tests with GO and GEO (P-GO and P-GEO) in the degradation of 4-CP.

Conclusions

According with the results showed in this research, it can be concluded that GO and GEO are materials with sufficient capacity to degrade 4-CP present in water as contaminant. This fact promises a new trend in the application of carbon nanomaterials without doping as photocatalysts. UV determinations showed that the degradations of 4-CP in 92% and 97% using GO and GEO at 100 min respectively, are superior to photolysis (50%) during the same time, it was found that the reaction mechanism is favourable for 4-CP degradation with carbon oxides. The main by-products generated during the photolysis, and photocatalytic method with GO and GEO, correspond to aromatic compounds and carboxylic acids. In the photocatalytic process the by-products generated were lower in comparison with photolysis process, and better results were obtained with photocatalysis performed with GEO, in this case hydroquinone was not observed at the end of the reaction. Also, mineralization measured by COD indicates that up to 97% of organic matter is removed through photocatalysis using GEO. In addition, research findings show that nanometric size plays an important role in photocatalytic processes, reflected in the fact that GEO show better results in eliminating 4-CP than GO. Materials such as GO and GEO that have recently been used in photocatalytic applications such as water splitting [13,17] are showed in this research as an efficient alternative to eliminate 4-CP in water, using a small quantity of photocatalyst and a short reaction time. Thus, both materials are suggested as effective for their use in advanced oxidation processes. Thus, it can be concluded that, photocatalysis with GO and GEO is simple and effective, because, avoids the use of any oxidizing agent. Furthermore, their lower rates of recombination could be an important factor in this photocatalytic process. Therefore, the highly efficient degradation of 4-CP using GO and GEO as photocatalytic materials could be extended to other organic materials with aromatic rings, and thereby a new line of research in photocatalysis with carbon nanomaterials focused in the treatment of contaminated water, depending on the structural features of these materials, their electronic properties, dimensions and functional groups in the materials' surface.

Competing interests
The authors declare that they have no competing interests.

Authors' contributions
The authors contributed equally to this work. All authors read and approved the final manuscript.

Acknowledgments
The authors are grateful to Mr. Eduardo Martín del Campo for his assistance with the HPLC analyses. Ph.D. student Bustos-Ramírez Karina is thankful to CONACYT for grant no. 218707 and to Centro en Conjunto de Investigación en Quimica Sustentable UAEM-UNAM, especially to Dr. Gabriela Roa for the use of facilities in her laboratory. Also, Velasco-Santos Carlos appreciates the support of TecNM. Article in Memoriam Dr. Adolfo M. Espindola-Gonzalez.

Author details
[1]Centro Conjunto de Investigación en Química Sustentable, UAEM-UNAM. Km.12 de la carretera Toluca-Atlacomulco, San Cayetano 50200, Estado de México, México. [2]División de Estudios de Posgrado e Investigación, Instituto Tecnológico de Querétaro, Av. Tecnológico s/n Esq. M. Escobedo, Col. Centro Histórico, 76000 Querétaro, México. [3]Centro de Física Aplicada y Tecnología Avanzada, Universidad Nacional Autónoma de México, Boulevard Juriquilla 3001, 76230 Querétaro, México.

References
1. Hou Y, Li X, Zhao Q, Chen G. ZnFe2O4 multi-porous microbricks/graphene hybrid photocatalyst: facile synthesis, improved activity and photocatalytic mechanism. Appl Catal B-Environ. 2013;142–143:80–8.
2. Shinde SS, Bhosale CH, Rajpure KY. Photocatalytic oxidation of salicylic acid and 4-chlorophenol in aqueous solutions mediated by modified AlFe2O3 catalyst under sunlight. J Mol Catal A Chem. 2011;347:65–72.
3. Taherian S, Entezari HM, Ghows N. Sono-catalytic degradation and fast mineralization of p-chlorophenol: La0.7Sr0.3MnO3 as a nano-magnetic green catalyst. Ultrason Sonochem. 2013;20:1419–27.
4. Czaplicka M. Sources and transformations of chlorophenols in the natural environment. Sci Total Environ. 2004;322:21–39.
5. Seung Gun C, Yoon Seok C, Jae Woo C, Kyung-Youl B, Seok-Won H, Seung-Taek Y, et al. Photocatalytic degradation of chlorophenols using star block copolymers: removal efficiency by-products and toxicity of catalyst. Chem Eng J. 2013;215–216:921–8.
6. Benitez FJ, Beltran-Heredia J, Acero LJ, Rubio Javier F. Contribution of free radicals to chlorophenol decomposition by several advanced oxidation processes. Chemosphere. 2000;41:1271–7.
7. Olaniran OA, Igbinosa OE. Chlorophenols and other related derivatives of environmental concern: Properties, distribution and microbial degradation processes. Chemosphere. 2001;83:1297–306.
8. Tamer E, Hamid Z, Aly MA, Ossama TE, Bo M, Benoit G. Sequential UV-biological degradation of chlorophenols. Chemosphere. 2006;63:277–84.
9. Chen D, Ray KA. Photocatalytic kinetics of phenol and its derivatives over UV irradiated TiO2. Appl Catal B-Environ. 1999;23:143–57.
10. Pera-Titus M, Garcia-Molina V, Baños AM, Gimenez J, Esplugas S. Degradation of chlorophenols by means of advanced oxidation processes: a general review. Appl Catal B-Environ. 2004;47:219–56.
11. Muruganandham M, Suri RPS, Jafari Sh, Sillanpää M, Gang-Juan L, Wu JJ, et al. Recent Developments in Homogeneous Advanced Oxidation Processes for Water and Wastewater Treatment. Int J Photoenergy. 2014; doi:10.1155/2014/821674.
12. Ahmed S, Rasul MG, Martens WN, Brown R, Hashib MA. Heterogeneous photocatalytic degradation of phenols in wastewater: A review on current status and developments. Desalination. 2010;261:3–18.
13. Te-Fu Y, Jhih-Ming S, Ching C, Ting-Hsiang C, Hsisheng T. Graphite oxide as a photocatalyst for hydrogen production from water. Adv Funct Mat. 2010;20:2255–62.
14. Temel NK, Sökmen M. New catalyst systems for the degradation of chlorophenols. Desalination. 2011;281:209–14.
15. Amadelli R, Samiolo L, Maldotti A, Molinari A, Valigi A, Gazzoli D. Preparation, Characterisation, and Photocatalytic Behaviour of Co-TiO2 with Visible Light Response. Int J Photoenergy. 2008; doi:10.1155/2008/853753.
16. Avilés-García O, Espino-Valencia J, Romero R, Rico- Cerda J L, Natividad R. Oxidation of 4-Chlorophenol by Mesoporous Titania: Effect of Surface Morphological Characteristics. Int J Photoenergy. 2014; doi:10.1155/2014/210751.
17. Te-Fu Y, Jaroslav C, Chih-Yun C, Ching C, Hsishen T. Roles of graphene oxide in photocatalytic wáter splitting. Materials Today. 2013;16:78–84.
18. Te-Fu Y, Fei-Fan C, Chien-Te H, Hsisheng T. Graphite oxide with different oxygenated levels for hydrogen and oxygen production from water under illumination: the band positions of graphite oxide. J Phys Chem C. 2011;115:22587–97.
19. Sheath P, Majumder M. A Comparative Review of Graphene Oxide and Titanium Dioxide as Photocatalysts in Photocatalytic Systems [online]. In: Chemeca 2011: Engineering a Better World: Sydney Hilton Hotel, NSW, Australia, 18-21 September 2011. Barton, A.C.T.: Engineers Australia; 2011. p. 2346–57.
20. Jiang X, Nisar J, Pathak B, Zhao J, Ahuja R. Graphene oxide as a chemically tunable 2-D material for visible-light photocatalyst applications. J Catal. 2013;299:204–9.
21. Lling-Lling T, Wee-Jun O, Siang-Piao C, Mohamed RA. Reduced graphene oxide-TiO2 nanocomposite as a promising visible-light-active photocatalyst for the conversion of carbon dioxide. Nanoscale Res Lett. 2013;8:1–9.
22. Tingshun J, Zhangfeng T, Meiru J, Qian Z, Xiaoqi F, Hengbo Y. Preparation and photocatalytic property of TiO2-graphite oxide intercalated composite. Catal Commun. 2012;28:47–51.
23. Guardia L, Villar-Rodil S, Paredes JI, Rozada R, Martínez-Alonso A, Tascón JMD. UV light exposure of aqueous graphene oxide suspensions to promote their direct reduction, formation of graphene–metal nanoparticle hybrids and dye degradation. Carbon. 2012;50:1014–24.
24. Guoxin H, Bo T. Photocatalytic mechanism of graphene/titanate nanotube photocatalyst under visible-light irradiation. Mater Chem Phys. 2013;138:608–14.
25. Jianfeng S, Na L, Mingxin Y. Supramolecular photocatalyst of RGO-cyclodextrin-TiO2. J Alloy Compd. 2013;580:239–44.
26. Xiangang H, Li M, Jianping W, Qixing Z. Covalently synthesized graphene oxide-aptamer nanosheets for efficient visible-light photocatalysis of nucleic acids and proteins of viruses. Carbon. 2012;50:2772–81.
27. Cortes AD, Sanhueza L, Wrighton K. Removal of 4-chlorophenol using graphene, graphene oxide, and a-doped graphene (A 5 N, B): a computational study. Int J Quantum Chem. 2013;113:1931–9.
28. Bustos-Ramirez K, Martinez-Hernandez AL, Martinez-Barrera G, de Icaza-Herrera M, Castaño MV, Velasco-Santos C. Covalently bonded chitosan on graphene oxide via redox reaction. Materials. 2013;6:911–26.
29. Satuf ML. Photocatalytic degradation of 4-chlorophenol: a kinetic study. Appl Catal B-Environ. 2008;82:37–49.
30. Czaplicka M. Photo-degradation of chlorophenols in aqueous solution. J Hazard Mater-B. 2006;134:45–59.
31. Sharma S, Mukhopadhyay M, Murthy ZVP. Rate parameter estimation for 4-chlorophenol degradation by UV and organic oxidants. J Ind Eng Chem. 2012;18:249–54.
32. Elghniji K, Hentati O, Mlaik N, Mahfoudh A, Ksibi M. Photocatalytic degradation of 4-chlorophenol under P-modified TiO2/UV system: Kinetics, intermediates, phytotoxicity and acute toxicity. J Environ Sci. 2013;24:479–87.
33. Penghui S, Ruijing S, Shaobo Z, Mincong Z, Dengxin L, Shihong X. Supported cobalt oxide on graphene oxide: Highly efficient catalysts for the removal of Orange II from water. J Hazard Mater. 2012;230:331–9.
34. Li K, Xiong J, Chen T, Yan L, Dai Y, Song D, et al. Preparation of graphene/TiO2 composites by nonionic surfactant strategy and their simulated sunlight and visible light photocatalytic activity towards representative aqueous POPs degradation. J Hazard Mater. 2013;250–251:19–28.
35. Pino E, Encinas MV. Photocatalytic degradation of chlorophenols on TiO_2-325 mesh and TiO_2-P25. An extended kinetic study of photodegradation under competitive conditions. J Photochem Photobiol A. 2012;242:20–7.

36. Naeem K, Ouyang F. Influence of supports on photocatalytic degradation of phenol and 4-chlorophenol in aqueous suspensions of titanium dioxide. J Environ Sci. 2013;25(2):399–404.
37. Muhd JN, Bagheri S. Graphene supported heterogeneous catalysts: an overview. Int J Hydrogen Energ. 2015;40:948–79.
38. Gs P, Kambur A. Removal of 4-chlorophenol from wastewater: preparation, characterization and photocatalytic activity of alkaline earth oxide doped TiO2. Appl Catal B-Environ. 2013;129:409–15.
39. Apopei P, Catrinescu C, Teodosiu C, Royer R. Mixed-phase TiO2 photocatalysts: crystalline phase isolation and reconstruction, characterization and photocatalytic activity in the oxidation of4-chlorophenolfromaqueouseffluents. Appl Catal B-Environ. 2014;160–161:374–82.
40. Gs P, Kambur A. Significant enhancement of photocatalytic activity over bifuntional ZnO-TiO2 catalyst for 4-chlorophenol degradation. Chemosphere. 2014;105:152–9.

10

Performance of a single chamber microbial fuel cell at different organic loads and pH values using purified terephthalic acid wastewater

Seyed Kamran Foad Marashi and Hamid-Reza Kariminia*

Abstract

Background: Purified terephthalic acid (PTA) wastewater from a petrochemical complex was utilized as a fuel in the anode of a microbial fuel cell (MFC). Effects of two important parameters including different dilutions of the PTA wastewater and pH on the performance of the MFC were investigated.

Methods: The MFC used was a membrane-less single chamber consisted of a stainless steel mesh as anode electrode and a carbon cloth as cathode electrode. Both power density and current density were calculated based on the projected surface area of the cathode electrode. Power density curve method was used to specify maximum power density and internal resistance of the MFC.

Results: Using 10-times, 4-times and 2-times diluted wastewater as well as the raw wastewater resulted in the maximum power density of 10.5, 43.3, 55.5 and 65.6 mW m^{-2}, respectively. The difference between the power densities at two successive concentrations of the wastewater was considerable in the ohmic resistance zone. It was also observed that voltage vs. initial wastewater concentration follows a Monod-type equation at a specific external resistance in the ohmic zone.

MFC performance at three different pH values (5.5, 7.0 and 8.5) was evaluated. The power generated at pH 8.5 was higher for 40% and 66% than that for pH 7.0 and pH 5.4, respectively.

Conclusions: The best performance of the examined MFC for industrial applications is achievable using the raw wastewater and under alkaline or neutralized condition.

Keywords: Bioelectricity generation, Concentration effect, Microbial fuel cell, Petrochemical wastewater, pH effect, Purified terephthalic acid wastewater

Introduction

Microbial fuel cell (MFC) is a device that converts biochemically released energy from bacterial catalysis of organic and inorganic materials into electrical energy. In MFCs, electricity generation and wastewater treatment can occur, simultaneously. Therefore, MFCs are considered as one of the potential solutions to overcome the crises of energy shortage and environmental pollution. On the other hand, many challenges are still remained for commercialization of MFC technology. Designing a cost-effective system with high power generation is one of the most important challenges. For example, in order to achieve a high performance, expensive materials such as platinum as cathodic catalyst, carbon cloth as cathode or anode electrode, and also a suitable membrane such as nafion are inevitably necessary. Accordingly, more studies are required to find efficient materials both in terms of cost and power production [1].

In recent years, this technology has been studied by many researchers. Generally, different parameters including both operational and designing factors affect the MFC performance. Nature of the substrate, substrate concentration [2], temperature [3], microorganisms' species, alkalinity of anode and cathode chambers [4], external resistance [5] and residence time [6] are among the operational parameters. Anode and cathode material

* Correspondence: kariminia@sharif.ir
Department of Chemical and Petroleum Engineering, Sharif University of Technology, P.O. Box 11155–9465, Azadi Ave., Tehran, Iran

[7], type of membrane [8] and MFC architecture are among the designing parameters.

A wide range of different wastewaters have been examined in MFCs. For instance, domestic wastewater [3,9], landfill leachate [6], coking wastewater [2], confectionery wastewater [8] and cassava mill wastewater [10] can be mentioned. However, wastewaters from petrochemical industries have not been receiving much attention due to complications in their biodegradatiuon. Purified terephthalic acid (PTA) wastewater with a high strength organic content is generated during the production process. PTA is a raw material for manufacturing of many petrochemical products such as polyester textile fibers, polyethylene terephthalate bottles and polyester films. As much as 3–10 m^3 of such a wastewater is usually generated per one ton of PTA as product [11].

In our previous work, we studied the feasibility of utilizing PTA wastewater in a MFC for the first time [12]. In the present work, we investigate the effect of two main characteristics of the wastewater *i.e.* organic load and pH value that significantly influence the power generation. In the present research, we investigated the following issues:

1) Effect of wastewater concentration on power generation
2) Correlation between voltage and wastewater concentration
3) Effect of different pH values on power generation

Materials and methods

Wastewater and microorganisms

PTA wastewater was obtained from the PTA production plant of Shahid Tondgoyan Petrochemical Company, Mahshahr, Iran. It was kept at 4°C until use. This wastewater had the pH of 4.45 and pollution load of 8000 mg COD L^{-1}. It consisted of following components with given concentrations (mg L^{-1}): acetic acid (AA); 9850, benzoic acid (BA); 318, phthalic acid (PA); 400, terephthalic acid (TA); 389, *p*-toluic acid (*p*-Tol); 273, nitrate; 2234.7, and phosphate; 48.

Microorganisms, used in this research were obtained from the sludge of an up-flow anaerobic contact filter existing in the treatment plant of the abovementioned petrochemical company.

MFC assembly and operation

A typical membrane-less single chamber MFC as described previously [13] was used in this study (Figure 1). A stainless steel mesh (30 × 60 cm^2) and a carbon cloth (30% w/w wet proofed (type B-1B, E-TEK) using platinum as catalyst (0.5 mg Pt cm^{-2}) and four diffusion layers with projected area of 0.785 cm^2) were used as anode and cathode electrodes, respectively. Content of the MFC was mixed gently by a magnetic stirrer to reach a uniform concentration.

Analytical methods and calculations

To measure the voltage, a digital multimeter (m58217, Mastech) was used at specific time intervals. Current was calculated based on Ohm's law as $I = V/R$, where, I (mA), V (mV) and R (Ω) stand for current, voltage and external resistance, respectively. To calculate the current density, $i = I/A$ was used where, A (m^2) is the projected surface area of the cathode. Power density (P) was calculated using the following equation: $P = IV/A$. Reactions occurred in the cathode were considered as the basis to calculate current density and power density. To derive the polarization curve, the external resistance was changed from 400 KΩ to 300 Ω and the voltage was measured. Power density curve method was used to obtain maximum power density and internal resistance of the MFC [1]. Chemical oxygen demand (COD), nitrate, phosphate and pH were measured according to standard methods. The concentration of BA, PA, TA, *p*-Tol and AA was measured by a high performance liquid chromatography (HPLC, Agilent Technologies 1200 series, US) under isocratic conditions at the ambient temperature [12].

Results and discussion

Power production at different concentrations of wastewater

Effect of substrates' concentration required for the microbial activity in the anode chamber was investigated. The substrate as fuel was supplied in the following order, consecutively: 10-times diluted wastewater (C_1), 4-times diluted wastewater (C_2), 2-times diluted wastewater (C_3) and the raw wastewater (C_4). Figure 2 shows power density curves of the MFC at different concentrations of the wastewater. Maximum power density was 10.5, 43.3, 55.5 and 65.6 mW m^{-2} for C_1, C_2, C_3 and C_4, respectively. Internal resistance of the MFC was 5.6 kΩ for all concentrations except for C_3 that was equal to 3.2 kΩ.

Maximum power densities of C_3, C_2 and C_1 wastewaters were 84%, 66% and 16% of the maximum power density of the raw wastewater. Therefore, the maximum power density increased when more concentrated wastewater was used.

Current generated in a MFC is limited by two factors: (i) oxidization rate of substrate by bacteria and (ii) rate of electrons transfer to the electrode surface [1]. Substrate oxidation rate depends on the concentration of substrate which is assumed usually as a first order reaction. Therefore, it is expected to observe a higher current and power at higher concentrations. However, other factors such as mass transfer and biofilm layer thickness can suppress power production. The influence of such factors can be studied when the substrate

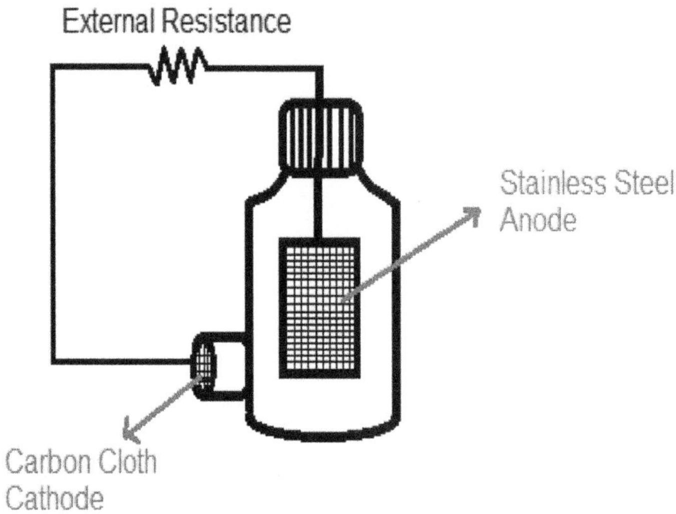

Figure 1 Schematic of the membrane-less single chamber MFC. The reactor was operated in a batch mode at room temperature (22–26°C). The working volume of the MFC was 250 mL. No mediator was added to the anode chamber.

concentration is high enough where oxidation rate is not limited. This observation has been further explained in the next section.

Power differences at different external resistances between two successive concentrations

Increase in the power density due to employing more concentrated wastewater in the anode, was correlated to the external resistance. Figure 3 indicates the difference between the power densities at two successive concentrations of wastewater at definite external resistances. The maximum power density difference was 32.7, 11.9 and 18.3 mW m^{-2} between C_2 - C_1, C_3 - C_2, and C_4 - C_3, respectively.

According to the polarization curve, mass transfer resistance zone and activation loss zone are observable at low external resistances and large external resistances, respectively. All three curves follow the same trend. The power density difference was negligible at higher external resistances while the cell operated in the activation loss zone. This is the same at very low external resistances when the cell operates in the mass transfer zone.

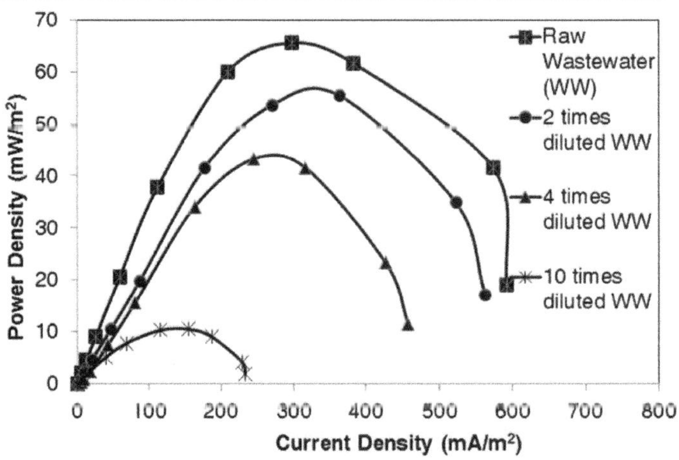

Figure 2 Power density curves at different concentration of PTA wastewater. Power density curves were obtained when the voltage reached to a stable value.

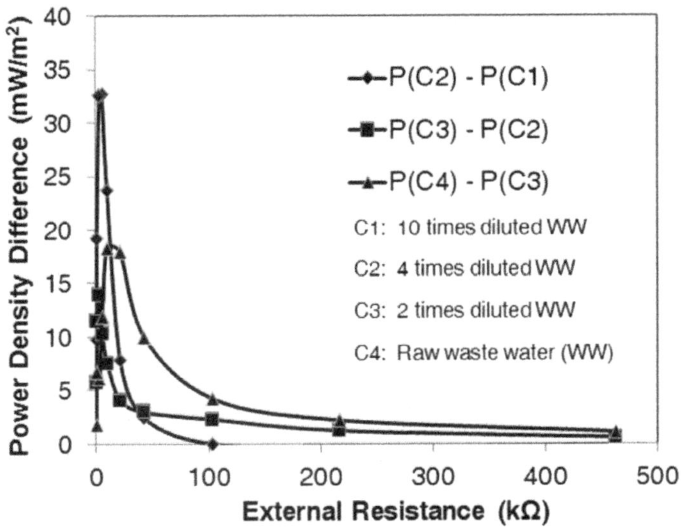

Figure 3 Power density difference between two successive concentrations of wastewater at different external resistances. Maximum power density was 10.5, 43.3, 55.5 and 65.6 mW m^{-2} for C_1, C_2, C_3 and C_4, respectively. The wastewater had the concentration of 8000 mg COD L^{-1}.

This shows that the substrate concentration has a minor effect in these zones. Accordingly, if a MFC is working with an external resistance which leads to operating, either in the activation loss zone or the mass transfer zone, increasing the substrate concentration would not have a significant effect on its performance. In contrary, a considerable power density difference was observed in the ohmic resistance zone. The power density difference reached a maximum value at an external resistance equal or close to the internal resistance of the MFC. Therefore, according to these observations, the maximum power production is reachable when the external resistance is near the internal resistance. Besides, the major positive effect of concentration increase is visible when the MFC works in the ohmic zone.

Generated voltage versus wastewater concentration in ohmic zone

In this section, the behavior of MFC in the ohmic zone is explored. The generated voltage at different concentration of wastewater for a certain external resistance (in the Ohmic zone) is exhibited in Figure 4. It was observed that the correlation between voltage and concentration is so that at higher concentrations, a little increase occurs in the voltage generation. For example, there is no significant difference between the produced,

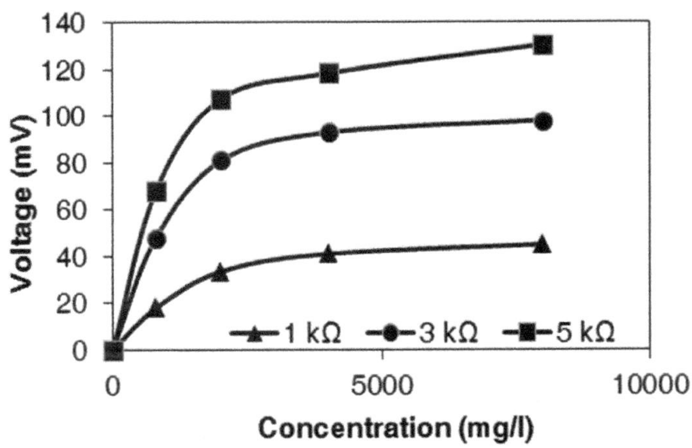

Figure 4 Generated voltage at different concentration of wastewater. Monod-type behavior of voltage against concentration.

Table 1 Calculated constants of Eq. 1 for different external resistances

R_{ext} (kΩ)	V_{max} (mV)	K_s (mg L^{-1})
1	45.0	1148.4
3	98.0	48.0
5	130.5	614.7

voltage when C3 or C4 was applied. One can say that the concentration increase effect is limited even in the ohmic zone which might be as a result of concentration inhibition that halts bacteria metabolism.

The voltages vs. concentration curves suggest a Monod-type equation as follows:

$$V = V_{\max}\frac{s}{K_s + s} \tag{1}$$

where, V (mV) and V_{max} (mV) stand for voltage and maximum voltage, respectively; S (mg L^{-1}) represents COD of substrates and K_s (mg L^{-1}) is the half-saturation constant. V_{max} and K_s were calculated for each curve as presented in Table 1.

Maximum achievable voltage versus external resistance follows a linear equation:

$$V_{\max} = 21.375\ R_{ext} + 27 \tag{2}$$

Not to be neglected that the above equation is valid only when the MFC operates at the ohmic zone.

Power production at different pH values

pH has a significant effect on the activity of bacteria in terms of removal efficiency and energy production. In order to study the influence of pH, the MFC was fed with 10- times diluted wastewater at three different pH values including 8.5, 7.0 and 5.4, periodically. These pH values were selected based on the optimal range of the pH reported for methane-producing bacteria. It has been observed that these bacteria are active in the pH range of 6.3-7.8 [14]. Presence of methane producers is very possible in our system. The power density curves for different pH values are shown in Figure 5. It was observed that the maximum power density was 12.5, 7.5 and 4.3 mW m^{-2} for the pH values of 8.5, 7.0 and 5.4, respectively.

In general, the higher the pH value, the higher the power density. The produced power at pH 8.5 was higher for 40% and 66% than that for pH 7.0 and pH 5.4, respectively. This observation is consistent with other previous studies [15,16].

Apparently, acidogenic bacteria are active in pH 5.5. Under this condition, hydrogen production would be the dominant mechanism which overcomes the pollutants degradation and a decreased removal rate is expected compared to the neutral or alkaline conditions [14]. Due to the low removal rate, fewer electrons are released and the power production is lowered, consequently. At pH 7.0, methane gas production is the dominant metabolic pathway. This would lead to a less number of released electrons that can contribute in electricity generation and a lower power density is observed, eventually. The increase in power density production at

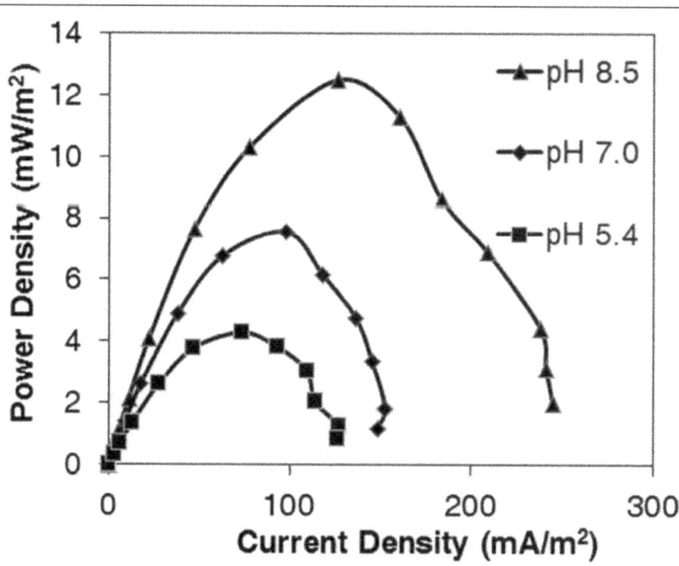

Figure 5 Power density curves at different pH values for 10-times diluted wastewater.

pH 8.5 might be due to the lower activity of methanogenic and acidogenic bacteria. As a result, the electrons released in the oxidation process of the substrates would contribute significantly in electricity generation. However, further studies are required to clarify the occurrence of these phenomena, more precisely.

It can be concluded from the trend of power production at different pH values that alkaline condition provides a favorable situation for the growth of electrogenic bacteria. Previous studies have shown that the electrochemical interaction of bacteria significantly increases under alkaline conditions [15,16], which ultimately leads to a higher power production.

Conclusion

The main purpose of this research was to provide more information and insight into the MFC operation that can pave the way towards practical utilization of MFC technology for the application of real wastewater. Bioelectricity generation using purified terephthalic acid wastewater from a petrochemical plant was successfully conducted in a single chamber microbial fuel cell with a stainless steel mesh as anode electrode.

The influence of wastewater concentration on the MFC performance showed that using the raw wastewater with the concentration of 8000 mg COD L^{-1} results in the highest power density (65.6 mW m^{-2}). Our observations suggest that the best performance is achievable when the MFC operates at the ohmic zone and has an external resistance which is equal to the internal resistance of the cell.

The voltage against different initial concentrations of the wastewater in the ohmic zone followed a Monod-type equation. This observation implies that the concentration increase has a positive effect of electricity generation but it cannot exceed a maximum value.

Performance of the MFC at different pH values was investigated and the highest power density was observed under alkaline condition (pH 8.5) due to inactivation of acidogenic and methanogenic bacteria in favor of more activity for electrogenic bacteria.

Competing interests

The authors declare that they have no competing interests.

Authors' contributions

SKFM carried out the experiments, analyzed the data and drafted the manuscript. HRK designed the study, participated in data analysis and reviewed the article. Both authors read and approved the final manuscript.

Acknowledgements

Authors wish to thank the research office of Sharif University of Technology for the financial support.

References

1. Logan BE. Microbial Fuel Cells. NewJersy: John Wiley & Sons; 2008.
2. Huang L, Yang X, Quan X, Chen J, Yang F. A microbial fuel cell–electro-oxidation system for coking wastewater treatment and bioelectricity generation. J Chem Technol Biot. 2010;85:621–7.
3. Ahn Y, Logan BE. Effectiveness of domestic wastewater treatment using microbial fuel cells at ambient and mesophilic temperatures. Bioresour Technol. 2010;101:469–75.
4. Zhuang L, Zhou S, Li Y, Yuan Y. Enhanced performance of air-cathode two-chamber microbial fuel cells with high-pH anode and low-pH cathode. Bioresour Technol. 2010;101:3514–9.
5. Lyon DY, Buret F, Vogel TM, Monier J-M. Is resistance futile? Changing external resistance does not improve microbial fuel cell performance. Bioelectrochemistry. 2010;78:2–7.
6. Greenman J, Gálvez A, Giusti L, Ieropoulos I. Electricity from landfill leachate using microbial fuel cells: Comparison with a biological aerated filter. Enzyme Microb Technol. 2009;44:112–9.
7. Popov AL, Kim JR, Dinsdale RM, Esteves SR, Guwy AJ. The effect of physico-chemically immobilized methylene blue and neutral red on the anode of microbial fuel cell. Biotechnol Bioprocess Eng. 2012;17:361–70.
8. Sun J, Hu Y, Bi Z, Cao Y. Improved performance of air-cathode single-chamber microbial fuel cell for wastewater treatment using microfiltration membranes and multiple sludge inoculation. J Power Sources. 2009;187:471–9.
9. Rodrigo MA, Ca˜nizares P, Lobato J, Paz CSa R, Linares JJ. Production of electricity from the treatment of urban waste water using a microbial fuel cell. J Power Sources. 2007;169:198–204.
10. Kaewkannetra P, Chiwes W, Chiu TY. Treatment of cassava mill wastewater and production of electricity through microbial fuel cell technology. Fuel. 2011;90:2746–50.
11. Joung JY, Lee HW, Choi H, Lee MW, Park JM. Influences of organic loading disturbances on the performance of anaerobic filter process to treat purified terephthalic acid wastewater. Bioresour Technol. 2009;100:2457–61.
12. Marashi SKF, Kariminia H-R, Savizi ISP. Bimodal electricity generation and aromatic compounds removal from purified terephthalic acid plant wastewater in a microbial fuel cell. Biotechnol Lett. 2013;35:197–203.
13. Marashi, SKF, Kariminia, H-R, Electricity generation from petrochemical wastewater using a membrane-less single chamber microbial fuel cell. Renewable Energy and Distributed Generation (ICREDG), 2012 Second Iranian Conference on (pp. 23-27). IEEE. doi:10.1109/ICREDG.2012.6190462
14. Zhu G-F, Wua P, Wei Q-S, Lin J-y, Gao Y-L, Liu H-N. Biohydrogen production from purified terephthalic acid (PTA) processing wastewater by anaerobic fermentation using mixed microbial communities. Int J Hydrogen Energy. 2010;35:8350–6.
15. Behera M, Jana PS, More TT, Ghangrekar MM. Rice mill wastewater treatment in microbial fuel cells fabricated using proton exchange membrane and earthen pot at different pH. Bioelectrochemistry. 2010;79:228–33.
16. Yuan Y, Zhao B, Zhou S, Zhong S, Zhuang L. Electrocatalytic activity of anodic biofilm responses to pH changes in microbial fuel cells. Bioresour Technol. 2011;102:6887–91.

Bacteriological quality of effluent submitted consecutively to a macrofiltration and ultraviolet light systems in the Tunisian conditions

Brahmi Mounaouer* and Hassen Abdennaceur

Abstract

This paper deals with the study of bacteriological quality of effluents that have undergone consecutively different macrofiltration system (pressure sand filter or disc filter used as a secondary treatment) and UV254 irradiation process (used as a tertiary treatment). These two successive systems of treatment were evaluated to determine their possible application as commonly alternatives to the conventional system of wastewater treatment and disinfection before wastewater reuse. They both combined systems of wastewater treatment released effluent of excellent bacteriological quality, with almost total absence of feacal coliforms, of *E. coli* and of *P. aeruginosa*). However, if the bacteriological quality of the effluent remained constant in the case of macrofiltration system (disc filter or pressure sand filter); the UV disinfection process showed to deeply depend on the quality of effluent, particularly with regard to UV transmittance. The daily bacteriological monitoring of the secondary effluent at the exit of the pressure sand filter by UV reactor and by using a dose of 96 mJ/cm^2, corresponding to an exposure of 16 min, showed an average rate of inactivation of around 3 U-Log, for feacal coliforms, *E. coli* and *P. aeruginosa*, respectively. Therefore, the average bacterial concentration remaining in the water at the exit of the UV reactor is less than 1000 cfu/100 ml for feacal coliform and *E. coli*. For *P. aeruginosa*, the remaining number is less than 100 bacteria/100 ml. These two last values coincide substantially with the range recommended by several standardized international guidelines. Therefore, numerous authors reported that *P. aeruginosa* is very resistant to UV irradiation compared to the other bacterial indicators. In contrast, our study revealed that feacal coliforms and *E. coli* were more UV light resistant than *P. aeruginosa*. This finding could be explained by the fact that *E. coli* and feacal coliform forms aggregates in the treated effluent, while *P. aeruginosa* exists either as discrete cells or as cell pairs.

Keywords: Wastewater, Macrofiltration systems, UV reactor, Disinfection, Reuse

Introduction

Reclaim and reuse of urban wastewater have increased in recent years, largely due to lack of water resources and inadequate economic structures, particularly in arid and semi-arid countries [1]. However, the contamination of urban wastewater with pathogenic microorganisms represents a significant risk to public health due to the possible presence of human enteric pathogens. Poor water quality can cause diseases such as gastroenteritis (characterized by vomiting, diarrhea and abdominal pain or fever) or upper respiratory (ear, nose, and throat) infections to exposed swimmers. Highly polluted water can occasionally cause serious diseases such as typhoid fever, dysentery, hepatitis, and cholera [2]. In this sense, to reduce the inconvenience, reuse must be safe to avoid damaging public health and the environment [1].

The usage of treated effluent is considered as an important alternative water resource. Although conventional treatment processes, i.e. primary treatment, disc filter and pressure sand filter (macrofiltration systems) well-known as secondary treatment and recognized to remove up to 99% of microorganisms, were not sufficient to achieve requirements for wastewater discharge and wastewater reuse [3]. The disinfection treatment is considered as the primary mechanism for the inactivation or destruction of pathogenic organisms, to prevent the spread of waterborne disease to downstream users and the environment.

* Correspondence: brahmounaouer@yahoo.fr
Water Research and Technology Center, University Tunis Cartage, Borj Cédria Science and Technology Park, P.O. Box 273, Soliman 8020, Tunisia

Nevertheless, the UV water disinfection efficiency depends on several factors: mainly an adequate contact time and UV intensity to guarantee a sufficient microbial pathogen lessening, In fact, the UV dose is defined as the product of intensity and exposure time [4].

To date, chlorination is the most widely employed ways to inactivate pathogenic microorganisms in waster and it is considered as the primary process for preventing water-borne infectious diseases throughout the world [1]. However, several studies have reported that the effectiveness of the process is reduced by the water turbidity conditioned by suspended solids and nitrogen compounds such as ammonia and nitrite concentrations [3]. Furthermore, the use of chlorine in wastewater disinfection allowed rising the rate of undesirable and hazardous by-products in both to humans and the environment [5].

On the other side and at the present, UV irradiation is considered as one of the best alternatives to water, chemical disinfection, especially the water chlorination [6]. UV radiations act by interacting damagingly with nucleic acids and other vital cellular components, such as proteins and lipids [7]. The knowledge gained in this field demonstrates that the use of UV for disinfection is a fast, efficient, safe and cost-effective process [6]. The UV irradiation process has been practiced for many years in several countries to disinfect the water [7]. However, microbes have evolved repair mechanisms and can reactivate, once their DNA is partially denatured. Because of their broad wavelength spectrum, the UV lamps, only low or medium pressure, are capable of destroying cellular components such as proteins and enzymes, and so avoiding this reactivation. This fact is justified when the water to be treated must fulfil certain conditions to obtain an optimal effect of UV irradiation. This high failure can be avoided and solved by the application at the beginning of the process, a filtration system such as disc filter or pressure sand filter that assured a good lessening of the main physicochemical parameters such as water turbidity, hardness, suspended solids, iron, manganese, humic acids. All these last parameters were well known as important disruptive factors of UV disinfection [8].

In view of these considerations, the objective of the present work was to evaluate the bacteriological quality (based on the parameters E. *coli*, feacal coliforms and *Pseudomonas aeruginosa*) of different effluents from two macrofiltration processes (pressure sand filter and disc filter) were signaled by lots of authors as pre-treatment. In contrast, in our study, these systems worn as secondary treatment and ultraviolet technologies used as tertiary treatment, in order to ameliorate the physico-chemical and bacteriological characteristics of wastewater disinfection. On the other hand, the aim of this report was to determine the UV irradiation dosages required to destroy E. *coli*, feacal coliforms and *Pseudomonas aeruginosa* in a secondary effluent of a wastewater treatment plant (WWTP), for irrigation purposes.

Materials and methods

Scheme of the experimental system

Two forms of treatment were set in operation. The first form, constituted with a primary settling and followed by the two macrofiltration processes (pressure sand filter and disc filter), was established in parallel as shown in Figure 1. The second form consisted to a UV treatment process organized as an UV254 monolamp reactor. The pressure sand filter (i) was filled with silica sand of 1 and 3 mm in diameter, and an effective size of 0.8 mm and of high uniformity ($Cu = 1.6$). The filtration system operated with an upward flow at 5.0 m^3/m^2 h of hydraulic loading. Cleaning phase was manual, according to load loss (maximum 10 m) and using filtrated water mixed with 10 mg/l of chlorine. Disc filter (ii) was the Arkal battery 3 SKS 2" with an average pore size of 22 µm and an effective surface of 0.282 m^2, operating at a flow of 4 m^3/h. The system was equipped with an automatic cleaning system according to load loss (maximum 20 m), and using filtrated water. A cleaning phase using chlorinated (20 mg/l) filtrated water was carried out daily. Feeding of each process was carried out through independent pumping, using water from secondary settling effluent with a range of temperatures between 25 and 30°C.

Experimental methodology and analytical determinations

All the systems worked continuously, and samples of water were held daily. Feacal coliforms, *E. coli*, and *P. aeruginosa* were analyzed as bacteriological parameters in all water samples. For bacteriological analysis, water samples were collected in sterile glass bottles of 1 liter and often analyzed within the 48 h after sampling. The presence of thermo tolerant coliforms (feacal coliforms) and *E. coli* was studied using the membrane filtration procedure UNE-EN ISO 9308–1 [9]. Samples (100 ml or dilution) were filtered through Millipore sterile membrane filters (0.45 µm) placed in Petri dishes containing a double layer of tryptic-bile-agar and tryptic-soy agar (Difco), respectively. Petri dishes were incubated at 37 ± 0.5°C for 4 h and then at 44.5 ± 0.5°C for 18 h. The colony count was calculated from the arithmetic mean of three membrane filter counts.

All feacal coliforms isolated in the samples were taxonomically identified, using the bacterial identification system API 20 E (Bio Meriwux, Marcy d'Etoile, France).

Although conventional wastewater treatments are known to remove up to 90–99% of some microorganisms, they may not be sufficiently rigorous and reused effluents

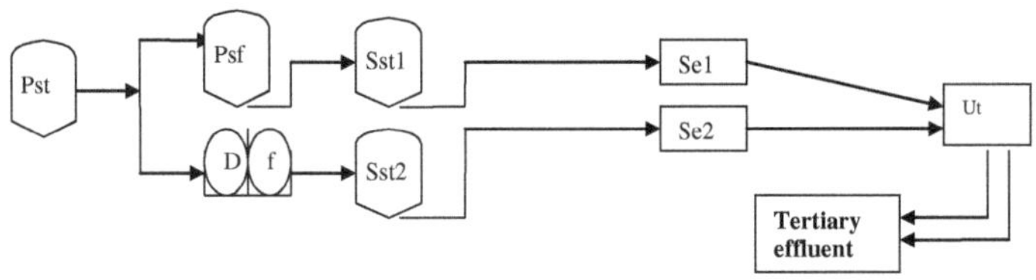

Figure 1 Pst: Primary settling tank (Influent); Psf: Pressure sand filter; Df: Disc filter; Sst1 and Sst2: Secondary settling tanks; Se1 and Se2: Secondary effluent; Ut: UV treatment.

may still contain high concentrations of pathogenic microorganisms.

A most-probable-number (MPN) technique was evaluated to detect and enumerate *Pseudomonas aeruginosa* as opportunist pathogen in water and wastewater. Asparagine and acetamid broths were employed as presumptive and confirmatory media in MPN tests, as described in the 13th edition of *Standard Methods for the Examination of Water and Wastewater* [10].

Sample collection and UV light treatments

Water samples from the secondary effluent at the exit of the disc filter or pressure sand filter were collected in sterile glass bottles for bacteriological analyses. The UV radiation was applied using a low-pressure UVC lamp of 7 Watts (400 mm length and 85 mm diameter), with a flow-rate from 500 to 1100 l/h, and a wavelength of 254 nm. The UV irradiation system was designed to be used with 1000 ml of volume sample and irradiation exposure times of 4, 8, 12, and 16 minutes. According to these conditions, the UV doses provided by the system were of 24, 48, 72, and 96 mJ/cm^2, respectively. In addition, among the objective of this study was to apply later the selected UV dose for each strain detected in water at the exit of the UV system in order to treat and compare their rates and kinetics of inactivation.

Results and discussions

Bacteriological determinations

UV radiation is the most commonly used alternative to chlorination, with thousands of installations throughout the world, containing open channels equipped with low or medium pressure mercury discharge lamps. The success of this system can be attributed to high disinfection efficiency for viruses and bacteria, a minimum of disinfection by-products and low cost [11]. As previously indicated, the efficacy of UV disinfection of freshwater and wastewater depends on the UV dose. Because the biological UV dose response data are generally log-normally distributed, these data are log-transformed [12]. Figure 2 showed the UV inactivation rates for *E. coli*, feacal coliforms and *P. aeruginosa* (log reduction) obtained, respectively, at the exit of the disc filter or pressure sand filter and at different dose UV. From these inactivation curves, the wide divergence noted for *E. coli* could be explained by the poor quality of the influent or the clogging phenomena occurred in the pressure sand filter. For the other two types of bacteria, feacal coliforms and *P. aeruginosa,* we did not remarked any meaningful differences. For this reason, it appeared useful to adopt the secondary effluent at the exit of the pressure sand filter as a model water sample during the bacteriological investigations of the three-selected case of bacteria, and its use in the daily bacteriological monitoring.

Figure 3 showed the log reduction tendency for feacal coliforms, *P. aeruginosa* and *E. coli* obtained, respectively, at the exit of the disc filter or of the pressure sand filter and at different dose UV. It could be observed that *P. aeruginosa* was more UV resistant than feacal coliforms and *E. coli,* because a higher log reduction of around 4 and 3 U-Log for *E. coli* and feacal coliforms, respectively occurred after an exposure of 16 minutes that corresponds to a dose of 96 mJ.cm^{-2}.

All inactivation processes showed a linear portion whatever the dose, despite the lowest correlation coefficient determined for some adjustments. In this sense, to improve some of these adjustments, a linear regression was calculated only with data obtained at lower UV doses (<48 mJ/cm^2). The correlation coefficient slightly improved for *E. coli*, from 0.87 up to 0.92, for feacal coliforms, from 0.55 up to 0.58, and for *P. aeruginosa*, from 0.97 up to 0.98, leading to a better fitting (results not shown). Authors [13] have identified a gradual flattening at higher UV doses, often attributed to existence of particulate solid matter in the effluent. This point is consistent with the need to apply UV radiations to wastewater previously clarified, in order to avoid the undesirable effect of solid particles [1].

Figure 4 showed the UV inactivation rates for the three types of bacteria studied, at the exit of the coupled composed systems, disc filter and UV irradiation or pressure sand filter and UV irradiation, respectively, and by using changed UV doses. The percentage of removal, for the three types of bacteria, increased as the UV time exposure increased. In this sense, effluent samples

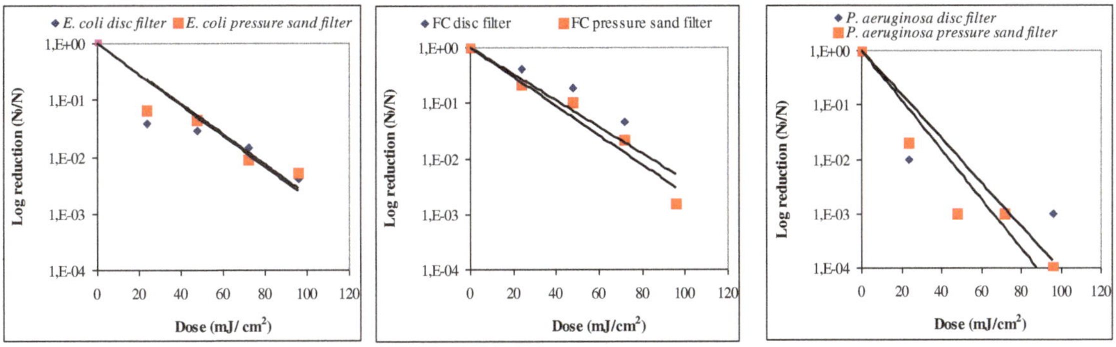

Figure 2 Comparison of UV inactivation rates for *E. coli*, feacal coliform and *P. aeruginosa* (log reduction) at the exit of the disc filter and of the pressure sand filter, respectively. y: Reduction = N/N_0 with *N*; Number of micro-organisms at the instant *T*; N_0; Number of micro-organisms at the instant *T* = 0; Dose (mJ/cm^2) = X = *It* = UV Intensity (mW. cm^{-2}). Time of contact(s).

irradiated during 4 min finalized a reduction of *E. coli*, of feacal coliforms and of *P. aeruginosa*, of around of 97, 94 and 78%, respectively. The removal percentages slightly improved for *E. coli*, from 94 up to 96%, for feacal coliforms, from 78 up to 80%, and for *P. aeruginosa*, from 97 up to 99%, and during 8 min of UV exposure. After 12 or 16 min, almost all of *E. coli*, feacal coliforms and *P. aeruginosa* appeared totally inactivated with any colonies on the growth media. The effect of UV dose on bacteria inactivation is shown in Figure 4. Data fitted to an exponential equation, with correlation coefficients of (0.78; 0.89) for *E. coli*, (0.96; 0.96) for feacal coliforms and (0.57; 0.66) for *P. aeruginosa*, for water samples taken at the exit of the filter disc and pressure San filter, respectively.

Figure 5 showed the inactivation rate of *E. coli*, of feacal coliform and of *P. aeruginosa* for effluent concentration for the disc filter, pressure sand filter and UV reactor, as a function of the *E. coli*, feacal coliform and *P. aeruginosa* concentration in the influent, as linear adjustment. Except for minor cases, a more or less acceptable correlation coefficient was observed in the other cases, showing that concentration of *E. coli*, feacal coliform and *P. aeruginosa* in the effluent is highly dependent with the bacterial concentration of influent. Similar slopes are observed for the majority of cases, with the macrofiltration systems (disc filter and pressure sand filter) presenting similar removal performance for *E. coli*, feacal coliform and *P. aeruginosa*. If the disc filter and the pressure sand filter presented an average retention of *E. coli*, feacal coliform and *P. aeruginosa*, with results of (64 and 62%), (50 and 50%) and (62.5 and 62.5%), respectively; UV represented high elimination percentages for *E. coli* with 87%, for feacal coliforms with 84% and *P. aeruginosa* with 87.5%, for 8 min UV exposure. After 12 or 16 min of UV exposure, *E. coli*, feacal coliforms and *P. aeruginosa* appeared almost all inactivated since any colonies looked in the agar growth media.

This ultraviolet dose is much higher than that reported by Gómez *et al.* [1], who indicated a value over 35 mJ/cm^2 for total removal ($N/N_0 = 0$) of feacal coliforms, of *E. coli*

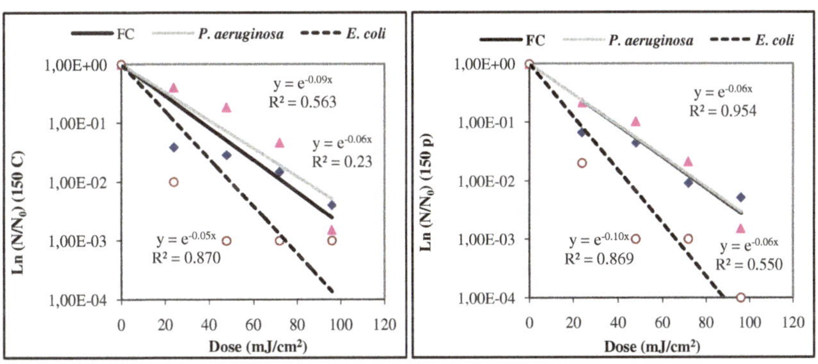

Figure 3 UV inactivation rates for *E. coli*, feacal coliform and *P. aeruginosa* (log reduction). y: Reduction = N/N_0 with *N*; Number of micro-organisms at the instant *T*; N_0; Number of micro-organisms at the instant *T* = 0; Dose (mJ/cm^2) = X = *It* = UV Intensity (mW. cm^{-2}). Time of contact(s).

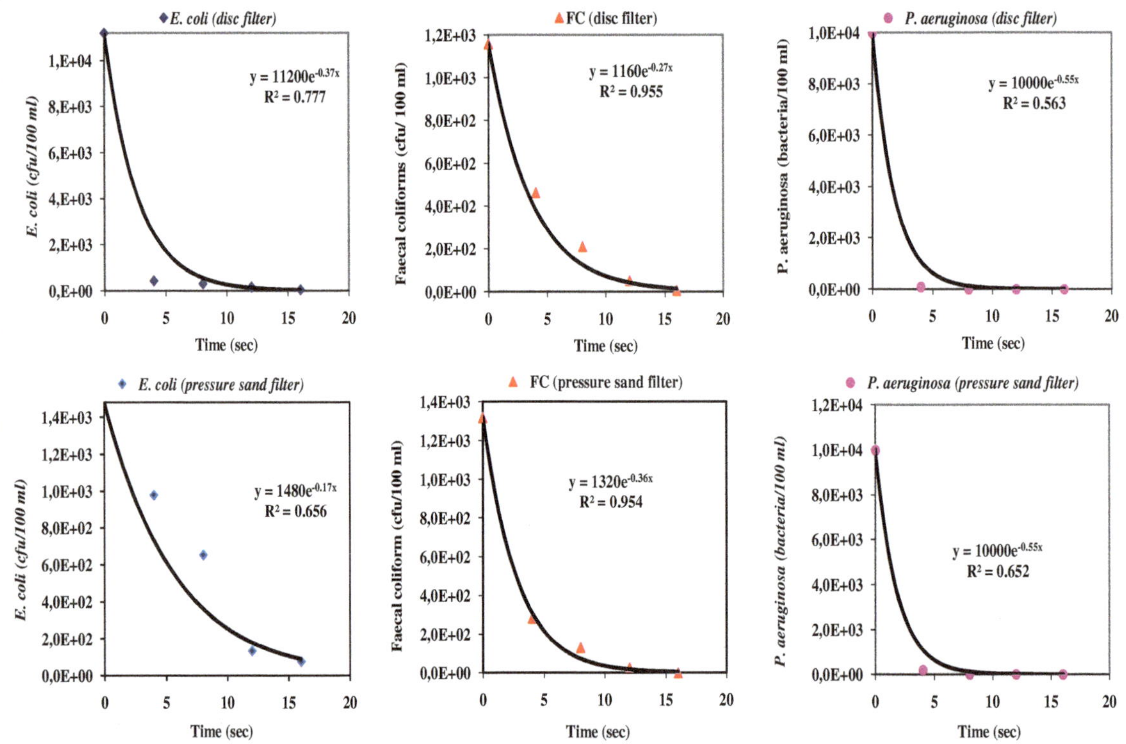

Figure 4 **UV inactivation rates for *E. coli*, feacal coliform and *P. aeruginosa* obtained on the exit of the disc filter or pressure sand filter, respectively, and at exposure different times UV.**

and of coliphages from municipal wastewater. These authors used a physicochemical coagulation-flocculation water clarification before UV disinfection, allowing an excellent effluents quality with a water turbidity of around 99%. In this study and basing on the Figure 3, a dose of 35 mJ/cm^2 would remove on average around 37.23 up 50% of *E. coli*, 27 up 37.5% of feacal coliform and 10 up 17.5% of *P. aeruginosa*. These results are also consistent with those reported by Andreakis *et al.* [13] who found a significant increase in the UV disinfection efficiency in sand-filtered water samples. The UV disinfection of water always required secondary effluents of the large degree of clarity by reducing suspended solids content and turbidity. Sharrer *et al.* [14] reported a complete inactivation of coliform bacteria at approximately 77 mJ/cm^2, in a recirculating salmonid culture system. However, these authors indicated that for total heterotrophic bacteria lessening in the recirculating system required in excess a UV dosage of 1800 mJ/cm^2 to achieve a quite 2 Log10 reduction. In our experiments, UV doses have been always less than 100 mJ/cm^2. According to Figure 4, a reduction down to 1000 cfu/100 ml for *E. coli and* feacal coliform and 1000 bacteria/100 ml for *P. aeruginosa* would need a dose over than 24 mJ/cm^2. An almost total elimination of these indicator bacteria from water would be achieved with doses over than 96 mJ/cm^2.

Bacteriological validation of Macrofiltration systems

Conventional wastewater treatments are traditionally known to remove up to 90–99% of microbes that may not be sufficiently rigorous for safe wastewater quality and for agronomic reuse. In this study, we preconized and considered useful a daily bacteriological monitoring of three customary microbes, namely feacal coliform, *E. coli* and *P. aeruginosa.*

All the bacterial counts were carried out for influent and effluent delivered by the two filtration systems under study. Figure 6 compared the result of the bacteriological concentrations (*E. coli*, feacal coliform and *P. aeruginosa*) in the influent and effluent of the disc filter and of the pressure sand filter, respectively, and indicated a substantial bacterial count reduction between the entrance and the exit of the two-macrofiltration systems. Therefore, these observed results demonstrated that both macrofiltration systems showed a high removal capacity that exceeds in some cases 4 U-Log for *E. coli and P. aeruginosa;* but for feacal coliform, their inactivation rate is around 3 U-Log.

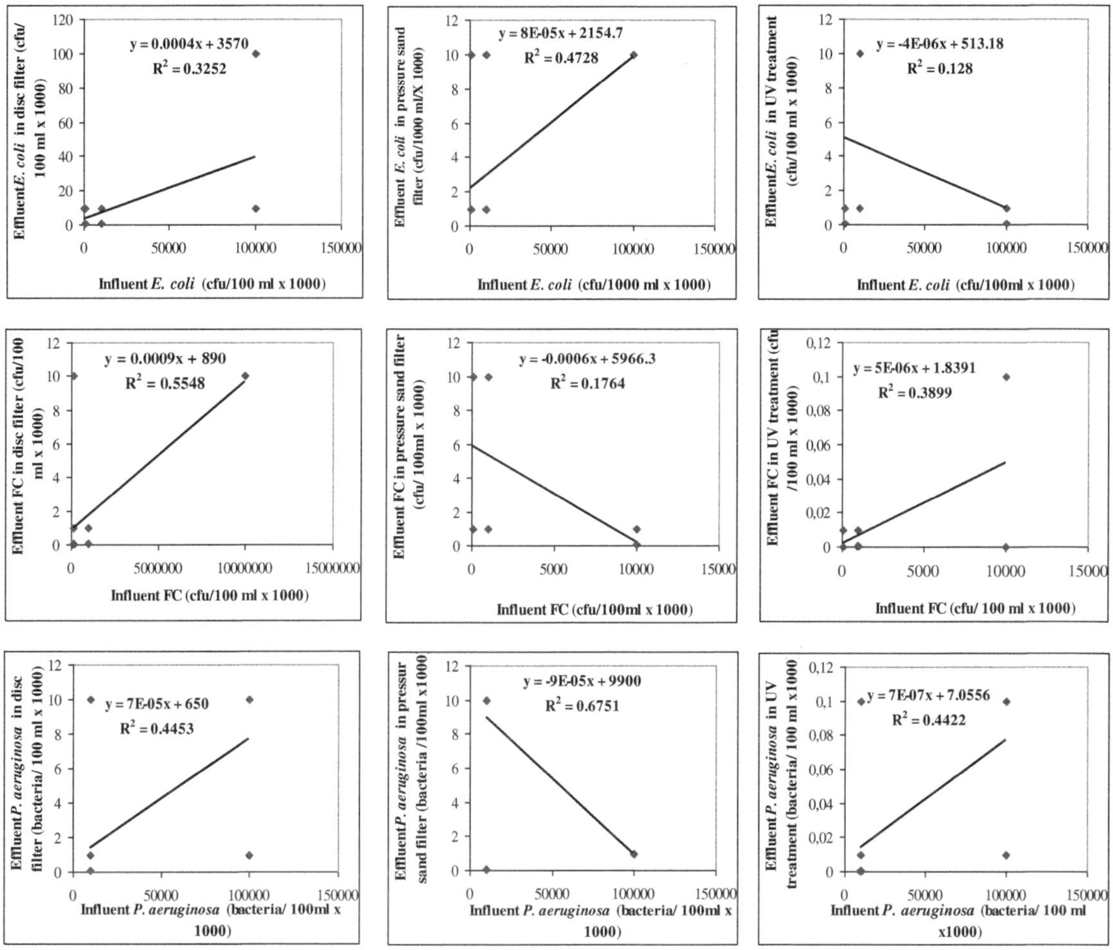

Figure 5 Effluent concentrations of *E. coli*, feacal coliform (FC) and *P. aeruginosa* in disc filter and pressure sand filter as a function of influent concentration of *E. coli*, feacal coliform (FC) and *P. aeruginosa* (Linear adjustment).

As stated in Figure 6, no important differences were found between counts in the effluent from disc filter and pressure sand filter for *E. coli*, feacal coliform and *P. aeruginosa*. Similarly, no significant differences were found between removal percentages of the two-macrofiltration systems. Despite this apparently good typical removal of 4 U-Log, it appeared on average for a N_o of 10^7 CFU/ml in the case of *E. coli* for example, the remaining number of 10^3 bacteria/ml could cause serious health and environmental problems.

Bacteriological validation of UV reactor

Because the UV dose delivered by the UV irradiation system is a complex function of many variables, the UV reactor validation was used to demonstrate the disinfection efficacy and performance. In addition, the disinfection performance of a UV system is determined based on a series of bacteriological challenges that are conducted on a pilot-scale UV reactor. During a validation, a UV system is evaluated under various operational conditions that may include flow rate, **UVT**, lamp power (or relative lamp output), water level, and number of operational lamps. During each test condition, water samples were collected at the entrance and the exit of the UV reactor to quantify the rate of inactivation of a target challenge bacteria associated to the specific operational conditions.

In this study and as shown in Figure 2, the UV bacterial inactivation rates for *E. coli*, feacal coliforms and *P. aeruginosa* (log reduction) obtained, respectively, at the exit of the disc filter or pressure sand filter and at different dose UV, did not noticed any meaningful differences. It seems useful to adopt the secondary effluent at the exit of the pressure sand filter as a basic sample for the bacteriological tests adopted for the three selected bacteria studied, and for future daily monitoring of the UV reactor.

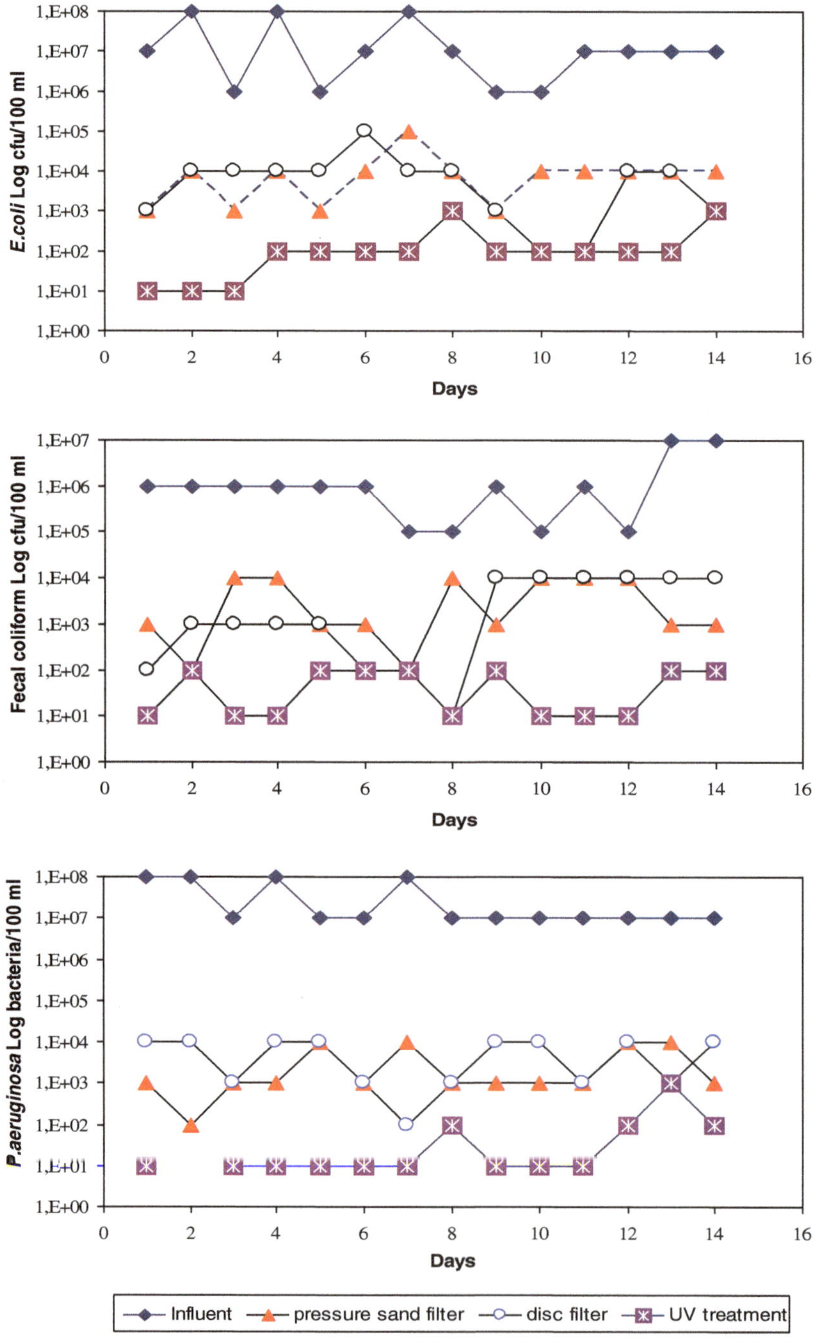

Figure 6 ***E. coli*, feacal coliform counts (Log cfu/100 ml) and *P. aeruginosa* counts (Log bacteria/100 ml) in influent from disc filter, pressure sand filter and UV treatment.** y: Reduction = N/N_0 with N; Number of micro-organisms at the instant T; N_0; Number of micro-organisms at the instant $T = 0$.

On the other hand, several standardized international guidelines stipulate that the reuse of wastewater requires a decrease in the number of indicator bacteria of about 3 U-log. However, the complexity of the present processes and requirements for environmental safety, microbiology, public health and even industry, need the introduction of advanced monitoring systems, based on monitoring methodologies built on the principle of analytical redundancy. For this reason, a second standard requires a reduction ratio of the number of *P. aeruginosa* of the order of 4 U-log for treated wastewater reuse [8].

As stated in Figures 4 and 5, an almost total elimination of these indicators would be achieved with UV doses over than 96 mJ/cm^2, corresponding to a UV exposure of 16 min. Therefore, the use of a dose of 96 mJ/cm^2 is necessary, firstly to calculate the performance of the UV reactor, and secondly to obtain water free from pathogen bacteria and meets the standards recommended by several standardized international guidelines.

In this sense, the daily bacteriological monitoring of the performance of the UV reactor by the use of a dose of 96 mJ/cm^2, corresponding to an exposure of 16 min and considering the wastewater at the outlet of pressure sand filter, was finalized and shown in Figure 6. It appeared from the Figure 6 that the rate of inactivation, on average achieved, were around 3 U-Log for *E. coli,* feacal coliforms and *P. aeruginosa*, respectively. Therefore, the average concentration remaining in the treated wastewater at the exit of the UV reactor is less than a 1000 cfu/100 ml of *E. coli and* feacal coliform. For *P. aeruginosa*, this rate left is less than 100 bacteria/100 ml. These values agree with the range recommended by several standardized international guidelines [8].

Also from the Figure 6, it seemed obvious that *E. coli* and feacal coliforms were signaled as the UV most resistant bacteria; contrariwise, *P. aeruginosa* was found to be the most sensitive. In dissimilarity, authors [15] and [16] reported that *P. aeruginosa* is very resistant to UV irradiation, which contradicts the above observations that *P. aeruginosa* is more sensitive to UV irradiation than *E. coli* and feacal coliform. This discrepancy in the results could be explained by the fact that *E. coli* and feacal coliform forms aggregates in the treated effluent, while *P. aeruginosa* exists either as discrete cells or as cell pairs. This self-aggregation ability provides an advantage to the *E. coli* and feacal coliform over *P. aeruginosa*, since the concentration of suspended matter and the state of aggregation could shelter and protect the bacteria from UV radiation in the effluent [17].

Conclusions

Results for the three categories of bacteria studied lead to similar conclusions. The macrofiltration systems (a disc filter or sand pressure filter) allowed a good removal of feacal bacteria (*E. coli,* feacal coliforms) and of *P. aeruginosa*, although the bacterial counts indicated the continued appearance and presence of these bacteria in the treated effluent. This result pleads and advocates the need for a disinfection treatment.

On the other side, the quality of wastewater acquired from a disc filter or sand pressure was dependent on the initial quality of the effluent to be treated. Consequently, bacteriological quality of water treated by macrofiltration will vary depending on the type of effluent used. It was consequently not possible to guarantee a specific quality of the effluents issued from the treatment of macrofiltration, and this fact affected some parameters such as turbidity and suspended solids [18]. Moreover, variability in the quality of macrofiltration effluent might affect seriously the performance of disinfection technologies, for instance UV radiation, which required a specific quality of effluent to be treated, particularly with regard to parameters such as turbidity, UV transmittance and suspended solids content [3,18].

A further consideration is that the UV radiation dose to be applied was affected by high variations in the number of microbes needful for elimination, as observed in the effluents under study, and this fact renders the treatment yet more problematic. This type of drawback may be avoided by employing an optimized good UV reactor as disinfection systems.

The use of a UV dose of 96 mJ/cm^2, corresponding to an exposure of 16 min of the secondary effluent at the exit of pressure sand filter, released water of a very good bacteriological quality and meets the standards recommended by several standardized international guidelines.

The greatest obstacle to these technologies remains to be the economic cost of both installations and system operation. In recent years, however, costs have fallen considerably due to technological improvements, particularly with regard to the macrofiltration systems and modular design. Macrofiltration systems followed by a UV reactor may now be seen as a practicable option for a large number of applications inside in the field of operations of wastewater reutilization [19].

Competing interests
The authors declare that they have no competing interests.

Authors' contributions
All authors designed the study, analyzed the data, drafted the manuscript, critically reviewed the article. All authors read and approved the final manuscript.

Acknowledgements
This study is financially supported by the European Union in the framework of Avicenna Project n° 93AVI054. We express great appreciation to all the team of the laboratory of Water Treatment and Recycling, Borj-Cedria techno-park that contributed to apprehend this work, particularly Mr Aissaoui, Mr Hachemi and Ms Mabrouki for their help.

References
1. Gómez A, Plaza F, Garralón G, Pérez J, Gómez MA. A comparative study of tertiary wastewater treatment by physico-chemical-UV process and macrofiltration-ultrafiltration technologies. Desal. 2007;202:369–76.

2. Deepali, Namita J. Problems of ground water contamination with focus on waterborne diseases, causes and prevention. App Sci Report. 2014;1(1):34–41.
3. Lazarova V, Savoye P, Janex MI, Blatchley III ER, Pommepuy M. Advanced wastewater disinfection technologies: state of the art and perspectives. Wat Sci Tech. 1999;40:203–13.
4. Chun-Chieh T, Chih-Shan L. Inactivation of virus-containing aerosols by ultraviolet germicidal irradiation. Aerosol Sci Technol. 2005;39(12):1136–42. doi:10.1080/02786820500428575.
5. Naddeo V, Cesaro A, Mantzavinos D, Fatta-Kassinos D, Belgiorno V. Water and wastewater disinfection by ultrasound irradiation -a critical review. Global Nest J. 2014;16(3):561–77.
6. Meiting GUO, Hongying HU, Wenjun LIU. Preliminary investigation on safety of post-UV disinfection of wastewater: bio-stability in laboratory-scale simulated reuse water pipelines. Int J Sci Technol Desalt Wat Purify. 2009;239:22–8.
7. USEPA: Voluntary National Guidelines for Management of Onsite and Clustered (Decentralized) Wastewater Treatment Systems. EPA, 832-B-03-001, 2003b.
8. Mounaouer B, Noureddine HB, Helmi H, Abdennaceur H. Modeling of secondary treated wastewater disinfection by UV irradiation: effects of suspended solids content. J Environ Sci. 2010;22:1218–24.
9. Asociación Española de Normalización y Certificación (AENOR). UNE 77079:2002. Water quality, Technical specifications of general character for continuous conductivity measurements instruments in industrial wastes. AENOR, 10 pages, November 2010.
10. Anita KH, Robert LA. Evaluation of a most probable-number technique for the enumeration of *Pseudomonas aeruginosa*. Appl Microbiol. 1975;30:596–601.
11. Marcucci M, Ciabatti I, Matteucci A, Vernaglione G. Membrane technologies applied to textile wastewater treatment. Ann N Y Acad Sci. 2003;984:53–64.
12. Tchobanoglous G, Burton FL, Stensel HD. Disinfection processes (Chapter 12). Wastewater engineering: treatment and reuse. Boston: McGraw-Hill; 2003. p. 1217–344.
13. Andreakis A, Mamais D, Christoulas D, Kabylafka S. Ultraviolet disinfection of secondary and tertiary effluent in the Mediterranean region. Wat Sci Tech. 1999;40:253–60.
14. Sharrer MJ, Summerfelt ST, Bullock GL, Gleason LE, Taeuber J. Inactivation of bacteria using ultraviolet irradiation in a recirculating salmonid culture system. Aquacult Eng. 2005;33:135–49.
15. Hassen A, Mahrouk M, Ouzari H, Cherif M, Boudabous A, Damelincourt JJ. UV disinfection of treated wastewater in a large-scale pilot plant and inactivation of selected bacteria in a laboratory UV device. Bioresour Technol. 2000;74:141–50.
16. Liberti L, Notarnicola M, Boghetich G, Lopez A. Advanced treatment for municipal wastewater reuse in agriculture. UV disinfection: bacteria inactivation. J Water Supply Res Technol AQUA. 2001;50:275–85.
17. Yael G, Eran F. UV disinfection of RBC-treated light grey water effluent: Kinetics, survival and regrowth of selected microorganisms. Water Res. 2008;42:1043–50.
18. Zhou H, Smith DW. Advanced technologies in water and wastewater treatment. J Environ Eng Sci. 2002;1:247–64.
19. Nicolaisen B. Developments in membrane technology for water treatment. Desal. 2002;153:355–60.

12

Enzymatic catalysis treatment method of meat industry wastewater using lacasse

K. Thirugnanasambandham and V. Sivakumar*

Abstract

Background: The process of meat industry produces in a large amount of wastewater that contains high levels of colour and chemical oxygen demand (COD). So they must be pretreated before their discharge into the ecological system.

Methods: In this paper, enzymatic catalysis (EC) was adopted to treat the meat wastewater.

Results: Box-Behnken design (BBD), an experimental design for response surface methodology (RSM), was used to create a set of 29 experimental runs needed for optimizing of the operating conditions. Quadratic regression models with estimated coefficients were developed to describe the colour and COD removals.

Conclusions: The experimental results show that EC could effectively reduce colour (95 %) and COD (86 %) at the optimum conditions of enzyme dose of 110 U/L, incubation time of 100 min, pH of 7 and temperature of 40 °C. RSM could be effectively adopted to optimize the operating multifactors in complex EC process.

Keywords: Enzymatic catalysis, Meat wastewater, Colour removal, Box-Behnken design, Model development, Process optimization

Background

Meat industry is the world's fastest growing sector due to ever increasing demand of its products. Meat processing industries use approximately 62 Mm^3/y of fresh water from river and canals [1]. Meat-based products have become an essential part of every day's life and its high demand has resulted in a large quantity of meat wastewater that needs to be treated in order to protect the environment and aquatic life [2]. The meat wastewater contains higher level of suspended solids and organic materials and these particles cannot be easily separated. For these reasons many attempts have been made to treat meat wastewater using conventional wastewater treatment methods [3]. There are a number of processes available for wastewater treatment such as chemical coagulation, electro coagulation, sedimentation precipitation, ozonation, evaporation, membrane filtration, adsorption, ion-exchange, oxidation and advanced oxidation, incineration, bio-degradation and biological treatment. Moreover, these conventional methods are also usually expensive and treatment efficiency is inadequate because of the large variability of the composition of meat wastewater [4].

Enzymatic catalysis using Laccase (EC) is one of the most practiced technologies extensively used on industrial scale wastewater treatment. Meanwhile, the EC treatment can be simpler and more efficient than the traditional physical-chemical treatments [5]. Laccase has the advantages over conventional chemical or microbial catalysts such as biodegradable, high level of catalytic efficiency, high degree of specificity, easily removed from contaminated streams, easily standardized in commercial preparations and absence of side-reactions [6]. These characteristics provide substantial process energy savings and reduced manufacturing costs. Nevertheless, the efficiency of EC process depends on several factors including the enzyme dose, incubation time, pH and temperature. The optimization of these factors may significantly increase the process efficiency [7].

Traditionally, optimization in wastewater treatment has been carried out by monitoring the manipulate of one factor at a time on an experimental response. While only one factor is changed, others are kept at a constant level. This optimization technique is called one-variable-at-a-time. Its major disadvantage is that it does not include the

* Correspondence: drvsivakumar@yahoo.com
Department of Chemical Engineering, AC Tech Campus, Anna University, Chennai 600 025TN, India

combined effects among the variables studied [8]. As a consequence, this technique does not depict the complete effects of the parameter on the response. Another disadvantage of the one-factor optimization is the increase in the number of experiments necessary to conduct the research, which leads to an increase of time, man power and operating cost [9]. In order to overcome this problem, nowadays optimization has been carried out by using multivariate statistic techniques. Among the most relevant multivariate techniques used in optimization process wastewater treatment is response surface methodology (RSM). RSM is a collection of mathematical and statistical techniques based on the fit of a polynomial equation to the experimental data, which must portray the performance of a data set with the aim of making statistical previsions. It can be well applied when a response or a set of responses of interest are influenced by several variables. In RSM, Box–Behnken design (BBD) is a statistical technique for designing experiments, building models, evaluating the effects of several factors, and searching optimum conditions for desirable responses. The main advantage of this method of other statistical experimental design methods is the reduced number of experiments trials needed to evaluate multiple parameters and their interactions [10].

An extensive literature survey shows that there is lack of knowledge regarding the optimization of EC paramerets to treat meat industry wastewater using RSM. Hence, in this present study an attempt was made to investigate the optimize the EC process parameters such as enzyme dose, incubation time, pH and temperature on the colour and COD removals from meat industry wastewater using four factors three level Box-Behnken design (BBD). The results will obtain shows the treatment efficiency of EC and its possibility to implement in industrial scale level by analyzing removal efficiencies of colour and COD.

Methods

Raw materials and chemicals

Wastewater used in this study was collected from a meat industry located in Erode, Tamilnadu, India and its physico-chemical properties was determined and shown in Table 1. In this present study, analytical reagent grade chemicals such as citrate hydrogen phosphate and disodium hydrogen phosphate were used to adjust the pH, which was supplied by Merck chemicals, Chennai. Commercial laccase formulation (DeniLite® IIS; 120 U/g) produced from genetically modified *Aspergillus oryzae* was purchased from local suppliers, Erode.

Table 1 Characteristics of meat industry wastewater

Characteristics	Value	Permissible values
pH	5.6	6–8
Colour (CU_s(Pt-Co)	223	5
COD (mg/l)	1658	500
Turbidity (NTU)	1568	10
Conductivity (mS/cm)	1.78	0.5
BOD (mg/l)	1685	100

Experimental setup

Jar-test experiments were conducted on meat wastewaters in different graduated glass beakers. A Jar containing 100 ml wastewater were tested at pH range between 5 and 9 with different enzyme dose (80–120 U/L). After each enzyme dose, sample was rapidly mixed at 180 rpm during 3 min and incubated (60–120 min) with different temperature (25–45 °C). After treatment, samples were centrifuged at 10,000 rpm for 15 min and analyzed for colour intensity and for COD.

Analytical method

Colour, COD, and conductivity were determined according to the standard methods described by American Public Health Association (APHA). Colour measurement was determined with standard dilution multiple method and by comparing absorbance to a calibration curve. Colour removal was determined by monitoring the decrease in the absorbance peak at the maximum wavelength (678 nm). Double beam UV-visible spectrophotometer (Shimadzu UV 1650 PC) was used in all experiments. COD was determined by open reflux method. The sample was refluxed in an acidic medium with a known excess of potassium dichromate ($K_2Cr_2O_7$) and the remaining dichromate was titrated with ferrous ammonium sulphate (FAS). Turbidity was measured using a turbidity meter (ELIKO, 456) in accordance with standard method via display. The conductivity was determined by conductivity meter (Lil120) via digital display. The removal efficiency (RE) of colur and COD was calculated by using the following equation [11]

$$RE = \left(\frac{c_0 - c_e}{c_0}\right) \times 100 \tag{1}$$

where, c_0 and c_e is the initial and final concentrations of colour and COD respectively.

Stastical experimental design

In this present study, Box-Behnken response surface experimental design (BBD) with four factors at three levels was used to optimize and investigate the influence of process variables such as enzyme dose (A), incubation time (B), pH (C) and temperature (D) on enzymatic catalysis process to reduce colour (Y_1) and COD (Y_2) from from meat wastewater. Process variables and their ranges (Table 2) were determined based on the preliminary

Table 2 Process variables and their ranges

Process variables	Level		
	−1	0	1
A (U/L)	80	100	120
B (min)	60	90	120
C	5	7	9
D (°C)	25	35	45

studies. Preliminary studies were carried out using Placket Burmann (PB) design. BBD design consists of 29 experiments with five centre points were designed and the data was analyzed by multiple regression analysis (Sequential sum of squares and model summary statistics) in order to study the ability of various mathematical models to express the enzymatic catalysis process [12].

All the statistical analyses were done with the help of Stat ease Design Expert 8.0.7.1 statistical software package (Stat-Ease Inc., Minneapolis, USA). Then the adequacy of mathematical model was analysed with various statistical analysis such as determination coefficient (R^2), adjusted determination of coefficient (R_a^2), predicted determination of coefficient (R_p^2), adequate precision (AP) and coefficient of variation (CV). Then, the individual and combined effects of process parameters on responses were studied by constructing three dimensional (3D) response surface plots from polynomial model [13].

Optimization of process variables for maximum colour and COD was carried out by derringer's desired function methodology. In this present study, goals of the operating conditions were selected as in a range and the responses goal was selected as maximize. After optimization, adequacy of the model equation for predicting the optimum response value was validated [14]. Triplicate verification experiments were performed under the optimal conditions and the average value of the experiments was compared with the predicted value of the developed model equation [15].

Results and discussions

In this present study, removal of colour and COD from meat industry wastewater are investigated using enzymatic catalysis method under various operating conditions such as enzyme dose, incubation time, pH and temperature. Four factors with three levels BBD response surface design (BBD) is used to examine and optimize the process variables. BBD experimental design consists of 29 experiments are carried out and the results are shown in Table 3.

Table 3 BBD experimental design with results

Run	A	B	C	D	Y_1	Y_2
1	120	90	5	35	85.48	69.83
2	100	90	7	35	89.42	79.85
3	120	120	7	35	89.36	79.79
4	120	90	7	25	84.42	74.85
5	80	90	5	35	59.42	55.85
6	120	90	7	45	90.36	80.79
7	100	60	5	35	42.12	39.55
8	100	60	7	25	34.56	24.99
9	100	90	7	35	89.42	79.85
10	80	90	7	25	49.72	48.15
11	100	90	9	25	55.66	50.09
12	100	60	9	35	44.74	39.17
13	100	90	5	45	73.03	67.46
14	100	90	9	45	96.42	86.85
15	100	120	9	35	74.42	67.85
16	80	60	7	35	31.94	22.37
17	100	90	7	35	89.42	79.85
18	100	120	7	45	73.36	63.79
19	100	90	7	35	89.42	79.85
20	100	90	7	35	89.42	79.85
21	80	120	7	35	63.92	50.35
22	100	60	7	45	64.46	54.89
23	100	120	5	35	77.72	66.15
24	100	90	5	25	68.72	59.15
25	80	90	7	45	74.42	66.85
26	120	90	9	35	77.42	67.85
27	120	60	7	35	59.38	49.73
28	100	120	7	25	75.42	65.85
29	80	90	9	35	64.42	50.85

Mathematical modelling

In order to select the suitable mathematical among various models such as linear, interactive, quadratic and cubic, BBD experimental data is analyzed by multi regression analysis namely the sequential model sum of squares and model summary statistics (Table 4). The obtained results indicates that, linear and interactive (2FI) models were exhibited lower R^2, adjusted R^2, predicted R^2 and also having high *p*-values, when compared with quadratic model. Cubic model was found to be aliased [16]. Therefore the quadratic model ischosen to describe the effects of process variables on the enzymatic catalysis treatment method. Mean while, second-order polynomial equation has been developed by fitting coefficient of process variables (individual and interactive) to the

Table 4 Sequential model sum of squares and model summary statistics for responses

Source	Sum of squares	DF	Mean Square	*F* Value	Prob > F	Remarks
Sequential model sum of squares for colour removal (%)						
Mean	146045.62	1	146045.62			
Linear	5202.01	4	1300.50	8.09	0.0003	
2FI	727.90	6	121.32	0.70	0.6548	
Quadratic	2998.97	4	749.74	80.57	<0.0001	Suggested
Cubic	129.16	8	16.15	86.70	<0.0001	Aliased
Residual	1.12	6	0.19			
Total	155104.77	29	5348.44			
Sequential model sum of squares for COD removal (%)						
Mean	112009.84	1	112009.84			
Linear	4385.38	4	1096.35	7.14	0.0006	
2FI	502.86	6	83.81	0.47	0.8186	
Quadratic	2934.27	4	733.57	41.62	<0.0001	Suggested
Cubic	191.83	8	23.98	2.62	0.1285	Aliased
Residual	54.92	6	9.15			
Total	120079.10	29	4140.66			
Source	Std.Dev.	R^2	Adjusted R^2	Predicted R^2	PRESS	Remarks
Model summary statistics for colour removal (%)						
Linear	12.6773	0.5742	0.5033	0.4257	5202.4046	
2FI	13.1851	0.6546	0.4627	0.2757	6561.6618	
Quadratic	3.0505	0.9856	0.9712	0.9172	750.4137	Suggested
Cubic	0.4315	0.9999	0.9994	0.9822	160.8996	Aliased
Model summary statistics for COD removal (%)						
Linear	12.3893	0.5435	0.4674	0.3806	4998.1928	
2FI	13.2937	0.6058	0.3868	0.1276	7039.4443	
Quadratic	4.1982	0.9694	0.9388	0.8239	1421.2648	Suggested
Cubic	3.0253	0.9932	0.9682	0.0200	7907.8116	Aliased

generalized quadratic model and the final model obtained in terms of coded factors are given below

$$Y_1 = 89.42 + 11.88A + 14.75B + 0.55C + 8.63D - 0.50AB - 3.27AC - 4.69AD - 1.48BC - 7.99BD + 9.11CD - 8.05A^2 - 20.41B^2 - 9.38C^2 - 6.76D^2 \tag{2}$$

$$Y_2 = 79.85 + 10.70A + 13.59B + 0.39C + 8.13D + 0.52AB + 0.75AC - 3.19AD + 0.52BC - 7.99BD + 7.11CD - 8.73A^2 - 20.33B^2 - 8.30C^2 - 5.42D^2 \tag{3}$$

Where, Y_1 and Y_2 are colour and COD removal (%) respectively; A, B, C and D are enzyme dose, incubation time, pH and temperature respectively.

Suitability of developed mathematical models

The predicting ability of the developed mathematical model are evaluated by constructing analytical plots (Fig. 1) such as residuals vs run, predicted versus actual plot to find out the connection between predicted and experimental values and also to know the fitness of the model. From the Fig. 1, it is observed that, residuals for the prediction of each response is minimum and it indicated a good adequate agreement between experimental data and the data predicted by model. This result confirms the normal distribution of the observed data and adequacy of the developed model [17]. Statistical significance of the developed mathematical model is examined using pareto analysis of variance (ANOVA) with corresponding *F* and *p*-values of process variables, which is shown in Table 5. The higher model *F* value and lower *p*-values ($p < 0.0001$) confirmed that, the developed model is significant. The goodness of fit of the model is also evaluated by the determination co-efficient of variance (CV), adequate precision (AP) and PRESS, which clearly stated that, the deviations between experimental and predicted values are low and confirms the reliability of the conducted experiments [18].

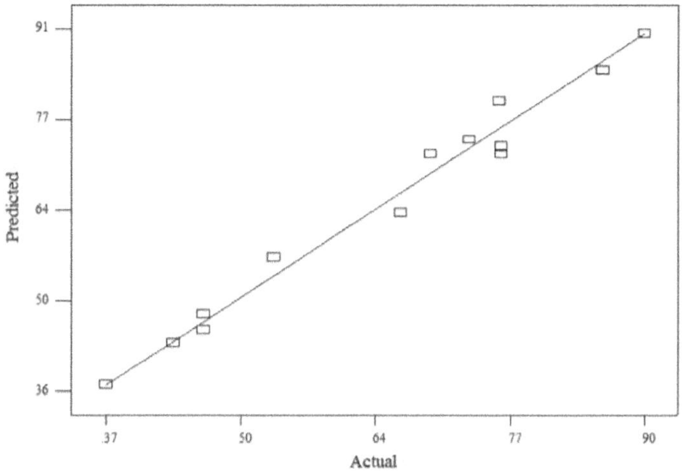

Fig. 1 Model adequacy plot

Influence of process parameters

Three dimensional (3D) response surface plots are plotted from the developed mathematical models in order to study the individual and combined effect of process variables on the responses to treat meat industry wastewater. In this present study, the model has more than two factors. So, the 3D plots are drawn by maintaining one factor at a constant level (in turn at its central level), whereas the other two factors were varied in their range, which are shown in Fig. 2.

Table 5 ANOVA results for responses

Source	Colour removal (%)		COD removal (%)	
	F-value	*P* value	*F*-value	*P* value
Model	68.54	<0.0001	31.70	<0.0001
A	182.05	<0.0001	77.98	<0.0001
B	280.55	<0.0001	125.75	<0.0001
C	0.39	0.5429	0.10	0.7529
D	96.02	<0.0001	44.99	<0.0001
AB	0.11	0.7479	0.06	0.8079
AC	4.58	0.0504	0.13	0.7245
AD	9.45	0.0082	2.31	0.1508
BC	0.94	0.3484	0.06	0.8079
BD	27.44	0.0001	14.49	0.0019
CD	35.69	<0.0001	11.48	0.0044
A^2	45.15	<0.0001	28.04	0.0001
B^2	290.24	<0.0001	152.04	<0.0001
C^2	61.38	<0.0001	25.38	0.0002
D^2	31.87	<0.0001	10.82	0.0054
C.V. %	4.30		4.85	
PRESS	754.08		596.54	
AP	27.65		31.54	

Effect of enzyme dose

Enzyme dose is one of the crucial parameter, which affects the performance of the enzymatic catalysis for treating meat wastewater significally. So that, experiments were carried out to study the effect of enzyme dose (80, 100 and 120 U/L) over the colour and COD removal and the results are shown in Fig. 2a–c. From the experimental results, it is observed that, the colour and COD removals were increased linearly with increasing enzyme dose upto 110 U/L. This is mainly due to the fact that by increasing the enzyme dose, an increase in the number of active sites takes place. At higher concentration of the enzyme the inhibitors will fall short. More active sites will reduce the colur and COD in the given period of time thus treatment efficiency is enhanced [19]. However, it is noticed that beyond enzyme dose of 110 U/L shows negligible effect on treatment efficiency.

Effect of incubation time

Incubation time is one of the important factor for the treatment of meat industry wastewater using enzymatic catalysis method. In order to investigate the effect of incubation time, experiments were carried out various incubation time (60, 90 and 120 min) and results are shown in Fig. 2a–d. From the results, it could be found that, the colour and COD removals were increased linearly with increasing incubation time upto 100 min. This is mainly due to the fact that, increase in enzyme dose would increase the reaction kinetic; this happens because free activation centers of the enzyme bind to free substrates thus removal efficiency are increased

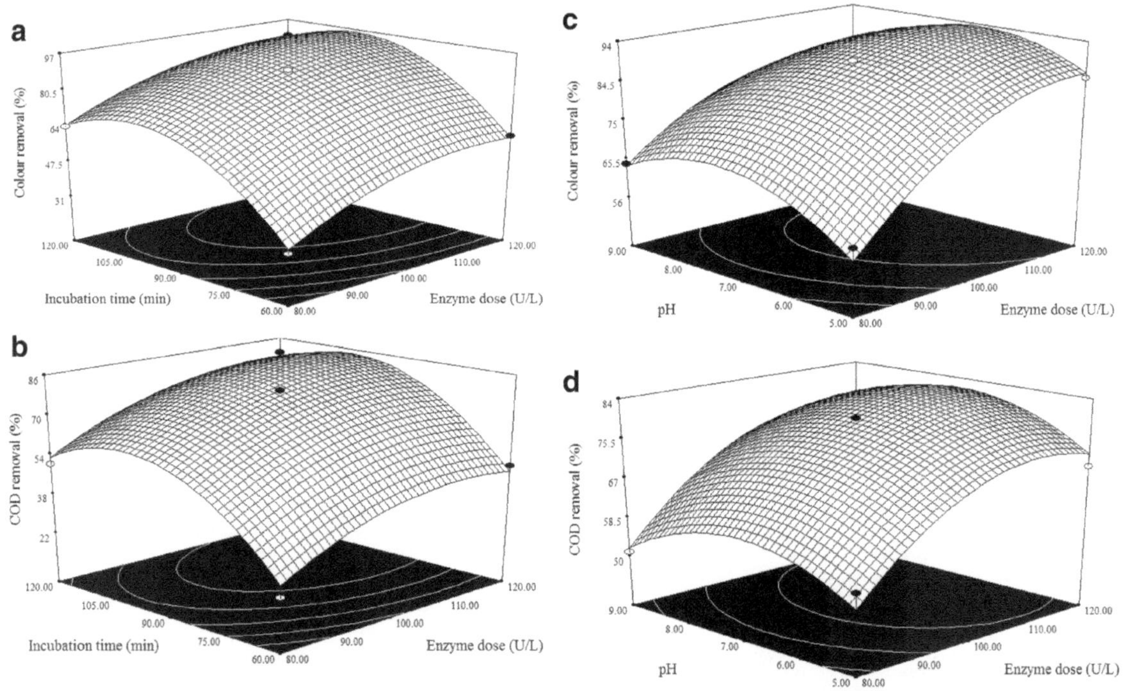

Fig. 2 Response surface plots representing the effect of process variables on the responses. **a** and **c**: Colour removal, **b** and **d**: COD removal

[20]. Thereafter, there is a negligible effect on the colour and COD removal efficiencies.

Effect of pH

The pH is also an important factor influences the treatment of meat wastewater using enzymatic catalysis method. The concentration of hydrogen ions in wastewater affects the enzyme activity. Each enzyme has maximal efficiency under an optimum pH otherwise there will be no enzymatic activity due to denaturation of enzymes. Therefore, in this study influence of pH on the colour and COD removal efficiencies was examined by varying its range (5, 7 and 9) and the results are illustrated in Fig. 3a–c. From the results, it is observed that, colour and COD removal efficiencies was increased with the increasing pH upto 8, due to the increase in the activity of enzyme and enhanced the treatment efficiency [21]. Beyond pH of 8 shows the negligible effect on removal efficiency of colour and COD.

Effect of temperature

Removal efficiency of colour and COD from meat waste water using enzymatic catalysis method is highly affectd by temperature and its influence on treatment efficiency is investigated by varying temperature (25, 35 and 45 °C) and the results are depicted in Fig. 3a–d. From the results, it is found that, colour and COD removal efficiencies were increased with the increasing temperature upto 40 °C and it can be explained the fact that, there are distinct temperature ranges under which enzymes operate and there is a specific temperature levels (optimum temperature) in which enzymes have maximum efficiency. Therefore temperature variations affect enzymatic activity and the kinetic of the reactions they catalyze. In addition, enzymes can be denatured under extreme temperatures and loses their catalytic activity [22]. These results indicates the key role of temperature on enzymatic catalysis method process for colour and COD removals.

Optimization and validation

For optimization, simultaneous optimization of the multiple responses is carried out using Derringer's desired function methodology in order to find out the optimum operating conditions for maximum removal efficiencies of colour and COD. This numerical optimization technique evaluates a point that maximizes the desirability function and optimum operating conditions were found to be as follows: enzyme dose of 110 U/L, incubation time of 100 min, pH of 7 and temperature of 40 °C. Under these conditions, the experimental results show that EC could effectively reduce the colour (95 %) and COD (86 %). Then, the suitability of optimum

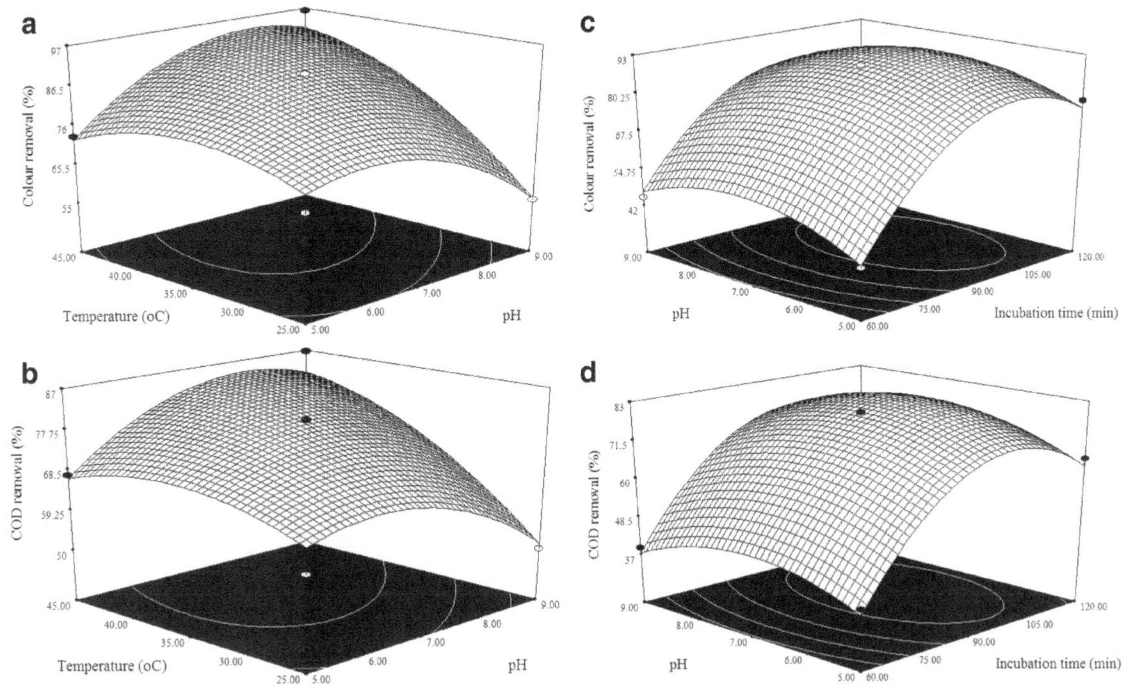

Fig. 3 Response surface plots representing the effect of process variables on the responses. **a** and **c**: Colour removal, **b** and **d**: COD removal

conditions for predicting optimum response value is tested based on above mentioned conditions. Triplicate experiments were performed under the optimized conditions and the mean value (95.35, 85.68 % for colour and COD removal respectively) obtained from real experiments, demonstrated the validation of the optimized conditions.

Conclusion

In this study, BBD was employed to study and optimize the process variables such as enzyme dose, incubation time, pH and temperature on the removal of colour and COD from meat wastewater using enzymatic catalysis method. From the results, it was observed that, all the process variables have significant effects on the treatment efficiency and quadratic model were developed for predicting the responses. Optimum set of the independent variables was obtained by derringer's desired function methodology in order to find out the maximum colour (95 %) and COD (86 %) removal efficiencies and it was found to be: enzyme dose of 110 U/L, incubation time of 100 min, pH of 7 and temperature of 40 °C. These results indicates that the proposed enzymatic catalysis process is an effective and economically viable method to treat meat industry wastewater.

Competing interests

The authors declare that they have no competing interests.

Authors' contributions

Both authors read and approved the final manuscript.

Acknowledgments

The authors are thankful to University Grant Commission (F.No:39-853/2010), Government of India, for financial support to fabricate and use the experimental setup.

References

1. Yi Jing C, Mei Fong C, Chung Lim L, Hassell DG. A review on anaerobic–aerobic treatment of industrial and municipal wastewater. Chem Eng J. 2009;155:1–18.
2. Eriksson E, Auffarth K, Eilersen AM, Henze M, Ledin A. Household chemicals and personal care products as sources for xenobiotic organic compounds in grey wastewater. Water SA. 2003;29:135–46.
3. Elmitwalli TA, Shalabi M, Wendland C, Otterpohl R. Grey water treatment in UASB reactor at ambient temperature. Water Sci Technol. 2007;55:173–80.
4. Shin HS, Lee SM, Seo IS, Kim GO, Lim KH, Song JS. Pilot-scale SBR and MF operation for the removal of organic and nitrogen compounds from greywater. Water Sci Technol. 1998;38:79–88.
5. Lesjean B, Gnirss R. Greywater treatment with a membrane bioreactor operated at low SRT and low HRT. Desalination. 2006;199:432–4.
6. Li Z, Gulyas H, Jahn M, Gajurel DR, Otterpohl R. Greywater treatment by constructed wetland in combination with TiO_2-based photocatalytic oxidation for suburban and rural areas without sewer system. Water Sci Technol. 2003;48:101–6.
7. Bektas N, Akbulut H, Inan H, Dimoglo A. Removal of phosphate from aqueous solutions by electro-coagulation. J Hazard Mater. 2004;106:101–5.
8. Adhoum N, Monser L, Bellakhal N, Belgaied JE. Treatment of electroplating wastewater containing Cu^{2+}, Zn^{2+} and Cr (VI) by electrocoagulation. J Hazard Mater. 2004;B112:207–13.

9. Sridhar R, Sivakumar V, Prince Immanuel V, Prakash Maran J. Treatment of pulp and paper industry bleaching effluent by electrocoagulation process. J Hazard Mater. 2011;186:1495–502.
10. Lai CL, Lin SH. Treatment of chemical mechanical polishing wastewater by electrocoagulation: system performances and sludge settling characteristics. Chemosphere. 2004;54:235–42.
11. Kobya M, Can OT, Bayramoğlu M. Treatment of textile wastewaters by electrocoagulation using iron and aluminum electrodes. J Hazard Mater. 2003;B100:163–78.
12. İnan H, Dimoglo A, Simşek H, Karpuzcu M. Olive oil mill wastewater treatment by means of electro-coagulation. Sep Purif Technol. 2004;36:23–31.
13. Fathollah GB, Amir HM, Simin N, Mohammad AF, Ramin N, Mahmood A. Application of immobilized horseradish peroxidase for removal and detoxification of azo dye from aqueous solution. Res J Chem Environ. 2011;15:73–8.
14. Olmez T. The optimization of Cr(VI) reduction and removal by electrocoagulation using response surface methodology. J Hazard Mater. 2009;162:1371–8.
15. Fathollah GB, Amir HM, Simin N, Mohammad AF, Ramin N, Mahmood A. Enzymatic treatment and detoxification of acid orange 7 from textile wastewater. Appl Biochem Biotechnol. 2011;165:1274–84.
16. Behbahani M, Alavi Moghaddam MR, Arami M. Techno-economical evaluation of fluoride removal by electrocoagulation process: Optimization through response surface methodology. Desalination. 2011;271:209–18.
17. Prakash Maran J, Manikandan S, Thirugnanasambandham K, Nivetha CV, Dinesh R. Box-Behnken design based statistical modeling for ultrasound-assisted extraction of corn silk polysaccharide. Carbohyd Polym. 2013;92: 604–11.
18. Sridhar R, Sivakumar V, Prince Immanuel V, Prakash Maran J. Development of model for treatment of pulp and paper industry bleaching effluent using response surface methodology. Environl Prog Sustain Energy. 2012;31:558–64.
19. Fathollah GB, Mohammad AF, Fatemeh NB, Amir HM. Oxidative degradation and detoxification of textile azo dye by horseradish peroxidase enzyme. Fresenius Environ Bull. 2013;22:1865–73.
20. Prakash Maran J, Sivakumar V, Sridhar R, Thirgananasambandham K. Development of model for barrier and optical properties of tapioca starch based films. Carbohyd Polym. 2013;92:1335–47.
21. Mahesh S, Prasad B, Mall ID, Mishra IM. Electrochemical degradation of pulp and paper mill waste water COD and color removal. Ind Eng Chem Res. 2006;45:2830–9.
22. Mayank K, Infant Anto Ponselvan F, Jodha Ram M, Vimal Chandra S, Indra Deo M. Treatment of bio-digester effluent by electrocoagulation using iron electrodes. J Hazard Mater. 2009;165:345–52.

13

Characterization of saline dust emission resulted from Urmia Lake drying

Akbar Gholampour[1,2], Ramin Nabizadeh[1], Mohammad Sadegh Hassanvand[1], Hasan Taghipour[1], Shahrokh Nazmara[3] and Amir Hossein Mahvi[3,4,5*]

Abstract

Compared with common dust storms, saline dust storms transport high concentrations of fine-grain saline and alkaline material. The saline dust storm differs from common dust storm, especially considering the sources of the suspended particulate matter (PM), chemical composition, grain size, and circulation processes. Atmospheric particulate matters (TSP, PM_{10}, $PM_{2.5}$, and PM_1) and their water-soluble ions were concurrently measured at two sites located at north and southeast part of Urmia lake from January 2013 to September 2013. Particulate matters (PMs) were measured using high volume sampler and HAZ-DUST EPAM-5000 particulate air monitors. In both of the sampling sites, the highest concentration of PM was observed during the summer season (521.6, 329.1, 42.6, and 36.5 for TSP, PM_{10}, $PM_{2.5}$, and PM_1, respectively). A total of 11 inorganic water-soluble ions in the TSP and PM_{10} were identified by ion chromatography (IC). No statistically significant difference was found between PM's ions concentrations of two sampling sites. The average of the total measured water-soluble ions in the sampling sites was 28.75 ± 12.9 μg/m^3 (11.9 ± 4.8% of total TSP mass) for TSP and 14.65 ± 7.1μg/m^3 (8.7 ± 4.4 of total PM_{10} mass) for PM_{10}. Among all detected ions, sulfate was the dominant constituent followed by nitrate and sodium. This study showed that the water soluble salts compose 3–20% of the total mass of TSP and PM_{10}. The PCA analysis showed that saline particulates formed from Urmia lake bed were the dominant source (57.6 %) of TSP. In addition, saline particulates together with crustal materials resulted from resuspension were the main source (59.9%) of PM_{10}.

Keywords: Urmia Lake, Saline dust, Particulate matters, Water-soluble ions, Source identification, Ions correlation

Background

Dust Storm phenomenon could change global climate and affect the economy and quality of human life [1]. In addition to contribution of the formation of gypcrete and calcrete, dust may lead to accumulation of more water soluble salts in soil profiles and thus contribute to salinization [2]. The saline dust storm differs from common dust storm, especially considering the sources of the suspended particulate matter (PM), chemical composition, grain size, and circulation processes. Saline dust storms are defined as "a kind of environmental disaster phenomenon in arid and semiarid regions that has been caused by dust deflated from the salt-rich sediments of dried lake beds and strongly salinized soils on the margins of lake floors" [3, 4]. Such a phenomena has been registered in many parts of the world, including the Aral Sea region in Kazakhstan and Uzbekistan, Lake Balkhash region in Kazakhstan, the Inner Mongolian region of China, southeastern Australia, and many other regions with arid and semiarid climate [5]. It was cleared that due to salt accumulation, sparse or absent of vegetation, and easily occurrences of wind erosion, these surface sediments will form a sleazy texture [3].

Compared with common dust storms, saline dust storms transport high concentrations of fine-grain saline and alkaline material, such as sodium sulfate, sodium chloride, and other potentially toxic components which could be threaten to the ecological security and humans health in the arid regions [3, 6, 7].

As mentioned above, chemical composition of saline dust storms is concerned to the characterization of region soil properties, and this redistribution leads to dual effects depending on the nature of transported

* Correspondence: ahmahvi@yahoo.com
[3]School of Public Health, Tehran University of Medical Sciences, Tehran, Iran
[4]Center for Solid Waste Research, Institute for Environmental Research, Tehran University of Medical Sciences, Tehran, Iran
Full list of author information is available at the end of the article

material. Based on studies, saline dust storms are rich in $CaCl_2$, NaCl, $MgCl_2$ and other chloride particles, which can be suspended in the atmosphere for long periods of time [8].

Urmia lake, located in northwest of Iran, is the second great saline lake in the world and the largest lake in Iran. In recent decade, the water level at Urmia lake has fallen more than 5 meters and the concentration of salt in this lake has increased from 185 to 220 g/L [9]. In addition to decrease in water level and increase in salt concentration, the unique ecosystem of the lake is being destroyed. As a result, a salt desert would be created with an area of more than 5000 km^2 (Fig. 1), overlaid with a 50–60 cm thick salt deposits [10]. In the warm season, wind could carry out these salts and transport those to adjacent areas as far as 300 km. The transported PM could damage agricultural lands, pollute the ecosystem and cause variety of diseases in nearby urban and rural areas [9].

Hitherto, no study has been conducted about atmospheric PM in Urmia Lake bed. The present study was therefore carried out to determine the mass levels of total suspended particulate (TSP), PM_{10}, $PM_{2.5}$ and PM_1 (aerodynamic diameter smaller than10, 2.5 and 1μm, respectively) along with the variations of water-soluble ionic species associated with TSP and PM_{10} in the floor of Urmia Lake.

Methods

Study area, sampling sites and schedule

Based on the region wind direction, two sites were selected (Fig. 2); 1) Tasuj site, located in the north of Urmia lake (38° 13' 17.8" N - 45° 24' 38.5" E), and 2) Ajabshir site, located in the southeast of Urmia lake (37° 31' 12.9" N - 45° 47' 53.0" E). The level of TSP, PM_{10}, $PM_{2.5}$ and $PM_{1.0}$ were measured 8 times every season in the period of January 2013 to September 2013. In total, 48 samples of TSP and PM_{10} were collected and analyzed during the study period.

PMs measurement

TSP and PM_{10} samples were collected by two high volume samplers manufactured by Graseby–Andersen at flow rates of 1.13–1.41 m^3/min for 24 h. Both TSP and PM_{10} were collected on a 20.3cm x 25.4cm Whatman glass micro fiber filter. Before and after sampling, filters were set under 40% relative humidity (RH) at 25°C for over 48h, afterward at room condition for 2 h; then were weighed three times using an A&D electronic balance with the reading precision of 0.1mg. $PM_{2.5}$ and $PM_{1.0}$ were measured using two portable HAZ-DUST EPAM-5000 particulate air monitors.

Chemical analysis

For water soluble ions analysis, one quarter of each filter was placed in a glass vial and then 40 mL ultra pure water (specific resistance ≥18 Ω cm) was added. The vials were

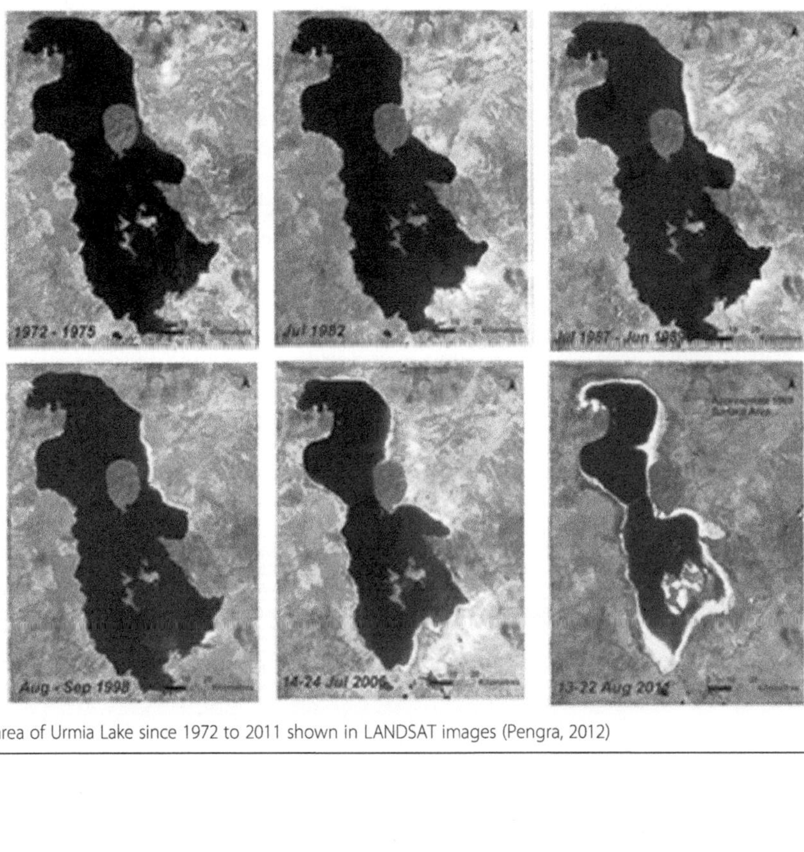

Fig. 1 Decreasing area of Urmia Lake since 1972 to 2011 shown in LANDSAT images (Pengra, 2012)

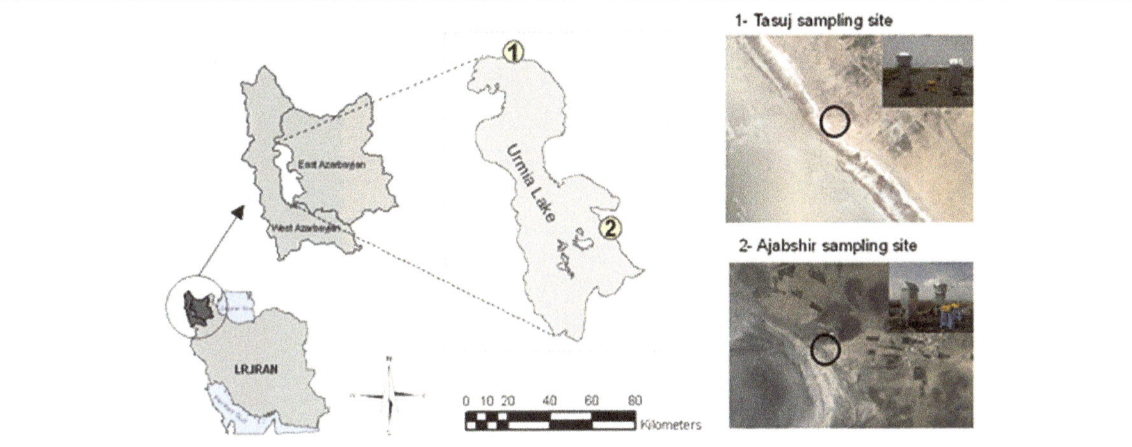

Fig. 2 Location of study area and sampling sites

shaken for 2h, and subsequently were ultra-sonicated for 30min. The extracted solutions were filtered through a micro porous membrane (with the pore size 0.45 μm) [11]. An ion chromatograph (Metrohm 850 Professional IC, Switzerland) with operating flow rate of 0.7 mL/min was used to analyze water-soluble ions. Field and laboratory blanks and spiked samples were analyzed along with the PM samples. For all ions, method detection limits (MDLs) were calculated by adding three standard deviations of the blank readings to the average of five replicates of the blank. The obtained MDLs and the recovery efficiencies for water-soluble ions are presented in Table 1.

Size and morphology

To determine the morphology and the elemental composition of the collected particles, TSP and PM_{10} samples were analyzed separately using the SEM-EDX system at the Razi Metallurgical Research Center.

Data analysis

Data were analyzed (with SPSS20 statistical software, SPSS Inc.) by means of the linear regression (for correlation coefficients among water-soluble ions), the bivariate correlations (to quantify the relation between the elemental concentrations), dimension reduction factor (for the quality principal components (PCs) of TSP and PM_{10}), and multivariate test (to quantify significance different between ions concentrations in Tasuj site vs. Ajabshir site). Differences and correlations were considered significant at the 0.05 level.

Meteorological data were obtained from the national climatic data center [12] and East Azerbaijan Meteorological Organization. The obtained data were examined for the missing values and outliers, and then were entered into WRPLOT View Freeware 7.0.0 to plot the wind-rose. The concentrations of PM were analyzed using Microsoft Excel 2010.

Results and discussion

Meteorological dates

Based on the collected meteorological dates, in both sampling sites, February was the coldest month with the monthly mean temperature of −1.0°C, while August was the warmest month with the mean temperature of 28.0° C. Also the RH varied from 25 to 72%. Dates of wind speed and the direction in both sampling sites revealed that in Ajabshir township, seasonal mean wind speed were 2.8, 2.72, 2.48 and 2.12 m/s, while in the Tasuj township were 2.36, 3.28, 3.25 and 1.97 m/s in winter, spring, summer and autumn, respectively. Annual wind rose plots for both sampling sites are shown in Fig. 3.

In Tasuj Township, the annual prevailing wind blew from South and South West with the speed of 0.5–13.6 m/s. The annual mean wind speed was 2.57 m/s. Calm wind (0 m/s) frequencies were 0.13, 0.6, 1.0, and 2.24% in spring, summer, autumn and winter, respectively. In Ajabshir

Table 1 MDLs and recovery efficiencies for water- soluble ions

Water-soluble ion	Na^+	NH_4^+	K^+	Mg^{2+}	Ca^{2+}	F^-	Cl^-	NO_2^-	NO_3^-	SO_4^{2-}	PO_4^{2-}
MDLs[a] (ng/mL)	95	6.3	4.4	12.5	5.3	3.7	6.5	3.6	52	45	6.1
MDLs[a] (μg/m³)	0.0025	0.0002	0.0001	0.0003	0.0001	0.0001	0.0002	0.0001	0.0014	0.0012	0.0002
Recovery efficiencies (%)	97–103	78–106	101–103	112–133	109–122	105–107	99–103	100–117	98–104	102–104	95–106

[a]Based on 3σ blank filters ($n = 5$)

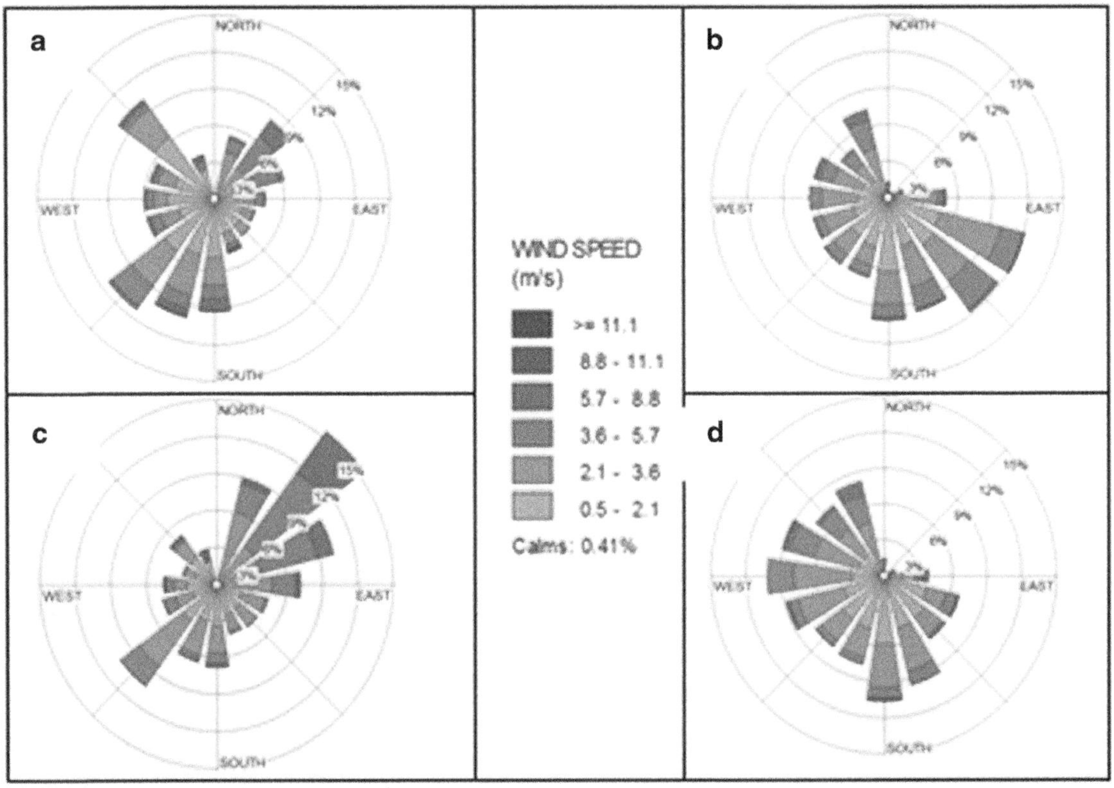

Fig. 3 Annual wind rose plots during the year of 2012 for (**a**) Tasuj and (**b**) Ajabshir and wind rose plots during June to January for (**c**) Tasuj and (**d**) Aajabshir

Township, wind speed varied from 0.5 to 11.12 m/s and annual mean wind speed was 2.57 m/s. In this region the annual prevailing wind blew from South and South East. Also, calm wind (0 m/s) frequencies were 0.5, 0.5, 2.9, and 1.0% in spring, summer, autumn and winter, respectively.

It was cleared that a drought associated with strong wind is regarded as the climatic background for the formation of dust storms [13, 14]. With respect to meteorological dates, June to September have the greatest potential to create dust storm, therefore, in order to predict the direction of probable saline dust storm, wind rose was plotted for mentioned months

(Fig. 3). As it can be seen in Fig. 3, in Tasuj sampling site prevailing wind blew from North East and South West during dry season; and in Ajabshir Township prevailing wind was from South to North and from

The PM mass concentrations and relations

Descriptive statistics of PM mass concentrations and the ratio of PMs' species in two sampling sites are presented in Table 2. According to Table 2, the average concentrations of TSP, PM_{10}, $PM_{2.5}$, and PM_1 in Tasuj sampling site were 230.1 ± 71.7, 140.3 ± 37.2, 28.3 ± 6.3, and 23.0 ± 5.6 μg/m^3, respectively. In Ajabshir sampling site the average concentrations were 291.4 ± 140.3, 220.1 ± 108.6, 31.8 ± 8.7, and 27.4 ± 7.6 μg/m^3 for TSP, PM_{10}, $PM_{2.5}$, and PM_1, respectively. In two sampling sites, the highest concentration of PM was observed during the summer season followed by spring.

Also, Table 2 represents the ratio of PMs' species in two sampling sites. The average of PM_{10}/TSP ratio in Ajabshir site (0.75) was higher than those for Tasuj site (0.64). Also the $PM_{2.5}/PM_{10}$ ratio for Ajabshir and Tasuj sampling sites ranged between 0.10–0.24 and 0.16–0.16, respectively. There was no significance difference between PM's ratios obtained from Tasuj and Ajabshir sampling sites (Wilks' Lambda value = 0.73, F = 0.65 and Pvalue = 0.65). Compared to our previous study on Tabriz urban and industrial suburban PM ratios, $PM_{2.5}/PM_{10}$ in Urmia lake region was smaller than urban (0.48) and industrial zone (0.38) of Tabriz [15]. It seems due to significant differences in particle sources and also some geographical and meteorological conditions the obtained results from one study could not be directly compared with the findings of other studies.

Table 2 Descriptive statistics for 24- hour PM mass concentrations (μg/m^3) and the ratio of PMs' species in Ajabshir and Tasuj sampling sites

Sampling sites		PM concentrations (μg/m^3)				The ratio of PMs' species			
		TSP	PM_{10}	$PM_{2.5}$	PM_1	PM_{10}/TSP	$PM_{2.5}/PM_{10}$	PM_1/PM_{10}	$PM'_1/PM_{2.5}$
Tasuj	Min	150.80	102.10	22.25	16.05	0.38	0.16	0.13	0.72
	Max	338.80	194.80	36.50	29.46	0.90	0.26	0.21	0.89
	Average	230.15	140.34	28.35	22.99	0.64	0.21	0.17	0.81
	SD	71.74	37.17	6.27	5.64	0.19	0.04	0.03	0.06
	Median	211.10	130.22	26.72	22.85	0.63	0.20	0.16	0.81
Ajabshir	Min	168.19	95.94	22.50	18.60	0.57	0.10	0.10	0.80
	Max	521.60	329.15	42.60	36.50	0.96	0.24	0.19	0.96
	Average	291.36	220.08	31.84	27.45	0.75	0.17	0.14	0.86
	SD	140.33	108.64	8.69	7.57	0.16	0.05	0.04	0.06
	Median	261.57	230.00	30.55	28.05	0.74	0.16	0.13	0.86

Ionic composition of PM

The statistical analysis of water soluble ions concentration in the TSP and PM_{10} showed that there was no significant difference between PM's ions concentrations at Tasuj and Ajabshir sites (Wilks' Lambda value = 0.022, F = 4.35 and Pvalue = 0.36 for TSP and Wilks' Lambda value = 0.019 F = 5.1 and Pvalue = 0.33 for PM_{10}). Therefore, the concentrations of water soluble ions were reported together as Urmia lake PM's ionic characterization.

The descriptive statistics of water-soluble ions concentration in TSP and PM_{10} collected from Urmia lake region are given in Table 3; expressed by cubic meter of sampled air (species in mass per volume units: μg/m^3) and by mg per g of sampled particles (species in mass/mass units: mg/g of TSP and PM_{10}). Also, the average of water-soluble ions concentration in TSP and PM_{10} are presented in Fig. 4(a and b); expressed by cubic meter of sampled air (μg/m^3) and percentage of species in the measured water soluble ions mass concentration.

The average of the total measured water-soluble ions in TSP was 28.75 ± 12.9 μg/m^3 (11.9 ± 4.8% of total TSP mass) and in PM_{10} was 14.65 ± 7.1μg/m^3 (8.7 ± 4.4 of total PM_{10} mass). As it can be seen in Fig. 4, about 90% of total detected water-soluble ions mass in PM_{10} included by SO_4^{2-} (29%), NO_3^- (21%), $Na+$ (14%), Cl^-(13%), and Ca^{2+}(100%) in TSP, and SO_4^{2-} (29%), NO_3^- (20%), Na^+(15%), Cl^-(12%), and Ca^{2+}(12%). Among all detected ions, sulfate was the dominant constituent followed by nitrate and sodium. These results are in agreement with the study by Hassanzadeh et al. [16] which Na^+, K^+, Ca^{2+}, Li^+, and Mg^{2+} were the main cations, while Cl^-, SO_4^{2-}, and HCO_3^- were the main anions in Urmia lake's water. The Urmia lake is a hyper-saline lake and the concentrations of Na^+ and Cl^- were roughly 4 times the concentration of natural seawater [16]. High concentrations of Na^+ and Cl^- (especially for TSP) could be caused by the higher and persistent on-shore winds which create abundant sea water droplets and marine aerosols.

Our study show that the water soluble salts compose 3–20% of the total mass of TSP and PM_{10}, while Abuduwaili et al. [3] stated that in the Ebinur region, the soluble salts compose 10–25% of the total mass of the saline dust, and salts are predominantly represented by sodium and calcium chlorides and sulfates. Gholampour et al. [15] reported that in the Tabriz urban and suburban region, that are the near to the Urmia lake, water soluble ions accounted for approximately 20 ± 10% of total TSP mass and 25 ± 12 of total PM_{10} mass. Low percentage of total ions in the PM mass could be due to the small amount of secondary ion, especially non sea salt sulfate and ammonium, in the PM of Urmia lake bed.

Despite of higher PM and ions concentration during warm season, the comparison of mass percentage of water soluble ions in the ambient air PM of Urmia lake during cold and warm seasons showed that there was no significant difference between the mass percentage of PM's ions in the various seasons (Wilks' Lambda value = 0.4, F = 1.64 and Pvalue = 0.2). Therefore, it could be concluded that in the Urmia lake region, the sources of PMs are same during various seasons.

Size and morphology of aerosol particles

SEM-EDX photographs for TSP and PM_{10} samples are shown as an example in Figs. 5(a) and 6(a); and the SEM-EDX spectra of those are shown in Figs. 5(b) and 6 (b), respectively. Quantitative estimates of the particulate's (TSP sample) elemental composition are given in Table 4. As shown in the table; Oxygen (30.7%) and Silicon (20.4%) are the major component of the analyzed particulate. However, other elements, such as Iron (8.7%), Magnesium (6.9%), Calcium (6.6%), Aluminum (4%), Sodium (1.2%), and Potassium (1%) are also of great importance. Also, elemental composition quantitative estimates of the PM_{10}

Table 3 Elemental analysis of Urmia lake TSF (PM_{10}) ($\mu g/m^3$ and mg/g) ($n = 48$)

	μg/m³					mg/g				
	Min	Max	Median	Mean	SD	Min	Max	Median	Mean	SD
Na^+	1.527 (1.114)	9.657 (4.524)	3.596 (1.793)	3.908 (1.994)	2.225 (0.875)	3.121 (2.720)	33.267 (25.982)	15.364 (12.817)	16.417 (12.858)	8.306 (6.966)
NH_4^+	0.184 (0.059)	4.664 (1.526)	1.645 (0.973)	1.787 (0.872)	1.288 (0.496)	0.516 (0.419)	15.701 (12.366)	5.628 (4.591)	7.357 (5.333)	4.701 (3.856)
K^+	0.229 (0.091)	1.700 (0.970)	1.195 (0.433)	1.074 (0.466)	0.476 (0.251)	0.438 (0.292)	9.142 (8.016)	4.457 (2.503)	4.753 (3.120)	2.563 (2.232)
Mg^{2+}	0.164 (0.094)	0.567 (0.267)	0.237 (0.157)	0.270 (0.166)	0.117 (0.052)	0.379 (0.339)	1.572 (1.645)	1.189 (1.077)	1.130 (1.021)	0.403 (0.432)
Ca^{2+}	1.822 (1.204)	4.769 (3.540)	2.687 (2.044)	2.763 (2.090)	0.842 (0.688)	5.533 (3.300)	22.560 (20.125)	12.349 (12.828)	12.006 (12.738)	5.068 (5.048)
F^-	0.000 (0.000)	0.489 (0.680)	0.014 (0.010)	0.152 (0.166)	0.211 (0.251)	0.000 (0.001)	2.481 (4.808)	0.072 (0.073)	0.555 (0.874)	0.805 (1.608)
Cl^-	2.227 (1.220)	5.506 (4.267)	3.307 (1.425)	3.553 (1.876)	1.223 (0.929)	4.350 (2.189)	29.619 (24.506)	14.420 (10.924)	15.316 (11.493)	6.726 (5.895)
NO_2^-	0.000 (0.000)	0.114 (0.039)	0.024 (0.005)	0.038 (0.009)	0.040 (0.012)	0.000 (0.001)	0.639 (0.194)	0.151 (0.048)	0.163 (0.052)	0.183 (0.057)
NO_3^-	1.334 (0.860)	13.281 (7.948)	5.174 (2.391)	6.199 (2.814)	4.251 (2.131)	5.800 (5.012)	62.317 (45.650)	27.651 (10.547)	25.539 (16.632)	16.400 (13.801)
SO_4^{2-}	2.400 (1.563)	20.572 (11.406)	6.014 (4.311)	8.694 (4.201)	6.346 (2.795)	9.119 (10.308)	79.699 (65.508)	36.516 (18.353)	34.815 (23.182)	21.675 (14.892)
PO_4^{2-}	0.000 (0.000)	0.830 (0.031)	0.184 (0.000)	0.316 (0.003)	0.332 (0.009)	0.001 (0.001)	3.839 (0.216)	0.923 (0.002)	1.250 (0.020)	1.361 (0.062)
Sum	15.595 (8.479)	49.267 (34.029)	24.080 (12.839)	28.753 (14.657)	12.941 (7.109)	30.176 (27.513)	227.127 (195.443)	124.526 (74.120)	119.301 (87.322)	48.723 (44.092)

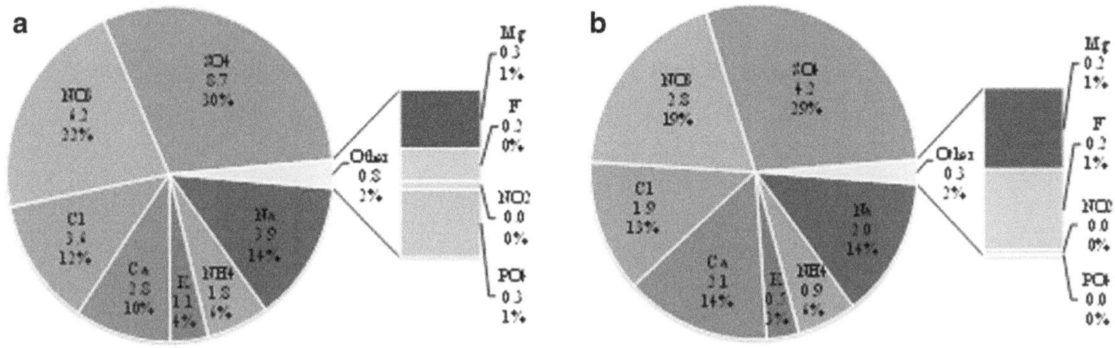

Fig. 4 Water-soluble ions concentration in TSP (**a**) and PM_{10} (**b**) collected from Urmia Lake

sample are given in Table 5. It can be seen that Oxygen (29.1%) and Silicon (14.4%) are the major component of the analyzed particulate. However, other elements, such as Aluminum (8%), Zinc (7.1%), Iron (6.7%), Carbon (3.6%), Magnesium (1.7%), Chlorine (1.6%), and Sodium (1.3) are with great importance.

Comparison of the TSP and PM_{10} elemental composition with world average values revealed that amount of Silicon in the Urmia lake dusts is less rich (20.4% for TSP and 14.4% for PM_{10}vs. the world average of 59.9%). However, the TSP resulted from Urmia lake dusts are richer in Fe (8.7% vs. the world average of 6.85%), Ca (6.6% vs. the world average of 3.94%), Mg (6.9% vs. the world average of 2.60%),and sodium (1.2% vs. the world average of 0.5–1%) than the Saharan, Harmattan, Chinese, and North American dusts [2].

It is important to note that the concentration of Chloride in the world average values is negligible; whereas our results indicated that chloride is one of the main ions in the Urmia lake dusts. This finding indicates that sea salt particles contribute large to the total mass of the particles collected. On the other hand, crustal dusts have also major role in the composition of TSP and PM_{10} in Urmia lake region.

Ionic balance of PM

Often the ionic balance is employed to determine the potentially ions missing, which are not measured during the extraction and the detection. The plots of total cations versus the total anions equivalents (*neq/m*^{3}) are presented in Fig. 7. The slope of the regression line for PM indicated a value greater than unity (slope = 2.95, $R^2 = 0.79$ for TSP and slope = 2.22, $R^2 = 0.7$ for PM_{10}), which might be due to high level of carbonate and bicarbonate, which were not analyzed. The main ions that could not be detected by our used method are HCO_3^- and H^+.

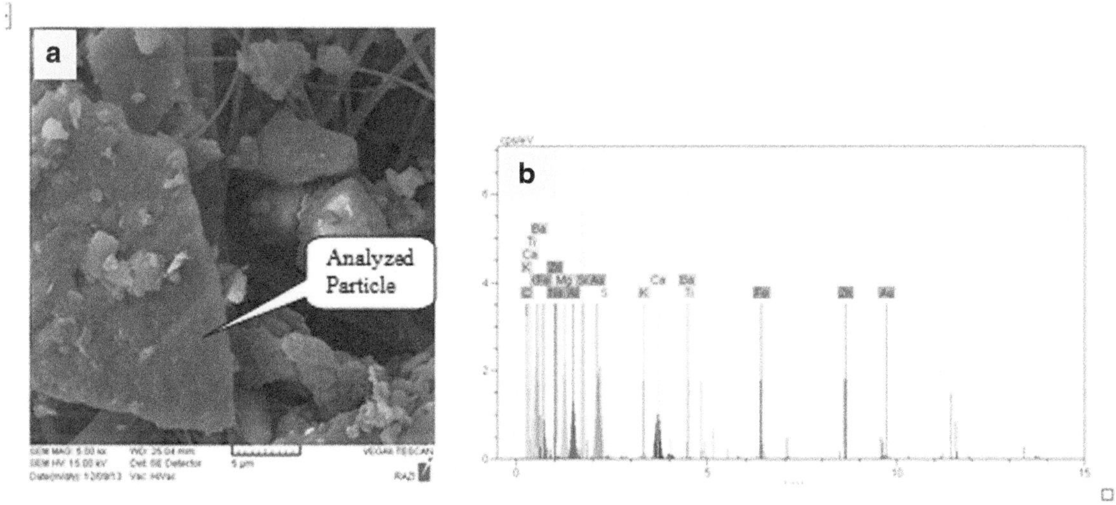

Fig. 5 SEM photograph (**a**) and X-ray spectra (**b**) of TSP sample

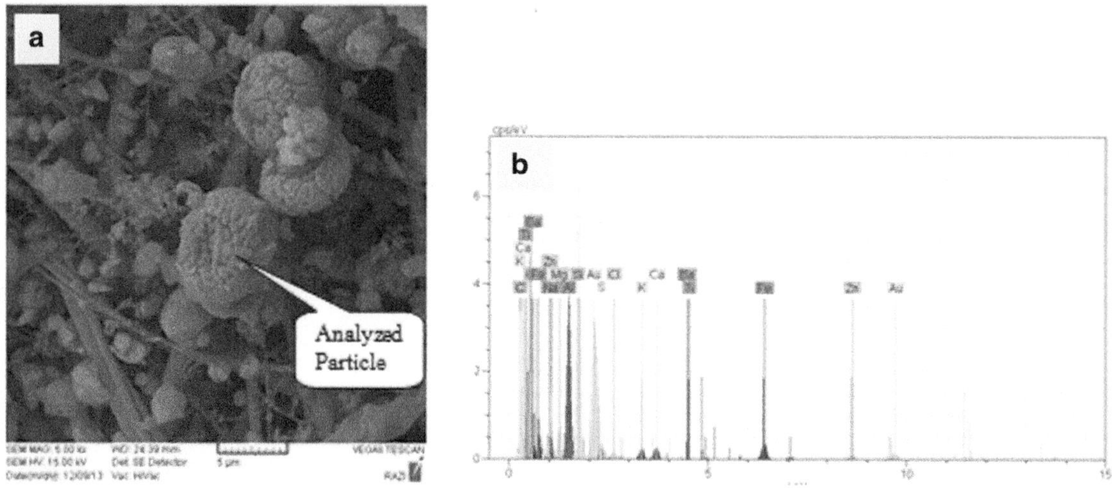

Fig. 6 SEM photograph (**a**) and X-ray spectra (**b**) of PM_{10} sample

On the other hand, as it was shown in Fig. 8, investigation of the relation between Cl^- with Na^+ and K^+ revealed strong correlation between Cl^- and Na^+ ($R^2 = 0.91$ and slope = 0.9 for TSP and $R^2 = 0.76$ and slope = 0.8 for PM_{10}) and Cl^- with K^+. But, the slope of relation between Cl^- with K^+ as smaller than Na^+. These results allow us to conclude that the main chlorinated compound in PM was NaCl followed by KCl.

Ionic correlation of PM

Ions correlation matrixes were calculated using bivariate correlations to quantify the relation between the elemental concentrations. As it is shown in Table 6, the number of significant correlations of the elements in PM_{10} is higher and also stronger than the TSP elements. Yatkin et al. [17] has stated that values of elemental correlations in $PM_{2.5}$ were much higher than PM_{10}. Therefore, it could be concluded that with decreasing the size of PM, the elemental correlation increases and it might show that the sources of smaller PM were limited compared to larger ones.

High level of correlations was obtained between the terrestrial elements in TSP and PM_{10}. For example, the correlation between Ca^{2+} and Mg^{2+} were 0.81 and 0.88 in TSP and PM_{10}, respectively ($P < 0.01$). These results

Table 4 Quantitative estimates of elemental compositions of TSP sample

Element	Series	unn. C [wt.-%]	norm. C [wt.-%]	Atom. C [at.-%]
Carbon	K series	1.01	1.05	2.4
Oxygen	K series	29.46	30.72	52.68
Sodium	K series	1.21	1.22	1.27
Magnesium	K series	6.61	6.89	7.78
Aluminium	K series	3.83	3.99	4.06
Silicon	K series	19.59	20.43	19.96
Sulfur	K series	0.33	0.34	0.29
Potassium	K series	0.95	0.99	0.7
Calcium	K series	6.35	6.63	4.54
Titanium	K series	0.08	0.09	0.05
Iron	K series	8.37	8.73	4.29
Zinc	K series	0.76	0.79	0.33
Barium	L series	0.01	0.01	0
Gold	M series	18.33	19.11	2.66
	Total:	95.90%		

Table 5 Quantitative estimates of elemental compositions of PM_{10} sample

Element	Series	unn. C [wt.-%]	norm. C [wt.-%]	Atom. C [at.-%]
Carbon	K series	3.87	3.58	8.46
Oxygen	K series	31.51	29.15	51.66
Sodium	K series	1.42	1.31	1.62
Magnesium	K series	1.86	1.72	2.01
Aluminium	K series	8.93	8.26	8.68
Silicon	K series	15.58	14.41	14.55
Sulfur	K series	1.06	0.98	0.86
Chlorine	K series	0.61	0.57	0.45
Potassium	K series	1.33	1.23	0.89
Calcium	K series	1.27	1.17	0.83
Titanium	K series	0.13	0.12	0.07
Iron	K series	7.27	6.72	3.41
Zinc	K series	7.71	7.14	3.09
Barium	L series	0.01	0.01	0
	Total:	108.10%		

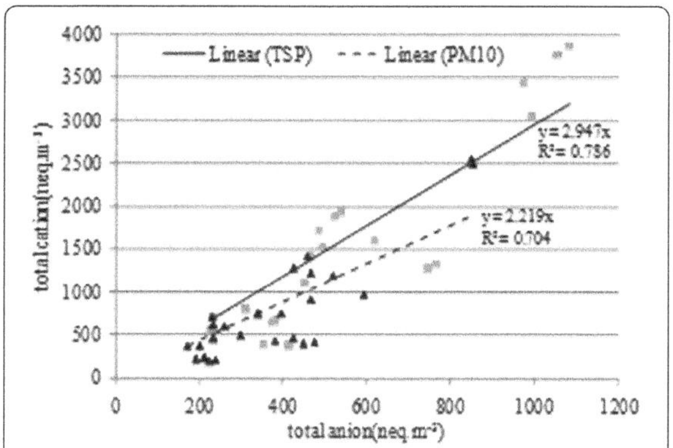

Fig. 7 The ionic balance for TSP and PM_{10} fractions in Urmia lake region

suggest that the sources of the terrestrial elements are most probably soil and soil-related activities. Also, the high and strong correlation between Cl^-, Na^+, Ca^+, Mg^{2+} and K^+ indicates that a main part of PM was originated from marine salt. Correlations between NH_4^+ with NO_3^- and SO_4^{2-} were weak; 0.35 and 0.46 in TSP and 0.31 and 0.46 for PM_{10}, respectively ($p > 0.05$). It could be concluded that secondary ions have a few roles in the formation of TSP and PM_{10} in the Urmia lake region.

The Cl^-/Na^+ equivalent ratio for the whole study period ranged from 0.85, in warm seasons, to 1.76, in cold seasons, for TSP. This ratio for PM_{10} was 0.67, in warm seasons, to 2.15, in cold seasons. These results reveal that the loss of particulate Cl^- during warm seasons caused by the formation of gaseous HCl from $NaCl$ and acidic gases [18]. The chloride loss may be illustrated by the reaction between HNO_3/or H_2SO_4 and NaCl in sea-salt particles generally formulated by:

$$HNO_3 + NaCl\ (sea\ salt) \rightarrow NaNO_3 (sea\ salt) + HCl$$

The $Cl^-/Na+$ ratio in Urmia Lake region is broader and higher than the measured ratio in PM of urban and industrial zones of Tabriz (0.41–1.07 for TSP and 0.42–0.78 for PM_{10}) [15].

Principal components analysis of PM

Three air quality principal components (PCs) for TSP and two PCs for PM_{10} with eigenvalues exceeding 1.0 were found. Based on Table 7, it was indicated that these PCs have a significant influence on the PM quality in Urmia Lake. For the TSP, the first PC showed high loading of Na^+, NH_4^+, K^+, Cl^-, F^-, NO_3^-, and SO_4^{2-} with a total variance of 57.6 %. These ions are saline particulates and formed from Urmia lake bed. The second PC showed the high loading of Mg^{2+} and Ca^{2+} with a total variance of 18.41%. Theses ions are typically associated with crustal materials in windblown dust and the resuspended dust from around lands. Finally the third PC showed high loading of NO_2^- and PO_4^{2-} with a total variance of 13.08 %. Application of chemical fertilizer in agricultural lands around sampling sites could be the origin of third PC.

As mentioned above, two PCs were found for PM_{10}. The first PC showed high loading of Na^+, K^+, Mg^{2+}, Ca^{2+}, Cl^-, F^-, NO_3^-, and SO_4^{2-} with a total variance of 59.9 %. These ions typically associated with saline particulates and crustal materials in windblown dust and resuspended dust from Urmia lake bed and sampling sites around lands. The second PC showed high loading of NH_4^+, NO_2^- and PO_4^{2-} with a total variance of 17.1%. High loading of these ions allows us to conclude that the main source of second PC was application of chemical fertilizer in agricultural lands around sampling sites.

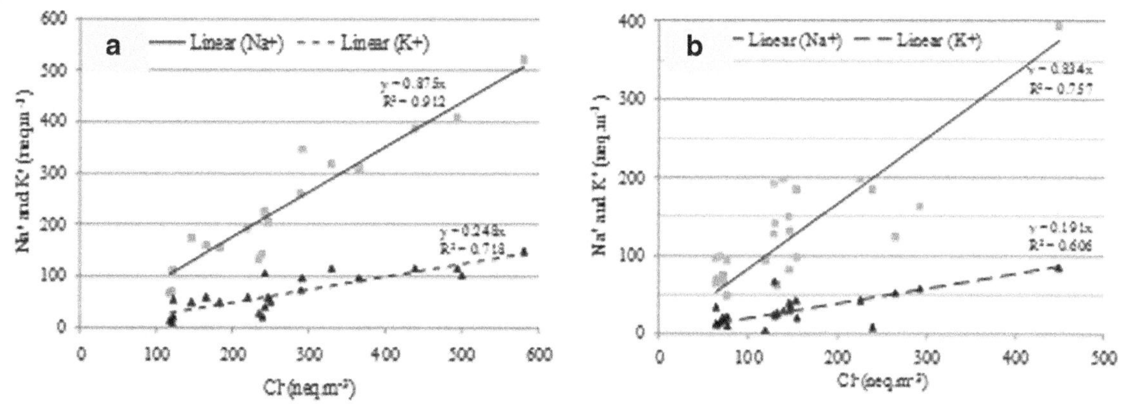

Fig. 8 Relation between Cl^- with Na^+ and K^+ for (**a**) TSP and (**b**) PM_{10} fractions in Urmia lake region

Table 6 The correlation matrixes of the elemental concentrations at urban site

	Na^+	NH_4^+	K^+	Mg^{2+}	Ca^{2+}	F^-	Cl^-	NO_2^-	NO_3^-	SO_4^{2-}
	TSP									
NH_4^+	**0.593****									
K^+	**0.856****	**0.602****								
Mg^{2+}	0.482*	0.368	0.464*							
Ca^{2+}	0.344	0.014	0.363	**0.806****						
F^-	**0.657****	**0.658****	0.487*	0.396	0.096					
Cl^-	**0.956****	**0.692****	**0.848****	**0.546****	0.270	**0.550****				
NO_2^-	0.253	0.464*	0.178	**0.600****	0.407	0.397	0.256			
NO_3^-	**0.708****	0.347	**0.569****	0.504*	0.301	**0.925****	**0.576****	0.406*		
SO_4^{2-}	**0.704****	0.457	0.547**	0.432*	0.266	**0.955****	**0.572****	0.444*	**0.958****	
PO_4^{2-}	−0.053	0.194	−0.167	0.239	0.388	0.334	−0.090	0.485*	0.426*	0.503*
	PM_{10}									
NH_4^+	**0.551****									
K^+	**0.749****	0.454*								
Mg^{2+}	**0.825****	**0.563****	**0.580****							
Ca^{2+}	**0.625****	0.257	0.441*	**0.875****						
F^-	**0.662****	0.187	**0.755****	0.547**	0.474*					
Cl^-	**0.882****	0.392	**0.795****	**0.814****	**0.753****	**0.834****				
NO_2^-	−0.087	0.345	−0.180	0.062	−0.120	−0.169	−0.293			
NO_3^-	**0.860****	0.316	**0.782****	**0.699****	**0.594****	**0.920****	**0.927****	−0.105		
SO_4^{2-}	**0.868****	0.464*	**0.712****	**0.805****	**0.618****	**0.796****	**0.902****	0.031	**0.920****	
PO_4^{2-}	−0.008	−0.386	0.211	0.019	0.190	0.549**	0.226	−0.199	0.306	0.030

$^{**}P < 0.01$ $^{*}P < 0.05$

Bold numbers represented the significant correlation

Table 7 Varimax rotated PCA loadings for water-soluble ions of TSP and PM_{10} in Urmia Lake

Variables	TSP			PM_{10}	
	PC1	PC2	PC3	PC1	PC2
Na+	**0.905**	0.31	−0.125	**0.926**	0.122
NH_4^+	**0.801**	−0.196	0.392	0.539	**0.707**
K^+	**0.881**	0.34	−0.184	**0.824**	−0.121
Mg^{2+}	0.36	**0.803**	0.335	**0.879**	0.217
Ca^{2+}	0.056	**0.952**	0.197	**0.743**	−0.047
F^-	**0.85**	−0.03	0.456	**0.825**	−0.424
Cl^-	**0.913**	0.246	−0.094	**0.967**	−0.171
NO_2^-	0.195	0.302	**0.777**	−0.082	**0.63**
NO_3^-	**0.806**	0.191	0.473	**0.934**	−0.204
SO_4^{2-}	**0.819**	0.092	0.537	**0.947**	0.113
PO_4^{2-}	−0.064	0.172	**0.897**	0.167	**0.808**
Eigenvalue	6.341	2.025	1.439	6.585	1.881
% of Variance	57.648	18.41	13.085	59.861	17.097
% of Cumulative	57.648	76.06	89.142	59.861	76.958

Bold numbers represented the significant correlation

Conclusion

The implemented prevention and control measures are mainly the diversion or conservation of water to recover dried lake beds to reduce wind erosion. However, water-saving potential is limited due to continuing social and economical development in arid regions. On the other hand, evaporative losses from lake surfaces are high because of intense sunshine, large water areas, shallow water depths, and vigorous evaporation from the water surface.

As mentioned above, the water level of Urmia Lake has been decreased up to 6 m during last decade. Along with decreasing of water level, a salt desert is created with area more than 5000 km^2. According to the dynamic characteristics of dust, grains with diameters smaller than 10 μm can be transported by wind for several thousands of kilometers under common wind power conditions, and those with diameters of 10–20 μm can be transported for hundreds or up to several thousands of kilometers with wind speeds > 15 m/s. Therefore, at Urmia Lake region and especially during the warm season, wind could carry on saline dust to adjacent areas as far as hundreds of kilometers.

The transported PM could damage agricultural lands, pollute the ecosystem and cause variety of disease in some state of Iran, Azerbaijan and other neighboring countries.

Competing interests
The authors declare that they have no competing interests.

Authors' contributions
All authors read and approved the final manuscript.

Acknowledgments
The authors would like to thank financial support for this research by Institute for Environmental Research (IER), Tehran University of Medical Sciences (grant number 92-01-46-21258). Also, we would like to acknowledge General Administration of Education at East Azarbayejan University of Medical Sciences for providing us with sampling locations.

Author details
[1]Center for Air Pollution Research, Institute for Environmental Research, Tehran University of Medical Sciences, Tehran, Iran. [2]School of Public Health, Tabriz University of Medical Sciences, Tabriz, Iran. [3]School of Public Health, Tehran University of Medical Sciences, Tehran, Iran. [4]Center for Solid Waste Research, Institute for Environmental Research, Tehran University of Medical Sciences, Tehran, Iran. [5]National Institute of Health Research, Tehran University of Medical Sciences, Tehran, Iran.

References

1. Okin GS, Mahowald N, Chadwick OA, Artaxo P. Impact of desert dust on the biogeochemistry of phosphorus in terrestrial ecosystems. Global Biogeochemical Cycles. 2004;18(2).
2. Goudie AS, Middleton NJ. Desert dust in the global system. Springer; 2006
3. Abuduwaili J, Liu D, Wu G. Saline dust storms and their ecological impacts in arid regions. J Arid Land. 2010;2(2):144–50.
4. Micklin P. The Aral sea disaster. Annu Rev Earth Planet Sci. 2007;35:47–72.
5. Gill TE. Eolian sediments generated by anthropogenic disturbance of playas: human impacts on the geomorphic system and geomorphic impacts on the human system. Geomorphology. 1996;17(1):207–28.
6. Small I, Van der Meer J, Upshur R. Acting on an environmental health disaster: the case of the Aral Sea. Environ Health Perspect. 2001;109(6):547.
7. Mu G, Yan S, Jilil A, He Q, Xai X. Wind erosion at the dry-up bottom of Aiby Lake. Sci China Ser D Earth Sci. 2002;45(1):157–64.
8. Liu D, Abuduwaili J, Lei J, Wu G. Deposition rate and chemical composition of the Aeolian dust from a bare saline playa, Ebinur Lake, Xinjiang, China. Water Air Soil Pollut. 2011;218(1–4):175–84.
9. Hoseinpour M, Fakheri Fard A, Naghili R, editors. Death Of Urmia Lake, a Silent Disaster Investigating Causes, Results and Solutions of Urmia Lake drying. 1st International Applied Geological Congress, Department of Geology, Islamic Azad University, Islamic Azad University-Mashad Branch, Iran; 2010.
10. Eimanifar A, Mohebbi F. Urmia Lake (northwest Iran): a brief review. Saline Systems. 2007;3(5):1–8.
11. Cheng M-T, Chou W-C, Chio C-P, Hsu S-C, Su Y-R, Kuo P-H, et al. Compositions and source apportionments of atmospheric aerosol during Asian dust storm and local pollution in central Taiwan. J Atmos Chem. 2008; 61(2):155–73.
12. NCDC. 2013. http://www7.ncdc.noaa.gov/CDO/cdoselect.cmd.
13. Fu P, Huang J, Li C, Zhong S. The properties of dust aerosol and reducing tendency of the dust storms in northwest China. Atmos Environ. 2008; 42(23):5896–904.
14. Ta W, Dong Z, Sanzhi C. Effect of the 1950s large-scale migration for land reclamation on spring dust storms in Northwest China. Atmos Environ. 2006;40(30):5815–23.
15. Gholampour A, Nabizadeh R, Naseri S, Yunesian M, Taghipour H, Rastkari N, et al. Exposure and health impacts of outdoor particulate matter in two urban and industrialized area of Tabriz, Iran. J Environ Health Sci Eng. 2014; 12(1):27.
16. Hassanzadeh E, Zarghami M, Hassanzadeh Y. Determining the main factors in declining the Urmia Lake level by using system dynamics modeling. Water Resour Manag. 2012;26(1):129–45.
17. Yatkin S, Bayram A. Elemental composition and sources of particulate matter in the ambient air of a Metropolitan City. Atmos Res. 2007;85(1):126–39.
18. Galindo N, Yubero E, Nicolas JF, Crespo J. Water-soluble ions measured in fine particulate matter next to cement works. Atmos Environ. 2011;45(12): 2043–9.

The study of CaO and MgO heterogenic nano-catalyst coupling on transesterification reaction efficacy in the production of biodiesel from recycled cooking oil

Kambiz Tahvildari[1], Yasaman Naghavi Anaraki[1], Reza Fazaeli[2], Sogol Mirpanji[1] and Elham Delrish[3*]

Abstract

Background: Fossil fuels' pollution and their non-renewability have motivated the search for alternative fuels. Some common example of seed oils are sunflower oil, date seed oil, soy bean oil. For instance, soy methyl and soy-based biodiesel are the main biodiesel. Biodiesel is a clean diesel fuel that can be produced through transesterification reaction. Recycled cooking oil, on the other hand, is one of the inexpensive, easily available sources for producing biodiesel.

Results: This article is aimed at production of biodiesel via trans-esterification method, Nano CaO synthesis using sol-gel method, and Nano MgO synthesis using sol-gel self-combustion. Two catalysts' combination affecting the reaction's efficacy was also discussed. Optimum conditions for the reaction in the presence of Nano CaO are 1.5 % weight fracture, 1:7 alcohol to oil proportion and 6 h in which biodiesel and glycerin (the byproduct) are produced. Moreover, the optimum conditions for this reaction in the presence of Nano CaO and Nano MgO mixture are 3 % weight fracture (0.7 g of Nano CaO and 0.5 g of Nano MgO), 1:7 alcohols to oil proportion and 6 h.

Conclusions: Nano MgO is not capable of catalyzing the transesterification by itself, because it has a much weaker basic affinity but when used with Nano CaO due to its surface structure, the basic properties increase and it becomes a proper base for the catalyst so that CaO contact surface increases and transesterification reaction yield significantly increases as well. This study investigates the repeatability of transesterification reaction in the presence of these Nano catalysts as well.

Keywords: Biodiesel production, Heterogenic Nano-catalyst, Recycled cooking oil, Transesterification reaction

Introduction

Today, the growing need for new energy sources in transportation is one of the primary challenges for different countries. Scientists are compelled to find alternatives to currently used fuels because of their decreased purification capacity; pollution caused by fossil fuels, their limited life span, and increased prices. Mono alkyl ester biodiesel is a clean diesel fuel that can be manufactured by fresh or used vegetable oils or even animal fats and waste oils. This fuel is made from renewable sources and is biodegradable [1–3]. Transesterification method or green process is one of producing biodiesels. In this method, vegetable oils are added to an alcohol (usually methanol) producing esters. It is noteworthy that glycerol is the byproduct of this reaction which greatly contributes to the pharmaceutical science and cosmetic products [4].

Parameters affecting transesterification procedure are: reaction temperature, alcohol-oil mole proportion, humidity, free fatty acids, mixing speed, alcohol type, reaction duration, catalyst type and amount [5–7]. Catalysts used in transesterification procedure are categorized into 3 groups: homogenic catalysts, heterogenic catalysts, and biocatalysts [8, 9]. The limitations of homogenic

* Correspondence: delrish.elham@gmail.com
[3]Nano-ophthalmology Department, Stem Cells Preparation Unit, Eye Research Center, Farabi Eye Hospital, Tehran University of Medical Sciences, Tehran, Iran
Full list of author information is available at the end of the article

catalysts have resulted in the dominant use of the heterogenic catalysts. Heterogenic catalysts and reactants are in separate phases and are divided into acidic and basic solid catalysts. ZrO and TiO are examples of acidic solid catalysts, while MgO and CaO are among the basic solid ones [10, 11]. It is worthy to mention that basic solid catalysts happen to be more effective than the acidic ones because they do not require high temperature and pressure, thus react more rapidly, have fewer side reactions, have no oxidation, and are more available and cost-effective [12, 13]. Heterogenic catalysts are beneficial in many ways: a) They decrease soaping problems and water usage, b) they do not mix with methanol or ethanol, c) they are easy to separate from biodiesel and glycerol, d) they are recyclable and can be reused many times, e) they are environmentally compatible and can be used in continuous and non-continuous procedures, f) they have low sensitivity to free fatty acids because of the stability of their surface microcrystal structure, and g) their quality of biodiesel is high, although they convert triglyceride to biodiesel rather slowly [14, 15].

In fact, the most important problem in producing biodiesel is its high cost which depending on the primal raw material can be 1.5 times the prices of petroleum diesel. Reports? almost 80 % of the total biodiesel cost comes from primal materials cost which are vegetable oils or animal fats. Thus, using burnt food oil decreases the related costs in producing biodiesel because of its availability and inexpensiveness. In addition, environmental pollution is lessened by recycling used cooking oils [16–18]. Used cooking oils have characteristics that make them different rather than vegetable oils or animal fats. High cooking temperature and food water hydrolyze triglycerides produce lots of free fatty acids. Reaction between these free fatty acids and water can form soaps and reduce biodiesel efficacy. Free fatty acids make up 0.5–15 % of used cooking oil weight, although the proper amount for transesterification reaction is less than 0.5 % of weight percentage [19, 20].

Basic heterogenic catalysts are divided into metallic oxides and their derivatives. CaO is one type of basic heterogenic catalysts which is most widely used for transesterification reaction because it is highly basic, and has a low solubility in methanol; it can be synthesized from inexpensive sources such as lime stone and calcium hydroxide and generates low bioenvironmental pollution. Nanocatalysts have high specific surface and degeneration activity. Other studies have shown that high specific surface and large porosity is beneficial for the catalyst to bond with the sub-layer which enhances the efficacy of transesterification reaction. One way to produce Nano CaO is to saturate lithium on CaO through wet method. It is suggested that a 12:1 proportion of methanol to oil at 65 C heat in 2 h using 5 % weight of the catalyst for esterification of jatropha oil has a yield over 99 % [21].

The first basic heterogenic catalyst in pilot scale used for transesterification reaction was MgO [18]. Other studies have indicated that MgO has a fine efficacy in non-continuous reactions. Production costs of biodiesel products in a discontinuous reactor decrease in the presence of MgO. MgO has a high yield in highly critical conditions and in a high proportion of methanol to oil [11, 22]. The following results are achieved in other studies concerning MgO catalyst (Table 1) [10].

Nano MgO exhibits a high yield for soy oil transesterification reaction in the presence of super critical methanol. This catalyst's solubility and penetration plays an essential role in enhancing the reaction efficacy, which also can be adjusted by mixing two catalysts. For instance, 90 % yield is achieved by soy oil in a 10-min reaction, using 36:1 methanol to oil ratio, 533 K temperature, 3 % weight catalyst, and 1000 rpm [23, 24].

Another tranesterification reaction was performed on cotton seed oil, in the presence of 14.4 % weight CaO-MgO catalyst, loaded on Al2O3, using 12:24 methanol to oil ratio, 95.63 °C temperature, and 97.62 % yield was achieved. Two types of commercial nanopowder calcium oxides were studied in order to discuss the transesterification reaction of canola oil: Nanopowder exhibiting a higher surface area (HSA nano-CaO) and nanopowder exhibiting a moderate surface area (nano-CaO). The effects of reaction temperature, catalyst/oil weight ratio, and methanol/oil molar ratio on the reaction's conditions were studied. The results claim that nanopowder CaOs present a higher activity than the other type, due to their larger BET surface areas. At 65 °C, 99.85 % biodiesel yield was obtained by 3 wt. % of the nano-CaO

Table 1 The efficacy of methyl ester using MgO as catalyst

Type of Oil	Surface Area (M^2/g)	Reaction's Temperature (° C)	Molar ratio Methanol/oil	Reaction's Duration (hour)	Catalyst concentration (% W/W)	Efficiency
Linseed Oil	300	Methanol-Reflux	75:1	22	10 %	64 %
Soybean Oil	36	180	12:1	1	5 %	72 %
Soybean Oil	229	180	12:1	1	5 %	90 %

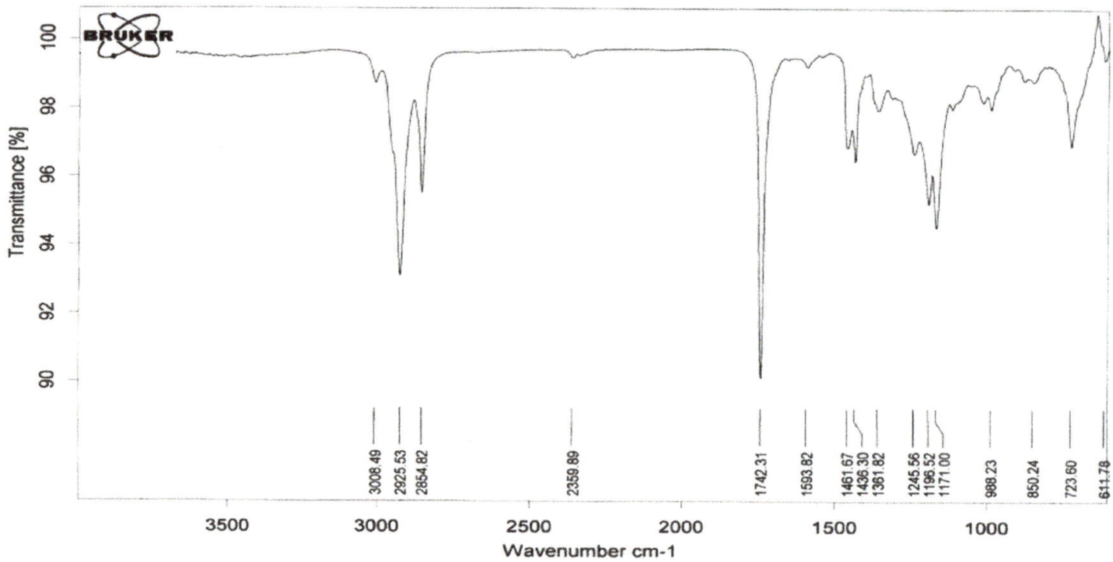

Fig. 1 Characteristics of synthetic Nano CaO: (**a**) SEM image; (**b**) XRD spectrum

catalyst, and 9:1 methanol/oil molar ratio, in 2 h. The required catalyst/oil weight ratio in order to achieve the same yield under the same conditions, was 10 times less in the HSA-nano-CaO catalyst's case [25].

In this study, Nano CaO and Nano MgO were synthesized, using sedimentation method and sol-gel self-combustion, respectively. While the next step was progressing, transesterification reaction was performed and examined in different ways with various proportions of catalyst weight and mole proportion of alcohol to oil. Also, catalyst repeatability was assessed. This study was aimed at comparing the efficacy of the reaction with and without catalysts by coupling Nano CaO and Nano MgO. Using a combination of 2 catalysts (MgO and CaO) results in an enhanced basic strength and contact surface. Subsequently, the reaction is performed more gently and is more repeatable.

Experimental

Materials

Analytical reagent (AR) grade calcium nitrate, ammonia, urea, sodium hydroxide, potassium hydroxide, magnesium sulfate, methanol, 2-propanol, and phenolphthalein were purchased from Merck. Co. Ethylene glycol and magnesium nitrate used in this study were obtained from Aldrich. Co. Moreover, home waste cooking oil was also provided. All other chemicals were obtained commercially and of analytical grade No additional purification was done on materials.

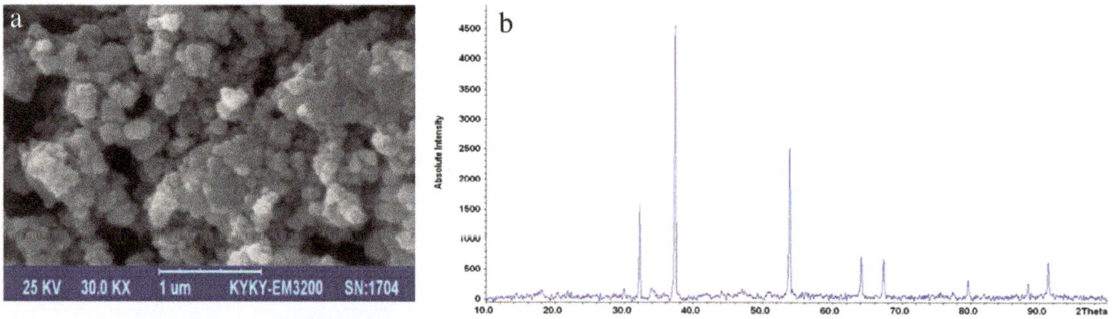

Fig. 2 Characteristics of synthetic Nano MgO: (**a**) SEM image; (**b**) XRD spectrum

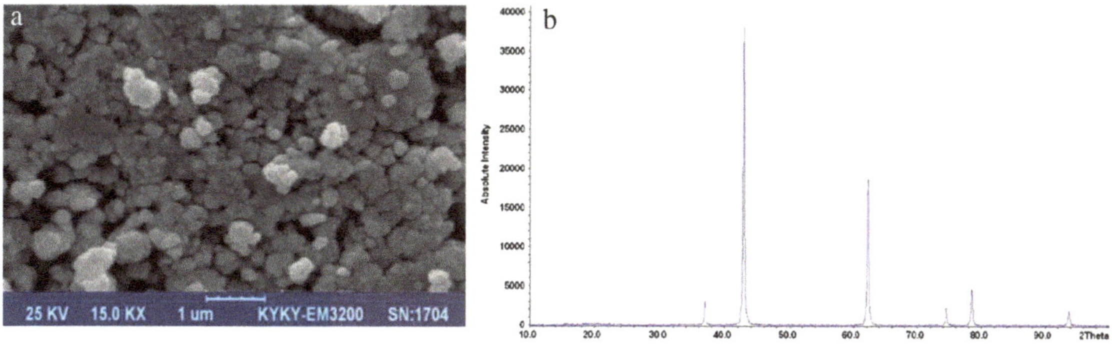

Fig. 3 Biodiesel FTIR spectrum in the presence of Nano CaO

Apparatus

Oven temperature programmed (up to 1200 C), X-ray diffraction (XRD) (STADI-P, STOE, Germany), scanning electron microscope (SEM) (Kyky 3200, China), field emission scanning electron microscope (FESEM) (S-4160, Hitachi, Japan), IKA-WERKE-EUROSTAR digital mechanical mixer (Germany, 50–2000 rpm), and Fourier transform infrared spectrometer (FTIR) (BRUKER, TENSOR2, Germany) were provided for conducting the study.

Catalyst preparation

Nano CaO synthesis using sol-gel method

Firstly, 11.81 grams calcium nitrate.$4H_2O$ was dissolved in minimum amount of water and then it was added to 25 ml of ethylene glycol being mixed by mechanical mixer. Two grams of NaOH was dissolved in 25 ml of purified water, added drop by drop, as the mixing took place. The produced mixture was mixed for 2 h so that a clear white gel was obtained. The white gel was kept still for 2 h for the reaction to complete. Then after 4 times of being washed with water, NaOH was excreted and pH was adjusted at about 10. After that, the gel was heated up to 80 °C for 2 h so that the water could be vaporized and the gel concentrated. The concentrated gel was placed in a desiccator for one hour to dry completely. The resulting dry gel was milled in the form of a white powder. The produced powder was put in the cruse and into the oven which was gradually heated up to 800 °C and stayed so for an hour for de-carbonization.

Nano MgO synthesis using sol-gel self-combustion with urea fuel

Initially, 21.58 g of magnesium nitrate.$6H_2O$ and 10.16 g of urea were dissolved in non-ionized water at the mole ration of 1:2. Ammonia was added drop by drop till pH of the mixture was 7. The system was placed in a 60–70 °C water bath and stirred by a mixer to allow the water and mobile materials present in the mixture to evaporate. As water vaporized, the solution was concentrated and became viscose. The resulting gel underwent self-combustion; as a result, it started boiling and surfaced the walls of the crucible. Subsequently, a thermo genic reaction took place and a lateritious gas was emitted. This reaction left a white porous mass. NO_3^- ions in the compound created an oxidative environment for the degradation of organic mixtures. In order to eliminate the remaining organic material, the powder from self-combustion reaction must be de-carbonized at higher temperatures. Next, the powder was fined and put in a furnace (600 °C for 2 h) to de-carbonize.

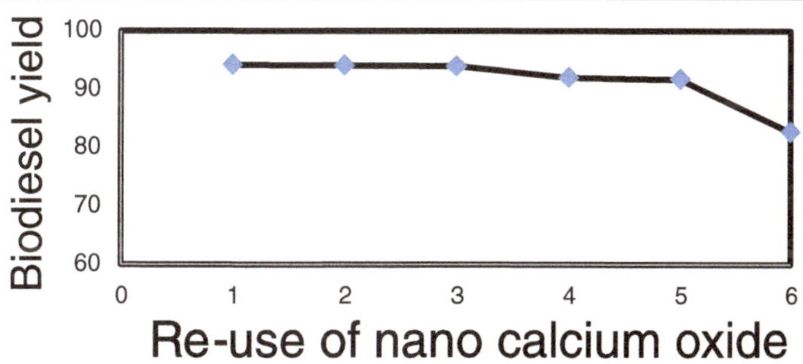

Fig. 4 The efficacy of biodiesel production in six repetitions of Nano CaO

Catalyst characterization

To investigate the structure and crystallinity of the catalysts, the X-ray diffraction analysis was conducted. Morphology and the mean particle size of the catalysts were analyzed by SEM and XRD spectrums. In addition, the microstructure was characterized by field emission scanning electron microscopy.

Transesterification reaction of cooking waste oil using methanol in presence of synthetized Nano CaO

The yield for waste cooking oil transesterification reaction in the presence of Nano CaO catalyst has been examined according to previous studies [16, 17].

Overall, 40 g of waste oil was filtered using Buchner funnel in vacuity and then 0.5 g MgSO4 was added while mixing to trap the Water mixed with oil. After filtering the waterless oil was poured into a 100 ml flask using stirrer and it was heated to 55 °C for 20 min. Then 0.4, 0.6, and 1.2 g of the catalyst and 8.76, 10.22, and 11.69 g of methanol were added to it. The heater was warmed to 75 °C so that methanol reflux was engaged. After 4 and 6 h, the mixture was moved to a decanter and over time 2 phases were shaped.

The final products of this reaction are biodiesel and combined glycerin with Nano CaO.

The upper phase was biodiesel and the lower was combined glycerin with Nano CaO.

The phases were separated and the biodiesel was returned to the decanter for washing. Then, 40mls of the 80° water was added to the biodiesel so that its pH reached 7. Moreover, the water used in this process was clear and neutral after the first washing. The produced biodiesel had some amount of water and magnesium sulfate was used to absorb it. Then the waterless biodiesel was separated from $MgSO_4$ by centrifuge. In order to check the purity, IR spectrums of biodiesel and oil were compared (Fig. 1).

The tranesterfication reaction of cooking waste oil using methanol in the presence of synthetized Nano MgO via self-combustion method

The yield for waste cooking oil transesterification reaction in the presence of Nano MgO catalyst using self-combustion was studied with alcohol-oil proportions of 1:30, 1:20, 1:12, 1:7, and 1:6 and 1.5, 3, 5 and 10 % weight catalyst during 6 and 12 h. It should be noted that yield was not sufficient in any of these conditions. Ten grams of waste oil was filtered using Buchner funnel in vacuity and then 0.5 g of magnesium sulfate was added while mixing to trap the oil water. After filtering the waterless oil was poured in a 100 ml flask with a magnet, it was heated to 55 °C for 20 min. Then 0,0.5, 1, 0.5, and 3.1 g of the catalyst and 2.2, 4.28, 10.7, 14.61, 55.19, and 95.4 g of methanol were added to it. The heater was warmed to 75 °C so that methanol reflux was engaged. After 12 h, the mixture was moved to the decanter but only a single yellow oily phase was formed under which was the catalyst.

It showed that transesterification reaction hadn't made any progress significantly in the presence of the catalyst.

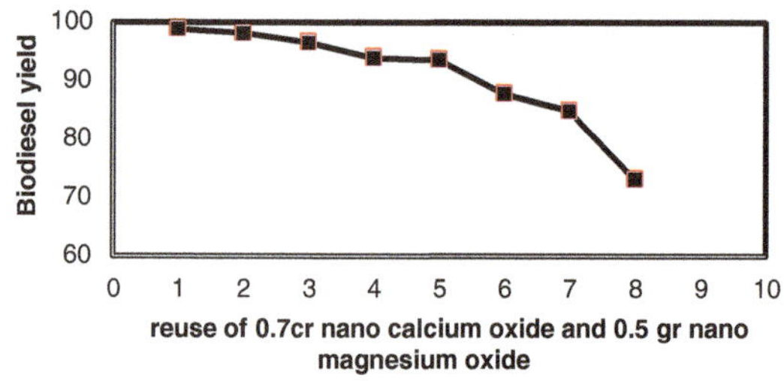

Fig. 5 The efficacy of biodiesel production in eight repetitions of CaO (0.7g)+MgO (0.5g) Nanocatalysts

The trasnesterification reaction of cooking waste oil using methanol in the presence of a combination of Nano CaO and MgO prepared by self-combustion method

The protocol for preparing oil was the same as what was explained earlier in this article only with the difference that here, 3 % weight of self-combustion combination of the catalysts, MgO and CaO, and 7:1 oil to alcohol proportion were used. The 3 % weight meant 1.2 g of the catalysts mixture which was generated by changing the mass proportion of the two catalysts of the transesterification reaction.

Recycling of catalyst

Recycling Nano CaO catalyst and evaluating its repeatability in waste cooking oil transesterification reaction

After transesterification reaction and separation of the biodiesel from glycerol and the catalyst, the remaining catalyst was washed away with n-Hexane and placed in a 70° oven for 2 h to dry. In the next step oil preparation and the reaction procedure were done as described. The catalyst could be used up to six times.

Table 2 The three main agent groups of biodiesel

Frequency (cm^{-1})	The Functional Group	Type of Vibration	Intensity
1436	-O-CH_3	Bending	Moderate
1196.52	-O-CH_3	Rocking	Moderate
1171	-C-O-(CH_3)	Stretching motions symmetric	High

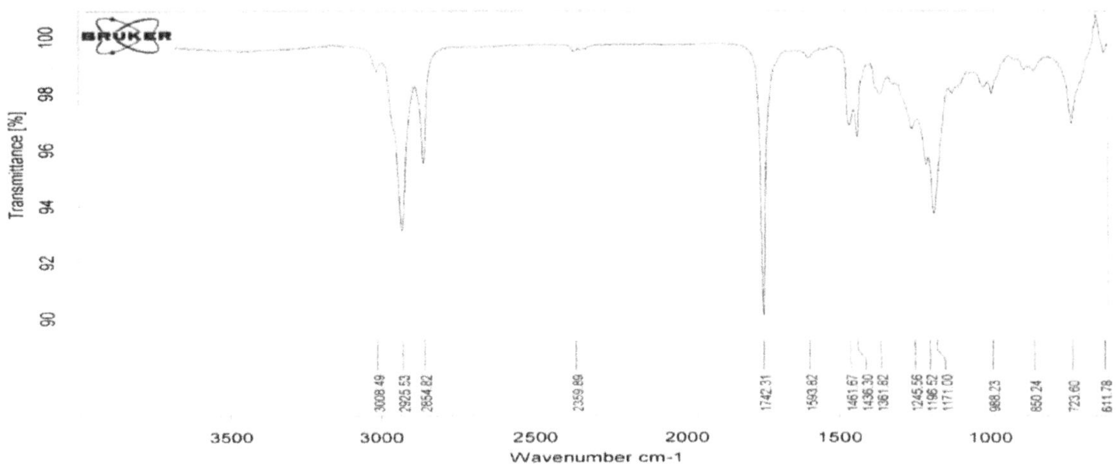

Fig. 6 Biodiesel FTIR spectrum in the presence of 0.7g of Nano CaO and 0.5g of Nano MgO

Recycling the catalysts Nano CaO (0.7 g) and self-combustion Nano MgO (0.5 g) and their repeatability in waste cooking oil transesterification

After transesterification reaction and separation of the biodiesel from glycerol and the catalyst, the remaining catalyst was washed away with n-hexane and it was placed in a 70° oven for 2 h to dry. In the next step, oil preparation and the reaction procedure were done as described earlier in this article. The catalyst mixture presented a repeatability of up to eight times.

Results

Catalyst characterization

SEM images indicated a spherical shape for the Nanoparticles (NPs) and CaO and MgO NPs were determined to be 65 and 70 nm in size. The application of XRD showed that the crystal structure of the particles was cubic. Additionally, the comparison of the obtained peaks and source peaks indicated that the Cao NPs were synthesized and average particle size was calculated 61 nm according to Scherer's equation (Fig. 2a, b). Also, the comparison of the obtained peaks and source peaks indicated that the Mgo NPs were synthesized and average particle size was calculated 69 nm according to Scherer's equation (Fig. 3a, b).

Effect of Catalyst Compound on biodiesel yield

Waste cooking oil transesterification reaction yield in the presence of synthesized Nano CaO catalyst

As described earlier in Section 2.5.1, this reaction was performed using different proportions of methanol to oil and various catalyst weight percentages. The results showed that 1:7 mol proportion for alcohol to oil and 1.5 % weight catalyst over 6 h are the optimum conditions for this reaction. Biodiesel production mass yield is 94.37 % in these optimum conditions (Table 3).

Waste cooking oil transesterification reaction yield in the presence of synthesized Nano MgO catalyst

Following the methods described in Section 2.5.2, this reaction was performed using different proportions of methanol to oil and various catalyst weight percentages. Nevertheless, transesterification reaction did not significantly progress in the presence of this catalyst.

Table 3 The efficacy of biodiesel production in the presence of synthetic Nano CaO catalyst

The Amount of Oil (gr)	The Catalyst Compound	Alcohol: Oil Mole Ratio	Mass Percent of the Catalyst Compound	Reaction's Duration (hr)	Mass Efficiency
40	CaO	6:1	1 %	4	78.35
40	CaO	6:1	1.5 %	4	80.12
40	CaO	6:1	3 %	4	80.18
40	CaO	7:1	1.5 %	4	92.39
40	CaO	7:1	3 %	4	92.33
40	CaO	8:1	1.5 %	4	92.36
40	CaO	7:1	1.5 %	6	94.37

Table 4 The efficacy of methyl ester using CaO as catalyst for 15 min

Type of Oil	Reaction's Temperature (° C)	Molar ratio Methanol/oil	Catalyst concentration (% W/W)	Efficiency
Linseed Oil	Methanol-Reflux	4.5 : 1	0.8	10 %
Linseed Oil	192	41.1 : 1	3	50 %

Waste cooking oil transesterification reaction yield in the presence of 3 % combined Nano CaO and self-combustion Nano MgO catalysts and alcohol to oil mole proportion of 1:7

Waste cooking oil transesterification reaction yield in the presence of combined oxide catalysts was studied and it indicated that by combining Nano CaO and self-combustion Nano MgO with the 3 % weight percentage and alcohol to oil mole proportion of 1:7 over 6 hours, biodiesel production mass yield rose by increasing CaO mass proportion to MgO. These studies show that although self-combustion Nano MgO does not help the transesterification reaction while combined with Nano CaO, it increases the biodiesel production mass yield. The optimum mass proportion for CaO to MgO is 0.7:0.5 that gives a mass yield of 98.95 %. Results given in Table 3 show the progressive biodiesel production mass yield increased with Nano CaO to self-combustion Nano MgO with mass proportion change (Table 5).

Recycling of catalyst

Waste cooking oil transesterification reaction with Nano CaO repeatability

After transesterification reaction in the presence of CaO the catalyst was separated from the main products and washed away with n-hexane and put in a 70° oven to dry. Then in optimum conditions of the reaction, repeatability was evaluated. The results and the number of repetitions are shown in Fig. 4.

Waste cooking oil transesterification reaction repeatability with Nano CaO and Nano MgO catalyst by the proportion of 0.7–0.5 g

When the optimum mass proportion for CaO to self-combustion MgO was determined and transesterification was over, the combination of the catalysts was separated from the main product and washed with n-hexane, then it was placed in a 70° oven to dry. Eventually, repeatability was determined for the catalyst mixture in optimum conditions. The results and number of repetitions are shown in Fig. 5.

FTIR analysis

IR spectrum for methyl esters (biodiesel) is somewhat similar to oil spectrum and it rarely has some differences in the finger print area. As the only change in oil structure is the exit of glycerol and substituting methanol in hydrocarbon chain, methyl ester IR spectrum is much like triglyceride oils and the most variations are in 1000–1500 area by which can be verified by the complete synthesis of the biodiesel. The three main effective groups are shown in Table 2.

In addition, the lack of -OH spectrum near 3500 region implies that the transesterification reaction is performed completely and lack of intermediate compounds like free fatty acids and mono and diglycerids can be also rationalized (Fig. 5). The resulting spectrum showed that transesterification did not make any progress much in the presence of Mgo Nanocatalyst and the three main effective groups were not recognizable in the spectrum. Additionally, transesterification in the presence of catalyst mixture progressed completely and the three main effective groups emerged in the spectrum (Fig. 6).

Discussion

During the first step of tranesterification reaction in the presence of Nano CaO, proton is absorbed from methanol by means of basic sections available in Nano CaO structure. This reaction results in meth oxide anion formation. Meth oxide group holds an oxygen molecule within its structure which attacks carbon from triglyceride-fatty acid's carbonyl group, resulting in alkoxycarbonyl formation as an intermediate structure. Alkoxycarbonyl transfroms itself into more stable products: fatty acid methyl ester and diglyceride. As the transformation continues, diglyceride converts to monoglyceride and fatty acid methyl ester. During the third step, monoglyceride undergoes the same reaction and produces glycerin and fatty acid methyl ester. In conclusion, fatty acid tri-methyl ester and glycerin are the final products of the reaction. The summarized version of reaction is provided below:

R1,R2,R3 = fatty acid carbonic chain

Table 5 The efficacy of biodiesel production in the presence of CaO + MgO Nanocatalyst

The Amount of Oil (gr)	The Catalyst Compound	Alcohol: Oil Mole Ratio	Mass Percent of the Catalyst Compound	Reaction's Duration (hr)	Mass Efficiency
40	CaO + MgO	7.1	0.5 g CaO+ 0.7 g MgO = 3 %	6	90.85
40	CaO + MgO	7:1	0.6 g CaO+ 0.6 g MgO = 3 %	6	96.22
40	CaO + MgO	7:1	0.7 g CaO+ 0.5 g MgO = 3 %	6	98.95
40	CaO + MgO	7:1	0.9 g CaO+ 0.3 g MgO = 3 %	6	98.57

Table 6 Standard test results for biodiesel were produced from waste cooking oil in the presence of combined Nano CaO and self-combustion Nano MgO catalyst 0.7:0.5 compared to D675-01 ASTM and EN14217

Property	The Standard Value	The Permissive Range	The Measured Value
Flash Point	D93	Minimum Value:130	150 (° C)
Kinematic Viscosity in 40° C	D445	1.6–9	4.8 mm^2/s
Cetane Number	D613	Minimum Value:47	48
Saponification Number	D460	Indefinite	190.70
Freezing Point	-	-	−7 (° C)
Ignition Point	-	-	220 (° C)
Cloud Point	D2500	Indefinite	4 (° C)
Pour Point	ISO3016	Maximum Value:0	−5 (° C)
Iodine Number	EN14111	Maximum Value:130	124.48
Density	EN ISO 3675	0.86–0.89 (gr/cm^3)	0.89 (gr/cm^3)

Alcohol's alkali group = R4

Nano CaO provides us with a better efficacy and using waste cooking oil is more cost-effective [16]. Optimum conditions for this catalyst is 1:7 methanol to oil, in six hours and 1.5 % of catalyst's weight at which biodiesel production yield is 94.37 % of weight (Table 3).

In 2008, Kouzu M. released an article, concerning Calcium oxide as a solid base catalyst for transesterification of soybean oil and its contribution to biodiesel production.

Soy fatty acid methyl ester production yield in the presence of CaO is reported 93 % in one-hour time duration and methanol-oil mole proportion of 12:1 [26, 27]. In 2010, Man kee Lam provided an article, concerning Homogeneous, heterogeneous and enzymatic catalysis for transesterification of hight free fatty acid oil (waste cooking oil) to biodiesel.

It was observed that when using 0.85 g CaO and under same conditions, yield decreases to 66 % [28]. Results obtained from different studies for CaO indicate that (Table 4):

By comparing obtained results from this survey, and other conducted surveys, it can be concluded that Nano CaO can enhance trans esterification reaction's efficacy more than CaO owing to its high contact area. Repeatability of Nano CaO and the ability of reusing this catalyst were also discussed. As the results indicate, repeatability of this catalyst was satisfactory (Fig. 4).

Nano MgO is not catalyzing the transesterification by itself, but when used with Nano CaO transesterification reaction yield significantly increases. By enhancing MgO's catalytic strength and basic strength, the reaction is performed in more gentle conditions (Table 5).

The comparison of the obtained values with the standard tests indicates that they all fall within the normal range and as a result, this biodiesel is viable (Table 6).

Conclusions

As the results indicate, Nano CaO provides us with a better efficacy, reaction duration, repeatability, used catalyst weight percentage, methanol amount, and biodiesel production mass yield in comparison with self-combustion Nano MgO, due to its basic nature. Nano MgO is not capable of catalyzing the transesterification by itself, because it has a much weaker basic affinity but when used with Nano CaO due to its surface structure, the basic properties increase and it becomes a proper base for the catalyst so that CaO contact surface increases and transesterification reaction yield significantly increases as well. Needless to say that higher proportions of Nano CaO to Nano MgO lead to increase in biodiesel production mass yield. The optimum condition for this catalyst is 1:7 methanol to oil (the same ratio which is applied for Nano CaO), 6 h and 0.7 g of Nano CaO plus 0.5 g of Nano MgO which gives the yield of 98.95 % of weight. Moreover, combined catalyst repeatability is better than Nano CaO alone. In addition, using waste cooking oil is more cost-effective.

Competing interests

The authors declare that they have no competing interests.

Authors' contributions

KT have designed of the study and participated in its Conception, data analysis and interpretation, Obtained funding, and final approval of the article. YNA carried out the experiments and data collection and helped to draft the manuscript. RF participated in analysis and interpretation of data. SM participated in data collection. ED coordination and helped to data analysis, Writing the article, and Critical revision of the manuscript. All authors read and approved the final manuscript.

Acknowledgements

We gratefully acknowledge the Department of Chemistry of North Tehran Branch of Islamic Azad University for financial and technical supports.

Author details

[1]Department of chemistry, Islamic Azad University, North Tehran Branch, Tehran, Iran. [2]Modeling and Optimization Research Center in Science and Engineering, Islamic Azad University, South Tehran Branch, Tehran, Iran. [3]Nano-ophthalmology Department, Stem Cells Preparation Unit, Eye Research Center, Farabi Eye Hospital, Tehran University of Medical Sciences, Tehran, Iran.

References

1. Murugesan A, Umarani C, Subramanian R, Nedunchezhian N. Biodiesel as an alternative fuel for diesel engines A review. Renewable Sustain Energy Rev. 2009;13:653–62.
2. Xie W, Li H. Alumni-supported potassium iodide as a heterogeneous catalyst for biodiesel production from soybean oil. J Mol Catal A Chem. 2006;255:1–9.
3. Xie W, Peng H, Chen L. Transesterification of soybean oil catalyzed by potassium loaded on alumina as a solid-base catalyst. Appl Catal A Gen. 2006;300:67–74.
4. Singh Chouhan AP, Sarma AK. Modern heterogeneous catalysts for biodiesel production. Renew Sust Energ Rev. 2011;15(4):78–4399.
5. Feng Y, Zhang A, Li J, He B. A continuous process for biodiesel production in a fixed bed reactor packed with cation-exchange resin as heterogeneous catalyst. Bioresour Technol. 2011;102:3607–9. ISSN 0960-8524.
6. Agarwal AK. Biofuels (alcohols biodiesel) applications as fuels for internal combustion engines. Prog Energy Combust Sci. 2007;33:233–71.
7. Dossin TF, Reyniers MF, Marin FB. Kinetics of Heterogeneously MgOCatalyzed Transesterification. Appl Catal B Environ. 2006;62:35–45. ISSN 0926-3373.
8. Dossin TF, Reyniers MF, Berger RJ, Marin GB. Simulation of heterogeneously MgO-catalyzed transesterification for fine-chemical and biodiesel industrial production. Appl Catal B Environ. 2006;67:136–48. ISSN: 0926-3373.
9. Wen G, YAN Z. Transesterification of soybean oil to Biodiesel over kalsilite catalyst. Chem Sci Eng. 2011;5(3):325–9.
10. Diserio M, Tesser R, Pengmei L. Heterogeneous catalysts for biodiesel production. Energy Fuel. 2008;22:207–17.
11. Dossin TF, Reyniers MF, Marin GB. Simulation of heterogeneously Mgo-Catalyzed transerterification for fine chemical andbiodiesal industrial production. Appl Catal B. 2006;67:136–48.
12. Lam MK, Lee KT. Homogeneous, heterogeneous and enzymatic catalysis for transesterification of hight free fatty acid oil (wast cooking oil) to biodiesel: Areview. Biotechnol Adv. 2010;28:500–18.
13. Kovacheva P, Arishtirova K, Vassilev S. MgO/NaX zeolite as basic catalyst for oxidative methylation of toluene with methane. Appl Catal A Gen. 2001;210:391–5. ISSN 0926-860X.
14. Yan S, DiMaggiom C. Advancements in Heterogeneous Catalsysis for Biodiesel Synthesis. Top Catal. 2010;53:721–36.
15. Bournay L, Casanave D, Delfort B, Hillion G, Chodorge JA. New heterogeneous process for biodiesel production: A way to improve the quality and the value of the crude glycerin produced by biodiesel plants. Catal Today. 2005;106:190–2. ISSN 0920-5861.
16. Zhang Y, Ma D, Mclean DD, Kates M. Biodiesel Production from waste cooking oil. Bioresour Technol. 2003;90:229–40.
17. Demirbas A. Biodiesel from sunflower oil in supercritical methanol with calcium oxide. Energy Conv Manag. 2007;48:937–41.
18. Issariyakul T, Kulkarne MG, Meher LC, Dalai AK, Bakhshi NN. Biodiesel production from mixtures of canola oil and used cooking oil. Chem Eng J. 2007;140:77–85.
19. Encinar JM, Gonzalez JF. Biodiesel from used frying oil. Variables Affecting the yields and characteristics of biodiesel. Eny Chem Res. 2005;44:5491–9.
20. Gerhard knothe JVG, Krahl J. The biodiesel hand book. Champaign: AOCS Press; 2004.
21. Kaur N, Amjad A. Lithium ion impregnated calcium oxide as Nano catalyst for the biodiesel production from karanj a and jatropha oils. Renewale Energy. 2011;36:2866–71.
22. Diserio M, Tesser R, Nasatasi M. Synthesis of biodiesel via homogeneous lewis acid catalysts. J Mol Catal. 2005;239:111–5.
23. Wang L, Yang J. Transesterification of soybean oil with noano-Mgo or not in super critical and subcritical methanol. Fuel. 2007;86:328–33.
24. Mahdavi V, Monajemi A. Optimization of operational conditions for biodiesel production from cottonseed oil on CaO–MgO/Al2O3 solid base catalysts. J Taiwan Inst Chem Eng. 2014;45(5):2286–92.
25. Zhao L, Qiu Z, Stagg-Williams SM. Transesterification of canola oil catalyzed by nanopowder calcium oxide. Fuel Process Technol. 2013;114:154–62.
26. Kouzu M, Kasuno T, Tajika M, Yamanaka S, Hidaka J. Calcium oxide as a solid base catalyst for transesterification of soybean oil and its application to biodiesel production. Fuel. 2008;87:2798–806.
27. Granados ML, Poves MDZ, Alonso DM, Mariscal R, Galisteo FC, Santamaria J, et al. Biodiesel from sunflower oil byusing activated calcium oxide. Appl Catal B Environ. 2007;73:317–26.
28. Mk L, Lee KT. Homogeneous, heterogeneous and enzymatic catalysis for transesterification of hight free fatty acid oil (wast cooking oil) to biodiesel: Areview. Biotechnol Adv. 2010;28:500–18.

15

Cadmium removal from aqueous solution by green synthesis iron oxide nanoparticles with tangerine peel extract

Mohammad Hassan Ehrampoush[1], Mohammad Miria[1], Mohammad Hossien Salmani[1*] and Amir Hossein Mahvi[2]

Abstract

Background: The adsorption process by metal oxide nanoparticles has been investigated an effective agent for removing organic and inorganic contaminants from water and wastewater. In this study, iron oxide nanoparticles were synthesized in the presence of tangerine peel extract as adsorbent for cadmium ions removal from contaminated solution. Iron oxide nanoparticles prepared by co-precipitation method and tangerine peel extract was used to prevent accumulation and reduce the diameter of the particles. Effect of various parameters such as contact time, pH, metal concentration and adsorbent dosage was determined on the removal efficiency.

Results: The different concentrations of tangerine peel had an impact on the size of nanoparticles. As, increasing the concentration of tangerine peel extract from 2 to 6 % the average size of synthesized iron oxide nanoparticles decreased 200 nm to 50 nm. The maximum removal of cadmium ions (90 %) occurred at pH of 4 and adsorbent dose of 0.4 g/100 ml. Adsorption of cadmium ions by synthesized iron oxide nanoparticles followed Freundlich adsorption model and pseudo-second-order equation.

Conclusion: The cadmium ions are usually soluble in acidic pH and the maximum removal of cadmium by green synthesis iron oxide nanoparticles was obtained in the pH of 4, so these nanoparticles can be a good adsorbent for the removal of cadmium from wastewater.

Keywords: Iron oxide nanoparticles, Cadmium removal, Tangerine peel extract

Background

Cadmium usually is a trace ion in the ground water and surface water. It may be hydrated ions, complexes - such as inorganic carbonate, hydroxide, chloride, sulfate, or as organic complexes with humic acids in water [1]. The high levels of cadmium in water may be existed in the plating and coating of pipes and fittings, soldering with silver-coated tubes places [2]. Cadmium is toxic for animals and human, and recently, much attention has been on the long-term risk factors for general population health that are affected by cadmium. Cadmium can be introduced to body via inhalation, ingestion or absorption through the skin and affects on the body organs. The effects of short-term exposure on cadmium include: nausea, vomiting, diarrhea, muscle cramps, dry mouth, impaired senses, liver damage, convulsions, shock and renal defects, influences on the lung and the cardiovascular system, liver, and nervous system [3, 4]. Long-term effects of exposure on cadmium include the impacts on the lungs, kidneys, bones, growth and carcinogenic. Plants, fruits and vegetables are grown in the fertile soil with superphosphate fertilizer relation to the soil has higher levels of cadmium. The daily intake cadmium for the average person weighing 70 kg was estimated 25–60 μg by The United States of America and Europe [5]. The WHO is recommended maximum allow of 10 μg/L cadmium ion in drinking water sources [6]. Therefore, in recent years, considerable attention has been devoted to the study of effective methods to remove low concentrations of cadmium in contaminated water.

When cadmium concentration in contaminated water is less than 0.5 mg/L, treatment of water by conventional methods such as precipitation with lime and treatment with alum and ferric sulfate is not suitable to remove it

* Correspondence: mhsn06@yahoo.com
[1]Department of Environmental Health, School of Public Health, Shahid Sadoughi University of Medical Science, Yazd, Iran
Full list of author information is available at the end of the article

and also is less effective [7]. Most researchers has proposed ion exchange, reverse osmosis, coagulation-filtration and adsorption processes as the best available technology for effective removal of cadmium to the 0.005 mg/L or 5 ppb [3, 8]. However, most of these methods have disadvantages such as expensive devices, production of toxic sludge or other waste materials, space and high energy requirements. Among these methods, adsorption has attracted the attention of many researches because it is a simple, low-cost, and effective for the removal of heavy metal ions in low and medium concentrations [9]. A number of minerals, clays, and waste materials were regularly used to remove heavy metals from water and wastewater [10]. Recently, it emphasized that the nanoparticles and nanostructure sorbents can be used as an efficient and convenient replacement instead of conventional adsorbents [11, 12]. Adsorption of metal ions on iron nanoparticles is an environmentally friendly technology that it has been studied as an effective agent for removing organic contaminants and heavy metal ions from water and wastewater [13–21].

Number various methods studied to synthesis of nanoparticles such as: co-precipitation, sol-gel synthesis, micro emulsion, and the oxidation of nanoparticles [22]. The chemical co-precipitation of ferric and ferrous ions in the alkaline solution is a commonly and large scale amount for synthesis of iron oxide nanoparticles [23]. During the separation of particles from bulk of solution, nanoparticle will lead to aggregation under Vander Waals force. The synthesis nanoparticles to agglomeration which converts a greater particles size in diameter. For prevention of agglomeration, it often used a surface modification using inorganic or organic material [24]. Most of water soluble polymers or surfactants can often be used a good dispersion or capping agent, but they are toxic for environment. In this study, tangerine peel extract a green material was applied to synthesis of iron oxide nanoparticles by co-precipitation methods and then these nanoparticles were used to remove cadmium ions from aqueous solutions. This method dose not required organic solvent for prevention of agglomeration that nanoparticles with an average diameter size of 50 nm can be produced in an aqueous peel extract solution. Also, this approach is entirely friendly environment and is not an environment pollutant.

Methods

Tangerine Peel Extract

Tangerine peel was collected from the local market at Yazd city. These washed with distillated water to clean the surface pollutants and dried in the air and absence of sunlight at the Lab. temperature (27 ± 2 °C). The dried peels were milled by electric milling and sieved to powders. 50 g of powders were introduced to 500 ml of distilled water in the beaker and heated to 80 °C for 15 min. After cooling to Lab. temperature filtered with 0.45 μ filter paper. This solution as capping agent was maintained in the refrigerator for further use.

Preparation of nanoparticles

The co-precipitation method was used to prepare nanoparticles [25, 26]. For this purpose, 5.35 g of $FeCl_3$ and 8.10 g of $FeCl_2.4H_2O$ were separately dissolved in 500 ml of different concentration of extract peel to form a solution with the concentration of 0.1 M for Fe(III) and Fe(II) in presence of extract peel as surfactant and stabilizer. Then two solutions were mixed a ratio of 40–60 ml and raised it to 80 °C using an electric heater. Finally, NH_4OH solution 25 % was dropped to this solution with extremely string at least 20 min until the final pH was came over than 9. The brown precipitate collected by magnetic piece and washed three times with distilled water. The treatment precipitant was dried at Lab. temperature at 1 week. Scanning electron microscopy (SEM) and dynamic light scattering (DLS) were used to specify nanoparticles size. These iron oxide nanoparticles were used to study of removal cadmium ions from aqueous solutions.

Adsorption process

To obtain different concentrations of working and standard solution of cadmium ions, the stock solution of 1 g/l of cadmium ions was prepared with pure cadmium nitrate Cd $(NO_3)_2.4H_2O$ and distilled water. Experiments were performed on four periods (15, 30, 60, 90 min), three levels of pH (2, 4, 6.5), four different concentrations of cadmium ions (5, 10, 15, 20 mg/l), and three levels of absorbent dose (0.2, 0.4, 0.6 gr/100 ml). Then cadmium ions solution contacted with the adsorbent, shake at specified time on the 120 rpm orbital shaker, separated by a piece of magnet, and centrifuged in the 5000 rpm. In the end of each experiment, the residual cadmium concentration in solution was determinate.

Data analysis

The remaining concentration of cadmium in clear solution was determined using of atomic absorption spectrometer (spectra model AA-20). For this purpose, different concentration (0.0, 2.0, 5.0, 8.0 and 10.0 mg/l) standard solutions of Cd^{2+} were prepared from stock solution of 100 mg/l and used for calibration of AA. Absorbance was recorded three fold at wavelength 228.8 nm and 0.5 nm in a standard mode and concentration of cadmium was calculated from Beer-Lambert equation. The removal efficiency of nanoparticles and adsorption capacity was calculated from experimental data as eqs. (1 and 2).

$$\% \text{ RE} = \frac{(C_0 - C)}{C_0} \times 100 \quad (1)$$

$$q_e = \frac{(C_0 - C)}{m} \times V \quad (2)$$

After determining of adsorption data, using linear equations related to isotherm and kinetic models, modeling of Cd^{2+} adsorption study on the synthesized iron oxide nanoparticles were determined.

Results and Discussion

Characterization of synthesized iron oxide nanoparticles

Iron oxide nanoparticles were prepared in the presence of various concentrations of tangerine peel extract (2, 4, 6, 8, and 10 %) that the size of them was controlled using scanning electron microscopy (SEM) and also the range size of produced particles was determined by dynamic light scattering (DLS). Average size of nanoparticles was about 200 nm at 2 % concentration of tangerine peel extract. As well as, the same average was obtained when tangerine peel extract increased to concentration of 4 %. While the tangerine peel extract reached to a concentration of 6 %, a significant decrease in the size of the iron oxide nanoparticles were appeared, so an average size was about 50 nm. Tangerine peel extract concentration of 10 % indicates severe aggregation and significant increasing in the size of the nanoparticles that the average size of nanoparticle was reached to 1 µ. Figure 1a, b shows the SEM and DLS of prepared nanoparticles at optimal conditions that was 6 % of tangerine peel extract.

Tangerine peel extract was used to prepare iron oxide nanoparticles as well as to reduce the impact on average nanoparticles size for increasing of its removal efficiency. The results showed that the concentration of tangerine peel extract can affect the nanoparticles size. So that with increasing concentration of tangerine peel extract from 2 to 6 %, the average size of nanoparticle reach out about 200 nm to 50 nm and the increasing

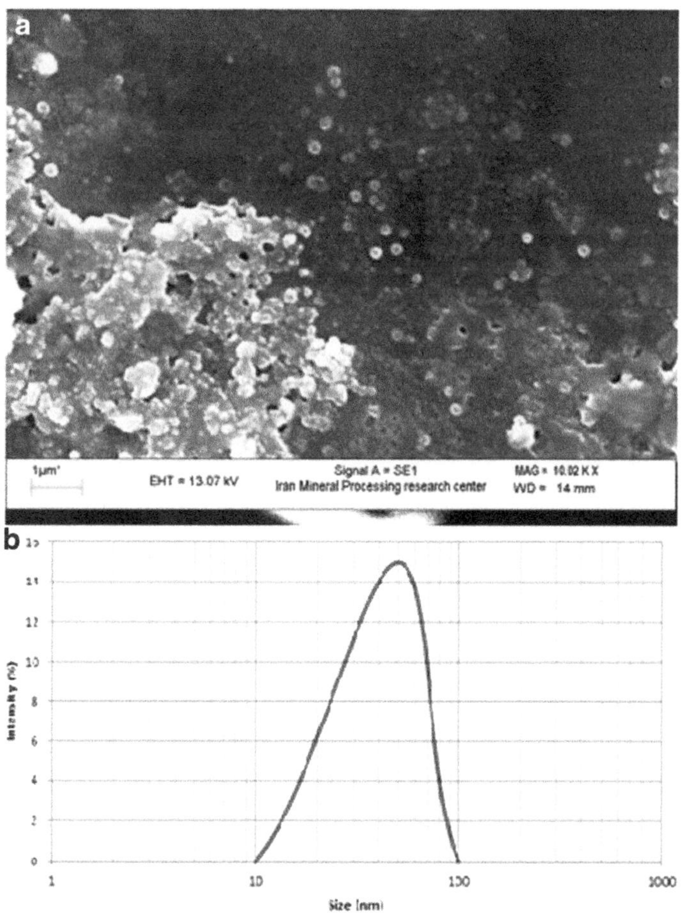

Fig. 1 Characterization of synthesized iron oxide nanoparticles **a**) SEM image **b**) Size distribution by DLS

concentration of tangerine peel extract continued up to 10 % the size of nanoparticles rose again due to the strong adhesion of nanoparticles. The tangerine peel extract concentration of 6 % is optimal for the production of iron oxide nanoparticles. Over the last few years, several synthetic methods have been focused on produce of controlled size nanoparticles and enhance to produce regular shape [27]. From SEM image predicted that iron oxide nanoparticles synthesized by tangerine peel extract of 6 % yield relatively uniform spherical shape in average range 50 nm that calculated from DLS micrograph. So, it seems that different agglomeration can occur depending on the used concentration of peel extract, which directly influences the size of particles.

Also, the synthesized iron oxide nanoparticles in presence of tangerine peel extract applied to remove of Cd^{2+} in aqueous solution. For obtaining the best condition, several experiments were done by variation of effective parameters such as contact time, pH, initial concentration and adsorbent dosage in a batch system.

The effect of contact time

The effect of contact time on cadmium removal efficiency by iron oxide nanoparticles synthesized in the presence of tangerine peel extract was investigated in an initial concentration of 5 mg/l of cadmium ions at 15, 30, 60 and 90 min. During this phase, adsorbent mass was 0.4 g/100 ml and the solution pH adjusted to 4. The effect of contact time is shown in Fig. 2. As observed, the removal rate increases with time so the optimal time is about 90 min for the best removal and this time was chosen to subsequent experiments.

According to Fig. 2, with increasing contact time, cadmium ion removal efficiency increases, because of cadmium ions are more opportunities for contact with the adsorbent surface when time increases. As can be seen from Fig. 2, the rate of cadmium ions removal was fast in the beginning times (first 15 min) due to the larger surface area of the adsorbent available. As time increases to 90 min, more amount of cadmium ions adsorb onto the surface of the adsorbent by attraction forces and cause a complete removal of cadmium ions. Therefor, the equilibrium time for this absorbent is about 90 min. Kosa et al. (2012) have been studied as heavy metals removal using carbon nanotubes modified with 8-hydroxyl-quinoline. Their results showed that removal efficiency was increased by enhancing the contact time between the adsorbent and cadmium ions. The maximum absorption occurred in the first 10 min that the results of this study are in line with the present study results [28].

The effect of solution pH on Cd^{2+} removal

pH is the most important factor in the absorption process. In this study, the effect of pH on cadmium removal efficiency by prepared iron oxide nanoparticles was determined in the absorption process at pH 2, 4, and 6.5. For each experiment, the 0.4 g of adsorbent was added into the 100 ml initial cadmium concentration of 5 mg/l at each above adjusted initial pH. After a contact time of 90 min, residual concentrations of cadmium ions in the solution were measured and the removal efficiency was calculated based on the results. The results are presented in Fig. 3. The optimum pH for removal efficiency of cadmium was 4 that were used in the following experiments.

Figure 3 revealed that the removal efficiency is lower at high acidic pH. It seems that the positive charge on the adsorbent is created in the acidic pH. So, there is an electrostatic repulsion between the adsorbent and cadmium ions in solution. The hydrogen ions instead of cadmium ions are placed in to the adsorbent sites when the amount of hydrogen ions increases in solution, and so the removal efficiency decreases. This study showed that changing of pH from 2 to 4, the removal efficiency increases but it has a decreasing trend. The similar observation was obtained in our previous study [29] . The zinc oxide nanoparticles were used for the removal of cadmium at high ionic strength solution that with a change in pH from 4 to 5, the removal efficiency of cadmium increased in a great deal, and when the pH increased to 7, the removal efficiency of cadmium has had

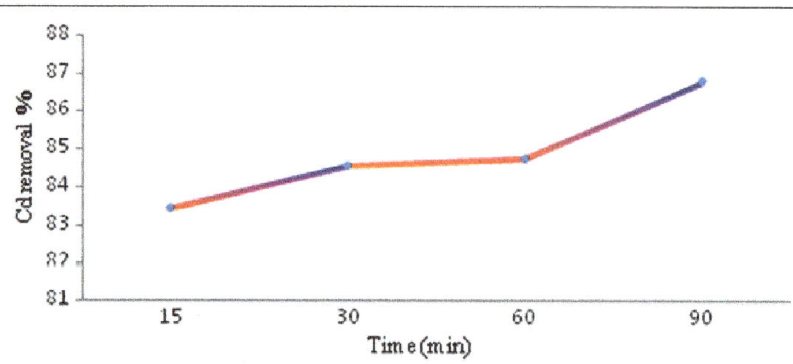

Fig. 2 The effect of contact time on the Cd removal efficiency

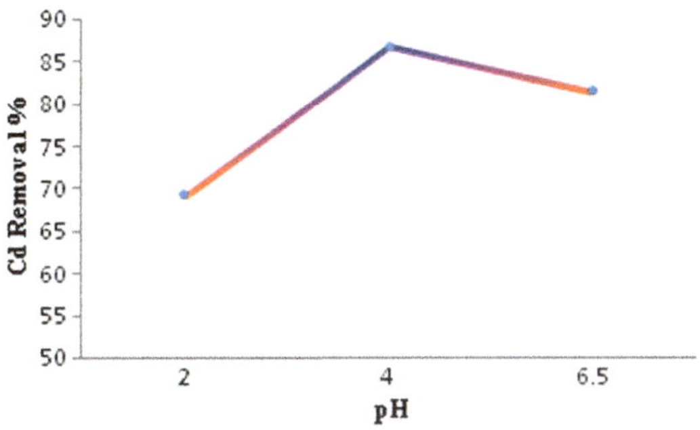

Fig. 3 The effect of pH on the Cd removal efficiency

a gradual increase. Thus, the highest removal efficiency gained in pH = 7 that was 89.6 %, and the lowest efficiency measured as 38 % in pH = 4.

A study conducted by Afkhami et al. (2010), The alumina nanoparticles modified with 2, 4-di-nitro phenyl hydrazine was used to remove heavy metals such as Pb (II), Cd (II), Cr (III), Co (II), Ni (II) and Mn (II). The specific effect of pH was determined to change of pH 1.5–5.5 ranges. The results showed that removal efficiency increases up to pH of 5 and then decreases with excess of pH up to 5. These results are in line with the present study [30]. The obtained results of the present study are in line with the mentioned research findings.

The effect of initial concentration on Cd^{2+} removal

Effect of initial cadmium concentration on the removal efficiency was investigated in the pH = 4, the mass of nanoparticles 0.4 g/100 ml solution with a concentration 5, 10, 15, and 20 mg/L of cadmium ions. The results are shown in Fig. 4. As observed, with increasing cadmium concentration of 5–20 mg/L, the removal efficiency is increased from 87 to 88.7 %.

An increased ratio of initial number of cadmium ions to the available surface area resulted in high concentration; hence fractional adsorption dependent on initial concentration. For a given adsorbent dose the total

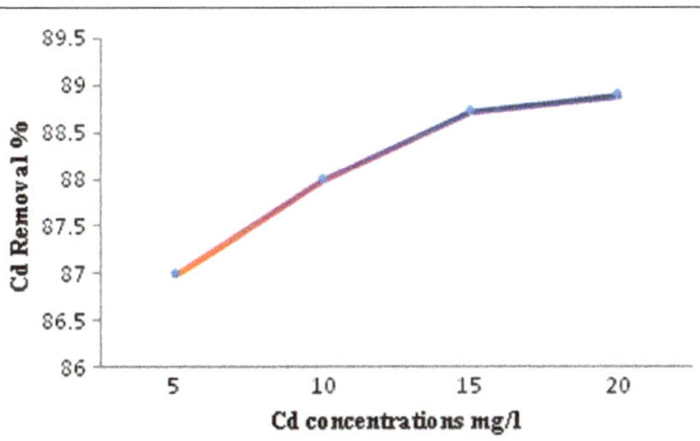

Fig. 4 The effect of initial concentration on the Cd removal efficiency

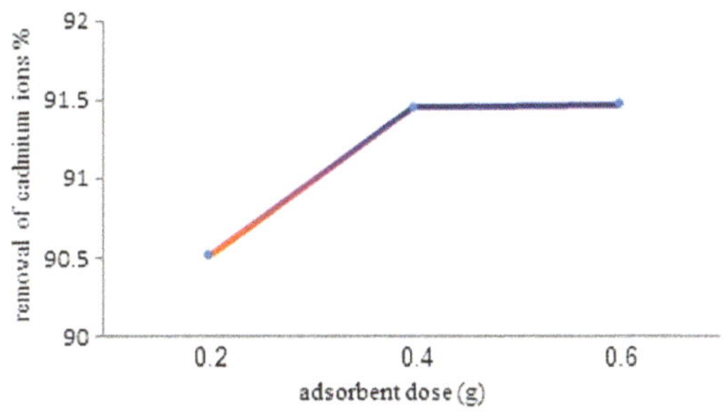

Fig. 5 The effect of adsorbent mass on the Cd removal efficiency

number of available adsorption active sites is constant thereby adsorbing almost the same amount of adsorbate, thus a decrease in the removal of adsorbate was resulted to an increase in initial concentration of cadmium. Similar results were also reported [31].

The effect of adsorbent mass on Cd^{2+} removal

In this study, the effect of iron oxide nanoparticles mass on the removal of cadmium was examined by changing of the mass of 0.2, 0.4, and 0.6 g at the 100 ml initial cadmium concentration of 15 mg/l. All suspensions were shacked 90 min, separated of adsorbent, measured the residual cadmium ions in solution and calculated the removal efficiency. The obtained results are presented in Fig. 5. The results showed the increasing of adsorbent mass from 0.2 to 0.6 g/ 100 ml the removal efficiency increased up to mass of 0.4 g and then remained constant. Hence value of 0.4 g/100 ml of adsorbent dosage was conducted as optimum value.

The influence of adsorbent dose on adsorption of cadmium ions was studied for obtaining the right adsorbent mass. Figure 5 shows, at the constant cadmium ions concentration, the adsorption percent of cadmium ions increases with increasing mass of the adsorbents. This is due to the existence of more available sites on surface of adsorbents at higher doses. When adsorbent dose was increased from 0.4 to 0.6 % w/v, the removal of cadmium ions had a low increasing. This effect may be due to the fact that some adsorption sites remain unsaturated during the batch adsorption process. This drop in adsorbed amount per unit mass of adsorbent is a routine behavior in the batch process.

Table 1 Linear equation and adsorption isotherm parameters for Cd^{2+} removal

Isotherm Linear equation	Langmuir			Freundlich		
	$\frac{1}{q_e} = \frac{1}{q_{max} K_l C_e} + \frac{1}{q_{max}}$			$\ln q_e = \ln K_F + \frac{1}{n} \ln C_e$		
Parameters	R^2	b	q_{max}	R^2	n	k_F
Obtained values	0.993	0.117	15.5	0.997	0.866	1.789

Table 2 Kinetic equation and obtained results for Cd^{2+} removal

	pseudo-first order		pseudo-second order	
model	$\log(q_e - q_t) = \log q_e - \frac{k_1}{2.303} t$		$\frac{t}{q_t} = \frac{1}{k_2 q_e^2} + \frac{1}{q_e} t$	
Equation	Y = −0.0352x-2.3298	$R^2 = 0.798$	Y = 0.9163 x + 0.9007	$R^2 = 0.999$
Obtained Value	$K_1 = 0.081$	$q_e = 4.7$	$K_2 = 1.119$	$q_e = 10.9$

Kinetic and isotherm adsorption

The adsorption data are usually described by adsorption equilibrium isotherms that indicate the effect of the initial concentration of pollutant on the adsorption quantity. In present study, the equilibrium adsorption of cadmium by iron oxide nanoparticles was explored at the contact time of 90 min., the adsorbent dose of 0.4 g/ 100 ml, cadmium initial concentrations in range of 5, 10, 15, 20 mg/L and the temperature of 25 °C. The *Langmuir* and *Freundlich* models were applied to determine the adsorption isotherm for cadmium removal by synthesized iron nanoparticles that the obtained results are presented in Table 1.

One of the most salient factors to design an adsorption system (to determine the optimum contact time) is anticipating the speed of the adsorption process that is controlled by isotherm and kinetic system. The common isotherm models are Freundlich and Langmuir that the linear equations are presented in 1. According to regression coefficient (Table 1), experiments data of cadmium adsorption on synthesized iron oxide nanoparticles followed Freundlich models better than those for the Langmuir model. Freundlich equation is an empirical adsorption isotherm equation that can be applied in case of low and intermediate concentration ranges. Freundlich isotherm gives the parameters, n, indicative of bond energies between metal ion and the adsorbent and K_F, related to bond strength [32]. The slope n and K_F from the linear equation was 0.866 and 1.789, respectively, satisfying of the condition for favorable adsorption.

In order to ascertain cadmium adsorption kinetic on iron oxide nanoparticles, the experiments were carried out under the optimized conditions and four different contact times as 15, 30, 60, and 90 min that were selected to obtain adsorption kinetic. *Pseudo-first order* and *pseudo- second order* equation were considered to determine the adsorption kinetic. The obtained results are presented in Table 2.

The pseudo-first-order and pseudo-second-order equations were applied to assess the suitability of the rate equation for the experiment data. The obtained rate equations were compiled in Table 2. The results show that the correlation coefficients for second order rate equations (0.999) were higher than those for the first order rate equations. Hence, the pseudo second order rate equation is more suitable to explain the cadmium adsorption on the iron oxide nanoparticles. In case of pseudo second order kinetics, the plot of (t/q_t) versus t gives a linear relationship that allows computation of q_e and K_2. The second order rate constant (k_2) value and equilibrium adsorption capacity (q_e) was 1.119 $g.mg^{-1}.min^{-1}$ and 10.9 $mg.g^{-1}$ for cadmium adsorption by synthesized iron nanoparticles in presence of tangerine peel extract.

Conclusion

The use of peel extracts as stabilizer agent for preparation of metal oxide nanoparticles is inexpensive, and eco-friendly. It is especially for preparation of nanoparticles that have been free of toxic contaminations. The peel extract can controlled the size and morphology of nanoparticles during synthesis process. Simple green synthesis of iron oxide nanoparticles through co-precipitation in alkali condition can exhibit an excellent adsorption for the cadmium ions that followed Freundlich adsorption model and pseudo-second-order equation. The obtained results of this investigation indicated that the synthesized adsorbent was more able to remove cadmium ions.

Competing interests

The authors declare that they have no competing interests.

Authors' contributions

The study was directed by MM who performed all the experiments. MHE is the first author read the manuscript. MHS (Corresponding author) advised the experimental methods and drafted the manuscript. AHM has given consultancy for the experiments and the English edition of manuscript. All authors have read and approved the final manuscript.

Acknowledgments

This project was financially supported by the Faculty of Public Health, Shahid Sadoughi University of Medical Sciences. The authors are grateful to the head of Environmental Chemistry Laboratory for his help.

Author details

[1]Department of Environmental Health, School of Public Health, Shahid Sadoughi University of Medical Science, Yazd, Iran. [2]Center for solid Waste Research, Institute for Environmental Research, Tehran University of Medical Science, Tehran, Iran.

References

1. Pan B, Qiu H, Pan B, Nie G, Xiao L, Lv L, et al. Highly efficient removal of heavy metals by polymer-supported nanosized hydrated Fe (III) oxides: behavior and XPS study. Water Res. 2010;44(3):815–24.
2. Mondiale B. Pollution prevention and abatement handbook-Toward cleaner production. Washington, DC: The World Bank; 1998. p. 457.
3. Mahvi A. Application of agricultural fibers in pollution removal from aqueous solution. Inter Environ Sci Tech. 2008;5(2):275–85.

4. Mbarek S, Saidi T, Mansour HB, Stéphane MP, Rostene W, Chaouacha-Chekir RB. Effect of cadmium on water metabolism regulation by Meriones shawi (Rodentia, Muridae). Environm Eng Sci. 2011;28(3):237–48.
5. Shils ME, Shike M. Modern nutrition in health and disease. Baltimore: Lippincott Williams & Wilkins; 2006.
6. WHO. Guidelines for drinking-water quality: recommendations. Geneva: World Health Organization; 2004.
7. Eddy M, Tchobanoglous G, Burton F, Stensel H. Theory and practice of water and wastewater treatment. New York: J. Wiley; 2003.
8. Ehrampoush MH, Masoudi H, Mahvi AH, Salmani MH. Prevalent kinetic model for Cd (II) adsorption from aqueous solution on barley straw Fresenius. Environ Bulletin. 2013;22(8):2314–8.
9. Fu F, Wang Q. Removal of heavy metal ions from wastewaters: a review. J Environ Manag. 2011;92(3):407–18.
10. Engates KE, Shipley HJ. Adsorption of Pb, Cd, Cu, Zn, and Ni to titanium dioxide nanoparticles: effect of particle size, solid concentration, and exhaustion. Environm Sci and Pollution Res. 2011;18(3):386–95.
11. Sheela T, Nayaka YA. Kinetics and thermodynamics of cadmium and lead ions adsorption on NiO nanoparticles. Chem Eng J. 2012;191:123–31.
12. Salmani MH, Ehrampoush MH, Aboueian-Jahromi M, Askarishahi M. Comparison between Ag (I) and Ni (II) removal from synthetic nuclear power plant coolant water by iron oxide nanoparticles. J Environ Health Sci Eng. 2013;11(21):1.
13. Xu P, Zeng GM, Huang DL, Feng CL, Hu S, Zhao MH, et al. Use of iron oxide nanomaterials in wastewater treatment: a review. Sci Total Environment. 2012;424:1–10.
14. Gong J, Wang X, Shao X, Yuan S, Yang C, Hu X. Adsorption of heavy metal ions by hierarchically structured magnetite-carbonaceous spheres. Talanta. 2012;101:45–52.
15. Mosaferi M, Nemati S, Khataee A, Nasseri S, Hashemi AA. Removal of Arsenic (III, V) from aqueous solution by nanoscale zero-valent iron stabilized with starch and carboxymethyl cellulose. J Environ Health Sci Eng. 2014;12(1):74.
16. Rafati L, Mahvi A, Asgari A, Hosseini S. Removal of chromium (VI) from aqueous solutions using Lewatit FO36 nano ion exchange resin. Inter J Environm Sci Tech. 2010;7(1):147–56.
17. Bazrafshan E, Mahvi AH, Naseri S, Mesdaghinia AR. Performance evaluation of electrocoagulation process for removal of chromium (VI) from synthetic chromium solutions using iron and aluminum electrodes. Turk J Eng Environ Sci. 2008;32(2):59–66.
18. Nouri J, Mahvi A, Bazrafshan E. Application of electrocoagulation process in removal of zinc and copper from aqueous solutions by aluminum electrodes. Inter J Environ Res. 2010;4(2):201–8.
19. Ebrahimi R, Maleki A, Shahmoradi B, Daraei H, Mahvi AH, Barati AH, et al. Elimination of arsenic contamination from water using chemically modified wheat straw. Desalin Water Treat. 2013;51(10–12):2306–16.
20. Mahvi A, Gholami F, Nazmara S. Cadmium biosorption from wastewater by Ulmus leaves and their ash. European J Sci Res. 2008;23(2):197–203.
21. Mahvi AH, Ebrahimi SJA-d, Mesdaghinia A, Gharibi H, Sowlat MH. Performance evaluation of a continuous bipolar electrocoagulation/electrooxidation–electroflotation (ECEO–EF) reactor designed for simultaneous removal of ammonia and phosphate from wastewater effluent. J Hazard Mater. 2011;192(3):1267–74.
22. Lu AH, Salabas EL, Schüth F. Magnetic nanoparticles: synthesis, protection, functionalization, and application. Angew Chem Int Ed. 2007;46(8):1222–44.
23. Nedkov I, Merodiiska T, Slavov L, Vandenberghe R, Kusano Y, Takada J. Surface oxidation, size and shape of nano-sized magnetite obtained by co-precipitation. J Mag and Mag Mater. 2006;300(2):358–67.
24. He F, Zhao D. Preparation and characterization of a new class of starch-stabilized bimetallic nanoparticles for degradation of chlorinated hydrocarbons in water. J Environ Sci & Tech. 2005;39(9):3314–20.
25. Berger P, Adelman NB, Beckman KJ, Campbell DJ, Ellis AB, Lisensky GC. Preparation and properties of an aqueous ferrofluid. J Chemical Edu. 1999;76(7):943.
26. Nassar NN. Rapid removal and recovery of Pb (II) from wastewater by magnetic nanoadsorbents. J Hazard Mater. 2010;184(1):538–46.
27. Duan H, Wang D, Li Y. Green chemistry for nanoparticle synthesis. Chem Soc Rev. 2015;44:5778–92.
28. Kosa SA, Al-Zhrani G, Salam MA. Removal of heavy metals from aqueous solutions by multi-walled carbon nanotubes modified with 8-hydroxyquinoline. Chem Eng J. 2012;181:159–68.
29. Salmani M, Zarei S, Ehrampoush M, Danaie S. Evaluations of pH and high ionic strength solution effect in cadmium removal by zinc oxide nanoparticles. J Appl Sci Environ Manag. 2014;191:123–31.
30. Afkhami A, Saber-Tehrani M, Bagheri H. Simultaneous removal of heavy-metal ions in wastewater samples using nano-alumina modified with 2, 4-dinitrophenylhydrazine. J Hazard Mater. 2010;181(1):836–44.
31. Kakavandi B, Jonidi AJ, Rezaei RK, Nasseri S, Ameri A, Esrafily A. Synthesis and properties of FeO-activated carbon magnetic nanoparticles for removal of aniline from aqueous solution: equilibrium, kinetic and thermodynamic studies. J Environ Health Sci Eng. 2013;10(1):19. doi:10.1186/1735-2746-10-19.
32. Li X, Li A, Long M, Tian X. Equilibrium and kinetic studies of copper biosorption by dead Ceriporia lacerata biomass isolated from the litter of an invasive plant in China. J Environ Health Sci Eng. 2015;13:37. doi:10.1186/s40201-015-0191-1.

Enhanced performance of non-thermal plasma coupled with TiO_2/GAC for decomposition of chlorinated organic compounds: influence of a hydrogen-rich substance

Kamaleddin Abedi[1], Farshid Ghorbani-Shahna[1*], Babak Jaleh[2], Abdolrahman Bahrami[1] and Rasoul Yarahmadi[3]

Abstract

Background: No study was found in the literature on the combination of TiO_2/GAC catalyst and non-thermal plasma for chlorinated volatile organic compounds abatement in air. This paper presents this hybrid process for the decomposition of chloroform (as a target compound) using a multi-pin to plate discharge reactor. The experiments were performed using a high frequency pulsed transformer as the power supply system to examine the effect of SIE, frequency, as well as initial concentration on the chloroform removal efficiency (RE). Toluene was added as a hydrogen-rich source to shift the reactions into the formation of environmentally desirable products.

Results: RE of around 60% was observed with the NTP-alone process at the highest possible SIE (3000 J L^{-1}), while it rocketed up to 100% (total oxidation) in the presence of TiO_2/GAC at SIE of 1000 J L^{-1}. About 100% O_3 destruction over TiO_2/GAC and both adsorption and catalytic activities of GAC may be considered as the reasons for better performance of the hybrid process. Toluene feeding diminished the chlorinated by-products such as Cl_2 and TCE significantly. The selectivity towards CO_2 was noticed to enhance noticeably, when both catalyst and toluene were introduced, regardless of the input concentration.

Conclusions: Our findings suggest that the hybrid of NTP with TiO_2/GAC will highly be effective in the abatement of chloroform, and the addition of toluene will successfully decline harmful chlorinated by-products.

Keywords: CVOCs removal, NTP-catalysis, TiO_2, Granular activated carbon, Hydrogen-rich source

Background

Most of the hazardous air pollutants listed by environmental protection agencies are volatile organic compounds (VOCs) particularly chlorinated hydrocarbons [1-3]. Prolonged exposure to chlorinated VOCs (CVOCs) and their emission into atmosphere has raised considerable public concern due to the fact that most of these pollutants can lead to harmful effects on human and some of them are known to be carcinogenic [4-6]. Moreover, most of these compounds persist a long time in the environment [7]. However, they are still widely used as solvents, refrigerants, etc. in industries and workplaces. Therefore, the removal of these toxic substances is an essential issue in environmental emissions, which requires efficient and low cost technologies. Due to the high energy consumption, conventional techniques are almost ineffective particularly when the pollutant concentrations are less than 100 ppm [8]. Among the new techniques, non-thermal plasma (NTP) seems to be a very attractive and promising method, and several researchers have investigated the destruction of CVOCs using NTP, indicating that it can highly be effective in the decomposition of these compounds [9-13]. However, wasting energy as heat is still a fundamental issue in all kind of NTP reactors [14]. Previous studies have demonstrated that using a pulsed power supply is highly beneficial for both enhancing removal and energy efficiency as compared to DC- or AC-energized systems

* Correspondence: fghorbani@umsha.ac.ir
[1]Department of occupational health engineering, Research center for health services, Hamedan University of Medical Sciences, Hamedan, Iran
Full list of author information is available at the end of the article

[14-18]. Furthermore, due to some limitations with the NTP-alone technology, special attention has recently been given to a hybrid use of pulsed NTP and heterogeneous catalysis, and previous works have shown that combining a metal oxide catalyst with NTP can be a preferred option [19-21]. But, because of low ability of metal oxide catalysts to adsorb organic compounds, owing to their polar structure, coating them on an adsorbent seems to enhance their efficiency resulting from the higher surface area and thereby higher residence time, yielding more oxidation and reduction rates [22]. Granular activated carbon (GAC) appears to be an extremely good adsorbent for the most of organic compounds.

In the present study, chloroform was chosen as the target CVOC which is widely used in industries, and despite its significant harmful effects, decomposition of this compound has rarely been reported in the scientific literature by plasma [11,23,24] and catalytic plasma [25]. In order to enhance catalytic reactions, GAC was employed in this work as the substrate for TiO_2 catalyst to improve the degradation efficiency of chlorinated compounds. According to previous studies, the production of undesirable by-products such as Cl_2 and $COCl_2$ during the conversion of CVOCs can be inevitable in particular when their molecular structure contain more chlorine than hydrogen atoms [26]. Introducing a hydrogen-rich molecule such as toluene in the gas stream seems to lead the reactions to the formation of desirable chlorine containing products which are water-soluble and can be conveniently removed using a wet scrubber. Toluene was therefore fed along with chloroform to the gas stream in this study to promote the selectivity towards favorable by-products. Hence, the aim of this study was to investigate the effect of SIE, catalyst incorporation, as well as toluene addition on the chloroform removal efficiency, with special focusing on diminishing harmful by-products.

Methods

Reagents

Chloroform, toluene, 2-propanol, and acetyl-acetone were purchased from Merck (Germany). They were all in analytical grade with purity higher than 99.9%, 99.9%, 99.8%, and 99%, respectively. Tetra-n-butyl titanate with purity higher than 98% was supplied from Fluka (Switzerland). Granular activated carbon (with a mean diameter of 1.5-2 mm) with highest purity available (extra pure) was also obtained from Merck (Germany).

Catalyst preparation and characterization

The catalyst was prepared by a dip-coating process using sol–gel technique. The detailed procedure has been discussed in Ref. [27]: 0.34 ml of tetra-n-butyl titanate was dissolved in a 6.1068 ml of 2-propanol and stirred for 1 h at room temperature, followed by the addition of acetyl-aceton (0.102 ml) and stirred again for 2.5 h at room temperature. By falling 2 or 3 droplets of HNO_3 in 1.8 ml of H_2O, an acidic solution with $pH = 2$ was resulted, which added completely to the former sol. The obtained mixture was then heated on a hot plate under reflux being placed in a water bath and stirred for 8 h at 75°C, resulting in a yellow transparent gel. Strict control of the reaction temperature is needed at this stage to avoid instant gelation. 0.125 grams of granular activated carbon was added in the resulting mixture (3 grams of GAC per 200 ml of sol [28]) and then subjected to vibrate in an ultrasonic bath for 0.5 h. The samples were then filtered, dried at room temperature, and calcined for 4 h at 300°C. Finally, the TiO_2/GAC was obtained.

Experimental system

The schematic diagram of the experimental set-up is shown in Figure 1. The experimental set-up consisted of an air supply system, a flow control and measuring unit, an injection unit, a corona discharge reactor, a catalyst reactor, an electric power supply, and some gas monitoring apparatus as shown in Figure 1. Normal air was supplied by using an air compressor with two pressure regulators. The air then passed through a mixed ceramic-activated carbon filter to be cleaned for water vapor and organic air pollutants and delivered into a mixing chamber, from which it could reach the plasma reactor. The total volumetric flow rate of gas stream was controlled to be in a range of 0.2-1 L min^{-1}. The corresponding residence time was then varied from 1 to 6 s. The gas flow rate was kept at a desirable value utilizing two control valves. All the experiments were carried out at atmospheric pressure and normal temperature. Two motor driving syringe pumps, JMS SP-510 (Japan), were used to inject the liquid substances (chloroform, and toluene) into the air stream at the liquid injection port, where the temperature was kept at 40°C to facilitate the vaporization of the volatile components. The injection rate of the liquid was calculated so that the initial concentration of the contaminants in the air stream was in a desirable range (100–700 ppm). After passing through the mixing chamber, polluted gas was fed into the plasma reactor. A high voltage pulse generator (HVPL-30 OCS Haiden laboratory inc.) with peak-to-peak voltage pulses in the range of 0-30 kV and a repetition frequency of 1-20 kHz was employed to generate NTP. A flow meter was connected before and after the plasma reactor to determine the influent and effluent stream. Finally, the gas stream leaving the reactor passed through a small home-made chamber, making it possible to monitor some inorganic by-products such as CO_x and NO_x directly. The experimental set-up was carefully inspected to be completely gastight.

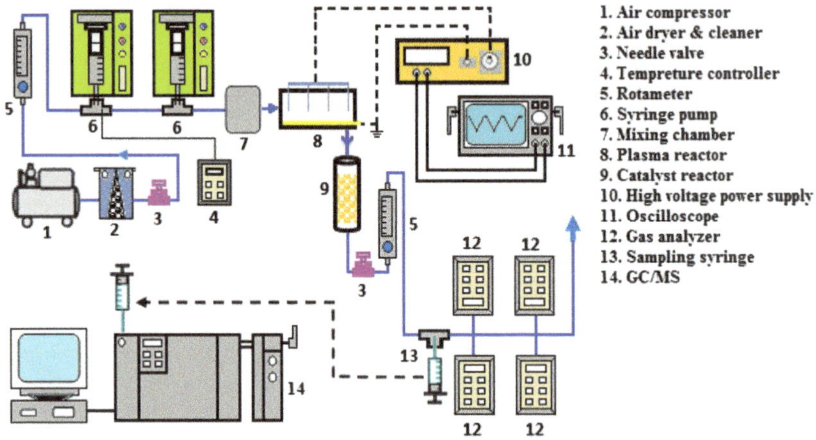

Figure 1 Schematic diagram of experimental setup.

Reactors configurations and electrical measurements

A rectangular corona discharge reactor was constructed of quartz with 20 × 15 × 200 mm dimensions as shown in Figure 2. An aluminum foil (200 mm length) was used as the inner electrode being placed along the floor of the reactor acting as the ground electrode. Furthermore, 6 thin stainless steel needles (each with an outer diameter of 1 mm, and a total length of 50 mm) were situated above the reactor perpendicularly against the aluminum plate acting as the discharge electrode. Then the discharge gap between ground and discharge electrodes was set to be 7 mm. The current was divided equally between electrodes using a resistance box. Small pieces of quartz were pasted inside the reactor near pin electrodes creating small tunnels along the rectangular tube so that the air stream was subjected to flow through these tunnels. This made the NTP more effective since the pollutant molecules were forced to pass as close as possible to energetic electrons. The discharge volume then became smaller and was estimated to be around 20 ml. A cylindrical glass tube, also made up of quartz, with an inner diameter of 15 mm and 100 mm length was used as catalyst reactor. About 3 grams of catalyst was placed inside the tube each time between 2 stainless steel screens. Small amounts of glass wool were also positioned in both ends of the tube to prevent particles escaping through the screens.

High frequency and high voltage (1–20 kHz, 8–22 kV) was applied between the electrodes to generate non-thermal plasma. Both the applied voltage and frequency were adjustable so that the plasma conditions could be optimized. A positive and negative pulsed voltage with a rising time of 200 ns and a duration time of 2 μs was applied to charge the discharge electrode. Typical voltage and current waveforms at applied voltage of 8 kV are shown in Figure 3. It can be seen from Figure 3 that each repetitive pulse appears in one division of oscilloscope screen, implying the duration of one cycle of waveform of 50 μS. Therefore, the pulse repetition frequency can be obtained 20000 Hz for the data shown in Figure 3. A good stability for discharge is also seen from the figure since the occurrence of voltage pulses and their corresponding current follows a logical and systematic process. The bipolar behavior of the the discharge current is also inferred from the data represented in Figure 3. The high voltage transformer was equipped with a diminishing system making it possible for applied current and voltage

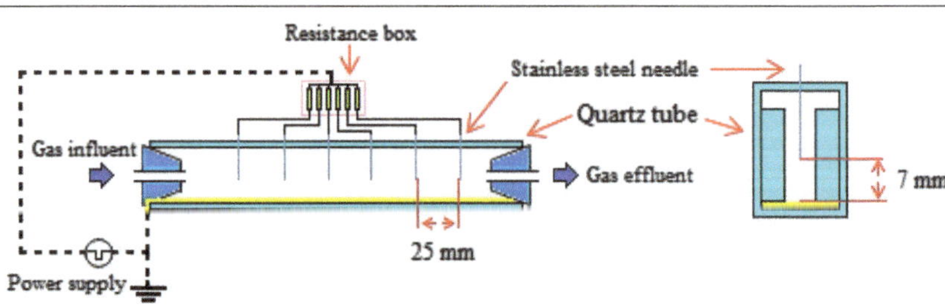

Figure 2 Schematic diagram of NTP reactor.

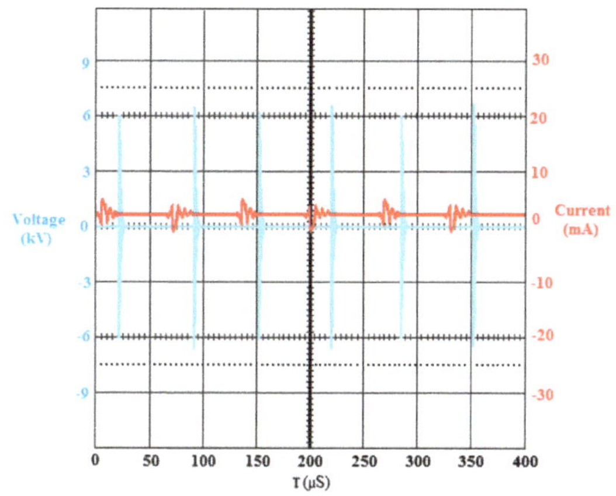

Figure 3 Typical voltage and current waveforms at applied voltage of 8 kV.

to be measured directly using an oscilloscope (HAMEG HM 203–7 Germany) without employing a high voltage probe. In order to evaluate the efficiency of the discharge reactor for decomposition of chloroform, we used specific input energy (SIE) as expressed by Eq. 1. The discharge power was calculated by integrating of the voltage and current products in a pulse time and then multiplying it by the pulse frequency as shown in Eq. 2.

$$SIE(^J/_L) = \frac{discharge\ power(^J/_S)}{gas\ flow\ rate(^L/_S)} \qquad (1)$$

$$Discharge\ power(^J/_S) = \left[\int |V(t) \times I(t)dt|\right](^J/_{Pulse}) \times Pulse\ frequency(^{Pulse}/_S) \qquad (2)$$

Gas analysis

The gas mixture of the outlet of the reactor was analyzed before and after the plasma catalytic process after having reached the steady-state conditions. Downstream products were collected into a gas-tight syringe through inline sampling ports and were injected into the gas chromatograph for analysis by using sample injection volume of 1 ml. The chloroform influent and effluent concentrations were averaged over three samples that were taken for each operating condition. When catalyst incorporated with the NTP, sampling was delayed until a stable breakthrough observed at the outlet. Gas analysis was conducted using a Varian 3800 GC equipped with a Saturn 2200 mass spectroscopy system (GC/MS). The GC was also equipped with a SGE capillary column with the inner diameter of 0.22 mm, film diameter of 0.25 μm, and length of 25 m. The supplying carrier gas was helium with a flow rate of 2 ml min^{-1}. Temperature programming was as follows: 60°C for 1 min and then increased by 15°C min^{-1} up to 180°C and kept constant there for 1 min. NO and NO_2 were measured using a NO_x analyzer (G750 polytector, Germany). Two single gas detectors were also employed directly in order to analyze CO (SGA91, U.K.) and CO_2 (Testo535, Germany). Ozone was monitored applying both KI titration method and an ozone analyzer (EST-1510, USA) for high and low concentrations respectively. Furthermore, a thermohygrometer (Testoterm, GmbH & Co., Germany) was used to record the temperature and humidity of the system before and after the plasma process. The difference of chloroform concentration before and after the catalytic plasma process was our indicator to determine the decomposition rate, and chloroform removal efficiency (RE) was then calculated as the following (Eq. 3):

$$RE(\%) = \left(1 - \frac{[chloroform]_{out}}{[chloroform]_{in}}\right) \times 100 \qquad (3)$$

Where $[chloroform]_{out}$ and $[chloroform]_{in}$ are the chloroform concentration in the effluent and influent gas respectively.

Also the selectivity towards CO_2 (S_{CO_2}) is given as (Eq. 4):

$$S_{CO_2}(\%) = \frac{[CO_2]}{[chloroform]_{in} \times RE} \times 100 \qquad (4)$$

Where $[CO_2]$ is the CO_2 concentration in the effluent gas after plasma and catalytic processes.

Results and discussion

Catalyst properties

Both GAC and TiO_2/GAC samples were subjected to XRD and SEM analysis. XRD and SEM profiles are shown in Figures 4 and 5, respectively. The only detected TiO_2 phase by XRD analysis was anatase as can be seen in Figure 4, and no rutile and brookite phase were observed. Major XRD peaks for TiO_2 particles were detected at 2θs of 25.1°, 47.6°, 53.7°, 54.7°, and 62.7°. A fairly high peak was also observed at $2\theta = 26.4°$ for GAC itself. The average size of TiO_2 particles was estimated to be in Nano scale, which was approved by SEM images, and Figure 5b shows that nanoparticles with a distribution diameter from ca. 50 nm up to several hundred nm were obtained. In our view, larger sizes of particles can be attributed to agglomeration, and despite the fact that the calcination temperature was relatively high around 300°C, agglomeration rate was also appeared to be significant. As can be seen in SEM images (Figure 5a and b), GAC had primarily a non-uniform, porous structure with small cavities and attached fine particles on its surface. It was then covered by TiO_2 particles (Figure 5b), becoming smoother, more

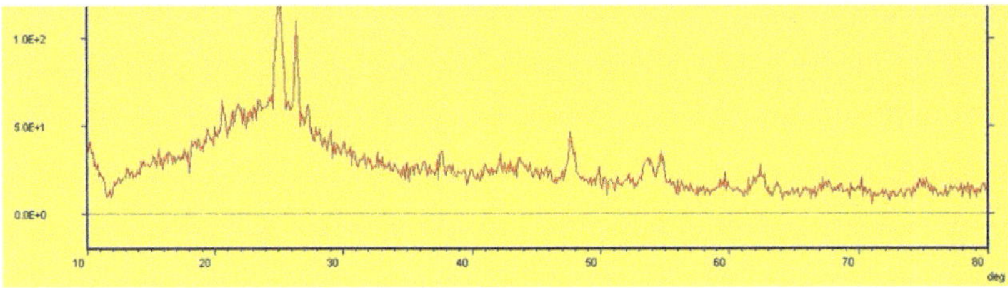

Figure 4 XRD pattern of TiO_2 nanoparticles coated on GAC.

even, and uniform. The BET surface area was also determined with the N2 adsorption data in the relative pressure (P/P_0) range of 0.05–0.577 K using a BELSORP-max nitrogen adsorption apparatus (Japan Inc.). The BET results are shown in Table 1. As can be seen in Table 1, the specific surface area was detected to be 969.1 and 935.2 $m^2\ gr^{-1}$ for GAC and TiO_2/GAC respectively. These findings revealed that the pore size of GAC was significantly affected by TiO_2 coating and it decreased about 35 $m^2\ gr^{-1}$ as TiO_2 particles were covered on GAC surface. The total pore volume was also decreased from 0.5724 to 0.5453 cc gr^{-1} as the substrate surface covered by TiO_2 nanoparticles. The reduction of surface area and total pore volume confirmed the SEM results. According to Figure 5, the deposition of TiO_2 onto GAC pores led to disappearance of holes from its surface, leaving a lower level of porosity which implies a lower surface area.

The effect of pulse repetition frequency on removal efficiency

The design of power supply system enabled us to adjust the applied frequency up to 20 KHz during this study. In order to examine the effect of frequency on chloroform conversion, pulse repetition frequency was varied between 1 and 20 KHz while applied voltage fixed at 18 KV. Figure 6 shows this impact on the chloroform decomposition rate for different initial concentrations. As it is seen, RE was strongly influenced by increasing frequency for various concentrations, and the rate of conversion achieved 56% for 100 ppm concentration at a frequency of 20 KHz. The frequency increment gave same trend of decomposition with other concentrations (Figure 6). Our observations revealed that increasing frequency resulted in a change in the voltage and current waveforms by raising the number of pulses per one division on oscillogram, which makes the discharge power much stronger, and as a result, more energetic electrons are released, and the number of spontaneous collisions is increased. Consequently, the rate of reactions between chlorinated carbons and active species available in plasma region goes up which is expected. Due to the beneficial effect of pulsed repetition frequency, it was fixed at its highest value (20 KHz) in our study, and kept constant during all experiments as an optimal condition.

However, the effect of applied frequency on the conversion rate is rather controversial. It has been reported in some studies that a dramatic enhancement is achieved in removal efficiency with increasing frequency from 50 to 150 Hz and also over 1000 Hz [5,29,30]. Furthermore, Kogelschatz argued that the preferred working frequency for a DBD reactor is ca. 10 MHz [31]. By contrast, Oda et al. reported a reverse effect in the decomposition of CVOCs with increasing frequency and stated that the highest level of decomposition was achieved at a frequency of 100 Hz [32]. It should be noted here that the most suitable frequency depends largely on various plasma parameters, particularly the type of applied power supply system and reactor configuration.

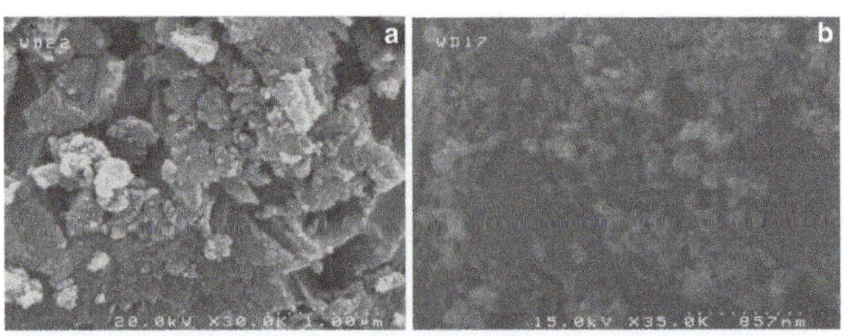

Figure 5 SEM micrographs of (a) GAC, and (b) TiO_2/GAC.

Table 1 The BET analysis data for GAC and TiO_2/GAC based on the nitrogen adsorption-desorption measurements

Sample name	GAC	TiO_2/GAC
Specific surface area (m^2g^{-1})	969.1	935.2
Total pore volume (cc g^{-1})	0.5724	0.5453

Plasma power effect on the decomposition of chloroform (SIE and catalyst introduction impact)

SIE was varied between 120–3000 J L^{-1} during the present study by changing the applied voltage from 8 to 22 KV at a frequency of 20 kHz, and also gas flow rate from 0.2-1 L min^{-1}. Figure 7 shows the conversion rate of 700 ppm of chloroform for SIE variation between 120 and 3000 J L^{-1}. It is seen from Figure 7 that the conversion of chloroform was strongly influenced by the SIE. This dependency is observed in various conditions with and without catalyst, and is more noticeable for both NTP-alone and NTP-GAC systems. The trend is obviously upwards with NTP-alone process and the gradual rise in RE from 10 to approximately 30% is followed by a sharper increase at SIEs higher than 1000 J L^{-1} reaching 61% at highest SIE. It is also observed that the combination of NTP with TiO_2/GAC is dependent on SIE to a lesser extent and even at SIE of 120 J L^{-1} the conversion rate rocketed to 95% with this coupling mode. This may be due to the fact that both TiO_2 and GAC have strong catalytic activity and a hybrid of these seems to produce a dramatic synergistic effect. However, when TiO_2/GAC was tested without NTP, no significant catalytic activity detected. Several studies have discussed the dependence of RE on energy density, supporting the observations made in the present study [33,34]. The main reason for this marked improvement may be the increased number of accelerated electrons due to higher input energy.

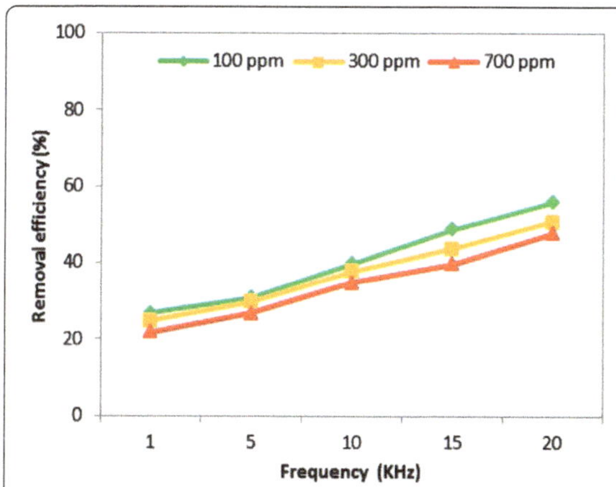

Figure 6 **The effect of frequency on chloroform removal efficiency with NTP-alone process (applied voltage of 18 kV).**

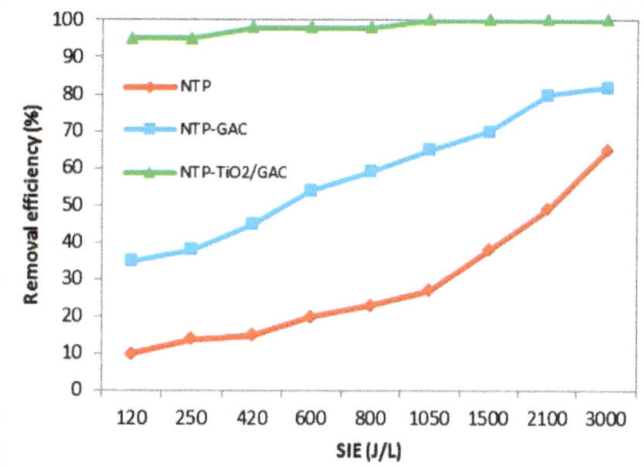

Figure 7 **Influence of SIE on chloroform removal efficiency (SIE 120–3000 J/L and 700 ppm of chloroform).**

The incorporation of TiO_2/GAC downstream of the NTP had a major effect on the chloroform conversion rate. 3 gram of TiO_2/GAC was used each time until catalyst deactivation occurred. As can be seen in Figure 7 chloroform decomposition is strongly enhanced with NTP-catalyst hybrid system and RE of 100% achieved at SIEs higher than 1000 J L^{-1} as compared to NTP-alone for which RE was about 60% at highest possible SIE. At the same time, ozone was considerably decomposed over TiO_2/GAC and reduced to less than 1 ppm in the effluent gas. These findings indicate that TiO_2/GAC plays a prominent role in both chloroform and ozone destruction and that decomposition of ozone is highly beneficial for chloroform conversion. This is attributed not only to the GAC or TiO_2 itself but also to the method of coating, because TiO_2/GAC preparation with another impregnation technique, did not yield same results. In the presence of catalyst other harmful by-products along with ozone were also decreased significantly. For instance, NO_2 that was 50 ppm for NTP-alone at SIE of 250 J L^{-1} was removed totally with NTP-TiO_2/GAC system. The absence of NO was also observed with this coupling system while its amount was more than 80 ppm with the NTP-alone process. Because a catalytic activity was also expected for GAC, NTP was coupled with bare GAC in a series of our experiments. As it is seen from Figure 7, our expectation came true and chloroform conversion increased about 20% when GAC introduced downstream of the NTP. A marked decline was also observed in ozone concentration and it decreased to ca. 100 ppm at SIE of 3000 J L^{-1}, whereas at the same SIE for NTP-alone it was as high as 700 ppm. NO, and NO_2 levels, however, remained the same as for NTP-alone process.

Since the gas temperature ranged between 30–40°C downstream of the plasma and catalyst reactor, dissociation of ozone by heat is ruled out. If the difference in ozone level with NTP-GAC and NTP-TiO_2/GAC is also considered, the role of TiO_2/GAC catalyst is obviously determined in ozone decomposition. It is in good agreement in previous studies that TiO2 contributes to ozone decomposition significantly and the OH radicals are considerably improved when O_3 passes over TiO_2 in the presence of H_2O [35-37]. OH radicals then can act as an oxidant agent in VOCs conversion as reported by Zhu et al. [37]. From these points we can conclude that TiO_2/GAC catalyst leads chloroform and its intermediate products to further reactions which results in the greater production of water vapor and carbon oxides subsequently.

The abatement of other plasma generating by-products such as NO and NO_2 over TiO_2/GAC can also been considered as chloroform removal efficiency promoting according to reactions (1) and (2) [38,39]:

(1) $NO_2 + HC \rightarrow HC_{oxidized} + 2NO$

(2) $HC_{oxidized} + 2NO \rightarrow N_2 + H_2O + CO_2$

Besides the removal of NOx, these redox reactions can be concluded as totally favorable reactions, since they contribute to the stable, safe, and desired end products. The lower level of CO which was obtained over TiO_2/GAC and will be discussed further in the following sections may be explained by the reaction (3) that is another crucial role for the TiO_2/GAC catalyst [40]. Simultaneous removal of unwanted by-products can be considered as one of the major advantageous of TiO_2/GAC.

(3) $2NO + 2CO \rightarrow N_2 + 2CO_2$

Effect of initial concentration

To investigate the influence of various concentrations on the performance of the reactor, initial concentration was varied between 100 and 700 ppm during this study. Table 2 shows RE for various concentrations with catalytic and non-catalytic plasma as a function of SIE. A higher amount of pollutant molecules causes a noticeable difference in gas composition in the plasma reactor, and the number of molecules available for decomposition grows per unit of discharge volume. This influences the energy density and also the quantities of active species produced in the plasma zone. Hence, the energy level that each individual molecule receives for the conversion decreases significantly which results in lower RE. This may be the reason why increasing initial concentration had a deleterious effect on chloroform conversion with NTP-alone system (Table 2). On the other hand, it seems that introducing more gaseous molecules into the plasma zone will generate a larger numbers of metastable and charged species especially when the feeding molecules are heavier and contain more atoms as in the case of toluene introduction. This effect reduced the voltage applied to the pin-to-plate reactor due to a corona-to-spark transition mode. With chloroform feeding, however, it did not affect the system even at higher concentrations (700 ppm). The effect of higher amounts of chloroform subjected to the reactor was not significant in the presence of TiO_2/GAC. As seen from Table 2, total oxidation (RE of 100%) was achieved over TiO_2/GAC at all SIEs when chloroform feeding was below 300 ppm, and RE dropped by only 5% with concentration of 700 ppm. A strong adsorption property of GAC is likely the reason of this better performance. For lower concentrations all of the species received from plasma medium can be adsorbed by GAC and hence higher residence time results in quite perfect catalytic reactions over TiO_2 surface while with increasing the initial gas feeding the breakthrough rises gradually, causing some compounds to leave the catalyst bed unconverted. The effect of higher gas feeding was also obvious when toluene was introduced into the reactor. A competition between toluene and chloroform molecules was observed to be in favor of toluene and its total oxidation was occurred with SIEs higher than 1000 J L^{-1}, while at the highest possible SIE (2100 J L^{-1}) some amounts of chloroform still remained unchanged. This may also be due to the fast deactivation of catalyst resulting from numerous carbons released from toluene molecules. Our findings are in good agreement with the previous works [7,41,42]. However, Magureanu [12] reported a higher level of decomposition for increasing input concentration, believing that secondary reactions triggered by secondary radicals and ions resulting from the initial decomposition of CVOC molecules causes such effect.

Selectivity towards CO_2 and CO_x

While passing through the discharge zone and catalyst bed, the chloroform vapor decomposed into a mixture of CO_2, CO, H_2O, and some chlorinated products. Since CO_2 is a desired final product, CO_2 selectivity was calculated and plotted in Figure 8a and b along with CO_x selectivity which can represent the carbon balance if the amount of hydrocarbon by-products is negligible. Figure 8a presents the selectivity towards CO_2, CO, and CO_x (CO_2 + CO) for 700 ppm chloroform at SIE of 3000 J L^{-1}. It is just evident from the figure that catalyst introduction influenced the products distribution effectively, and CO_2 selectivity increased about 44% in the presence of TiO_2/GAC, approaching almost 70%, whereas no result better than 20% was obtained with NTP-alone system. Although CO selectivity reduced substantially with TiO_2/GAC, but selectivity towards CO_x still remained high due to the high level of CO_2. Similarly, coupling NTP with bare GAC

Table 2 Influence of initial concentration on chloroform removal efficiency as a function of SIE with NTP-alone and catalytic NTP

SIE	Removal efficiency (%)							
	NTP-alone			NTP-TiO_2/GAC				
	100 ppm	300 ppm	700 ppm	100 ppm	300 ppm	700 ppm	Cloroform + Toluene	
							Chloroform (300 ppm)	Toluene (100 ppm)
120	15	12	10	97	97	95	92	94
250	20	18	14	100	100	95	92	94
420	22	20	15	100	100	96	93	95
600	30	24	20	100	100	96.5	93	95
800	36	29	23	100	100	97	94	98
1050	44	36	27	100	100	97	95	100
1500	58	44	38	100	100	98.5	95	100
2100	62	51	49	100	100	99	97	100
3000	69	63	61	100	100	99.5	-	-

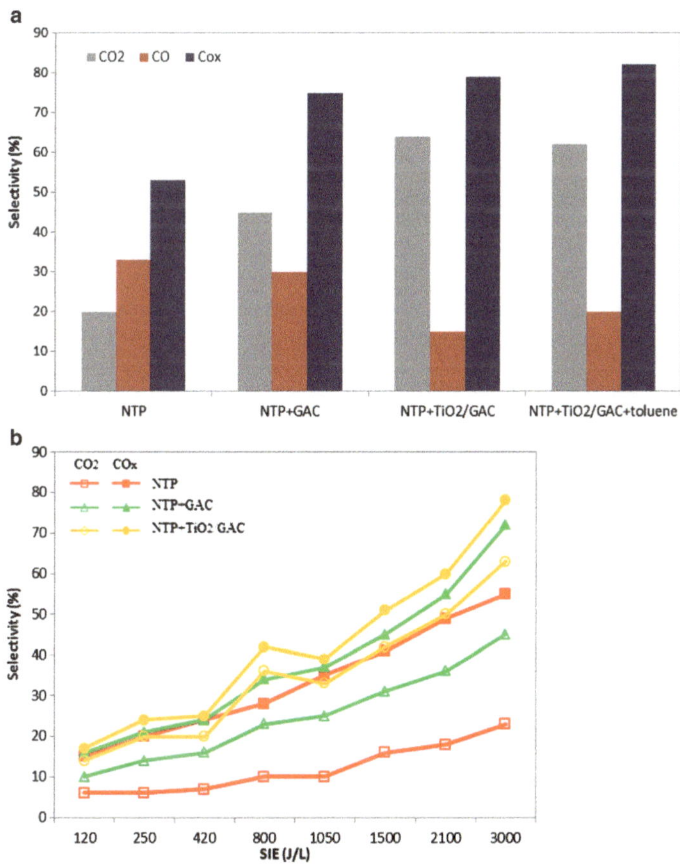

Figure 8 CO, CO_2, and CO_x selectivity (a) at highest SIE (3000 J/L), and (b) as a function of SIE.

showed a much better activity with regard to CO_x selectivity, soaring up to 75%, while the amount of CO stayed approximately as high as that of the NTP-alone system. The most CO_x selectivity was observed for NTP-TiO_2/GAC when toluene was added to the system, which was predictable due to the large quantities of carbon in toluene structure and also high quality of catalyst. Figure 8b shows CO_2 and CO_x selectivity resulted from the decomposition of 100 ppm chloroform as a function of SIE. The trend is obviously upwards with increasing SIE under all experimental conditions as can be seen from Figure 8b. There was a marked improvement especially in CO_x selectivity over catalysts for SIEs above 1000 J L^{-1}. From this result, it was recognized that ozone has a key role in improving the reactions towards both total oxidation and higher CO_x selectivity, because a dramatic increase was detected for ozone amount at these higher SIEs. Except for NTP-TiO_2/GAC process, a large gap is evident between the CO_2 and CO_x lines which is attributed to large quantity of CO produced under both NTP-alone and NTP-GAC conditions. No considerable influence of the chloroform initial concentration was observed on CO_2 selectivity in the present study. Strong adsorption property of GAC may be the reason again. Nevertheless, Magureanu et al. [41] reported that the selectivity towards CO_2 increases with lower gas flow rate and initial concentration, and argued that under these conditions higher residence time provides sufficient opportunity for the reactions to be carried out more efficiently. However, the dependence of CO_2 selectivity on SIE as observed in the present study is in good agreement with the previous works [41,43].

Mechanisms of chloroform oxidation and the formation of by-products

It was observed in several earlier studies that when the oxidation of chlorinated compounds occurs in a plasma reactor in an oxygen-rich environment such as air, a considerable amount of different chlorinated products can be produced, which could be more hazardous than the initial compound itself [44]. Among them, $COCl_2$, Cl_2, and CO seems to be the main harmful by-products [34]. The formation of products containing oxygen and chlorine is attributed to the reaction between chloride and oxygen atoms as described by Indarto et al., and Foglein et al. [23,24]. If the initial compound is chloroform, some amounts of HCl would also be produced along with $COCl_2$ [23,44]:

(4) $$CHCl_3 + O \rightarrow COCl_2 + HCl$$

The reaction pathways of chloroform decomposition in a discharge medium near room temperature in the presence of oxygen have been studied in several earlier researches [11,24,45]. Based on these experimental works, one can conclude that many active radicals such as $O^\bullet$, $OH^\bullet$, $Cl^\bullet$, $H^\bullet$, $CCl_3^\bullet$, $CHCl_2^\bullet$ etc. are generated during the short initial step of decomposition resulting from the electron collisions with the existed molecules. The products of the fast reactions of this step are mainly dominated by both $COCl_2$ and Cl_2 through numerous reaction pathways [45]. These chlorinated intermediates participate in subsequent reactions with O_2 to yield some peroxy radicals such as $CHCl_2O_2$, and CCl_3O_2, following by degradation into Oxy radicals, which in turn react with other radicals like $Cl^\bullet$ to form $COCl_2$ according to Mok et al. [11]. A series of chain reactions with various paths occur at later stages leading to the formation of final products. There is no agreement among the various studies on final products. Foglein et al. found that the end products are stable and eco-friendly compounds such as H_2O, CO_2, and HCl [24]. However, considerable amounts of CO, and $COCl_2$ were detected in the reactor outlet of other studies [11,23]. The production of Cl_2 and CCl_4 has also been noted in the literature [24,45].

Significant changes were detected for end products in the current study due to the catalyst and toluene incorporation. The final products detected during the present study under various conditions are listed in Table 3. In general, the decomposition products detected by GC/MS and other measuring apparatus during NTP-alone process included CO_2, CO, H_2O, Cl_2, TCBA (trichloro-benzaldehyde), TCAA (trichloro-acetaldehyde), TCE (tri-chladf67oro-ethylene), NO, NO_2, O_3, and $COCl_2$ as can be seen in Table 3. It is worth mentioning again that neither O_3 nor NO_x was observed with NTP-TiO_2/GAC while they were typical by-products in NTP-alone system. An interesting and favorable finding was also that no $COCl_2$ was observed with NTP-TiO_2/GAC with and without toluene addition. CO was detected with all conditions studied but its amount decreased over catalysts particularly with TiO_2/GAC. During the oxidative decomposition of chloroform, the favorable products are CO_2, H_2O and desired chlorinated compounds such as HCl and chloroaldehides which are water-soluble and can be removed easily using a wet scrubber. Among the chlorinated products, Cl_2 was the most abundant compound in the present study, followed by TCBA, TCAA, TCE, and $COCl_2$ with plasma-alone process. In the presence of TiO_2/GAC, however, $COCl_2$ was totally removed and the values of others changed dramatically. Figure 9a represents a GC/MS chromatogram for 300 ppm of chloroform at SIE of 2100 J L^{-1} with NTP-TiO_2/GAC. It is clearly evident from Figure 9a that the main chlorinated

Table 3 Main components of chloroform decomposition detected by analyzing apparatus

Compounds	m/z	NTP-alone	NTP-TiO_2/GAC	NTP-TiO_2/GAC + toluene
CO_2	40	√	√	√
CO	-	√	√	√
H_2O	-	√	√	√
Cl_2	74	√	√	√
TCBA	77-209	√	√	√
TCAA	148	√	√	√
TCE	97	√	√	√
NO	-	√	-	-
NO_2	-	√	-	-
O_3	-	√	-	-
$COCl_2$	98	√	-	-
HCl	-	-	-	-

by-products include TCAA, Cl_2, as well as TCE, which was followed by TCBA.

As mentioned earlier and represented in reaction (9), due to the great ability of TiO_2/GAC for decomposition of ozone, the production of O radicals is highly appreciated. Therefore, the $COCl_2$ removal over catalyst surface may be attributed to the reaction between $COCl_2$ and provided O radicals [46]:

$$(5) \quad COCl_2 + O^{\bullet} \rightarrow CO_2 + Cl_2$$

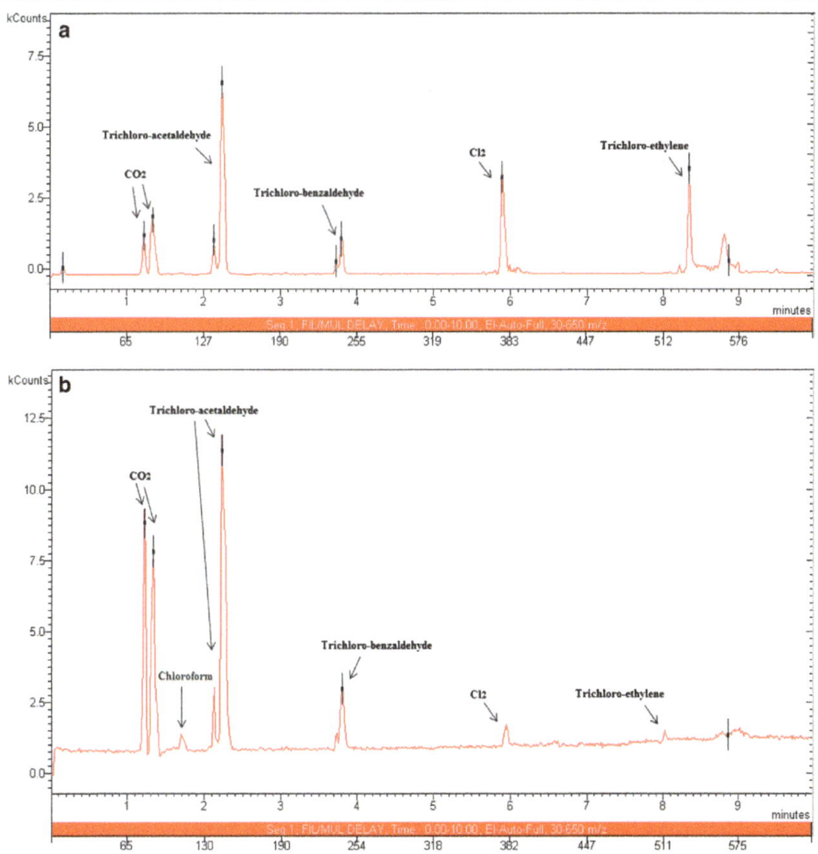

Figure 9 GC/MS chromatogram of chloroform products (a) without toluene, (b) in the presence of toluene.

As a result of this reaction, the selectivity towards CO_2 and Cl_2 can be considerably improved as observed with the NTP-TiO_2/GAC system.

We introduced a hydrogen-rich compound i.e. toluene into the gas stream to shift the reactions to HCl production in the present study. Two main reasons supported this Idea. First, when toluene introduces into the plasma medium, numerous $H^•$ radicals are predicted to generate along with $O^•$ and $Cl^•$, and the number of spontaneous collisions between these radicals is therefore enhanced significantly, resulting in more HCl and H_2O production. Second, there is a strong electronegativity between $H^•$, locating in the extreme left of the periodic table, and $Cl^•$, in the extreme right, offering more HCl production. Foglein et al. [24] also noticed that the presence of hydrogen results in a large number of active radicals such as $OH^•$, and $HO_2^•$ that lead to the subsequent decomposition of $COCl_2$ so fast that leaves it as an intermediate product. As mentioned earlier and shown in Table 3, toluene was converted totally itself but its presence decreased the decomposition of chloroform for the same SIE and initial concentration levels that were tested previously. It is likely related to consumption or deactivation of some radical intermediates present in the NTP reactor by toluene molecules. Table 3 represents the behavior of NTP-TiO_2/GAC system in the presence of toluene in relation to final products. The amount of H_2O was enhanced significantly after toluene introduction, and relative humidity reached up to 65% in the effluent gas at SIE of 2100 J L^{-1}. From these results, OH and HO_2 radicals may be appeared as two major active species generated under toluene feeding conditions but their amount seems to not exceeding that of ozone for which the concentration was still below 1 ppm downstream of the catalyst. Here, a synergy can be recognized between H radicals provided from toluene molecules and ozone that can act as an electron acceptor and donor over catalyst surface to generate $OH^•$ and $HO_2^•$ according to Einaga and Ogata [47]:

(6) $$O_3 + e^- \rightarrow O_3^{•-}$$

(7) $$H^+ + O_3^{•-} \rightarrow HO_3^•$$

(8) $$HO_3^• \rightarrow O_2 + OH^•$$

(9) $$O_3 + e^- \rightarrow O_2 + O^•$$

(10) $$O_3 + OH^• \rightarrow HO_2^• + O_2$$

(11) $$O^• + HO_2 \rightarrow 2OH^•$$

Although no peak was again observed for HCl on mass spectrograms, but a high HCl concentrations were detected using gas detector tubes. HCl was not possible to determine using GC/MS resulting from the interferences between hydrogen chloride and other chlorinated products [48]. However, using hydrogen chloride detector tubes, a favorable selectivity towards HCl was noticed. It seems that addition of hydrogen-rich molecules such as toluene shifts the reaction in both plasma zone and catalyst reactor and causes some reaction pathways to be dominant and contributes to the formation of more H_2O, and HCl [47,48].

(12) $$OH^• + CHCl_3 \rightarrow H_2O + CCl_3$$

(13) $$COCl_2 + H^• \rightarrow COCl^• + HCl$$

(14) $$HCOCl + Cl^• \rightarrow ClCO^• + HCl$$

During the toluene addition, a significant decline was also detected for Cl_2 and TCE, for which the total removal was not achieved but their peak area became negligible. The disappeared Cl_2 may be responsible for the further HCl production in the reaction with water vapor over TiO_2/GAC [49]:

(15) $$H_2O + Cl_2 \Leftrightarrow 2HCl + \frac{1}{2}O_2$$

Two chlorinated by-products that were observed to be increased in the presence of toluene were TCAA and TCBA. These results can be clearly seen in Figure 9b. It is evident from Figure 9b that with toluene feeding, the level of CO_2, TCAA, as well as TCBA increased obviously as compared for chloroform introduction alone (Figure 9a). These findings reveal that toluene addition is highly beneficial in relation to products distribution towards the less harmful by-products. Although these products are heavy aldehyde compounds but they are highly water-soluble and can be totally removed utilizing a wet scrubber downstream of the catalyst reactor. With toluene addition, these desirable results were obtained along with some limitations. First, the extent of other undesirable by-product i.e. CO also went up from less than 15 ppm to ca. 160 ppm for the highest SIE and Figure 8 shows that toluene introduction increased the selectivity towards CO about 5% which was expected due to higher quantities of C- atoms in the toluene structure. Adding hydrogen gas or H_2O may be a good alternative option in this regard. Second, because of higher concentrations and a major difference in the gas composition, the voltage at which corona-to-spark transition occurred, decreased substantially from 22 to 18 KV as toluene fed to the reactor and therefore supplying less energy was achievable. Another reactor configuration combined with other catalysts in the presence of toluene and H_2O is under investigation in order to overcome some of these limitations.

Conclusions

Influence of SIE, initial concentration, and toluene addition on chloroform removal efficiency was investigated in a catalytic plasma pin-to-plate corona discharge reactor. A much better performance was observed for hybrid process in both removal efficiency and COx selectivity compared to NTP-alone system. Ozone was noticed to have a powerful effect on chloroform destruction on TiO_2/GAC surface, and realized to play a key role in producing some active radicals which are helpful to remove hazardous by-products. Strong adsorption property of GAC affected the catalytic activity dramatically. Even though the toluene introduction was highly beneficial for shifting the reactions towards less harmful products, it slightly reduced the chloroform removal efficiency.

Competing interests
The authors declare that they have no competing interests.

Authors' contributions
All authors read and approved the final manuscript.

Acknowledgements
This work was part of Ph.D. thesis financially supported by Hamedan University of Medical Sciences (Grant no. 9107252600).

Author details
[1]Department of occupational health engineering, Research center for health services, Hamedan University of Medical Sciences, Hamedan, Iran. [2]Department of physics, Bu-Ali Sina University, Hamedan, Iran. [3]Department of occupational health, Occupational health research center, School of public health, Iran University of Medical Sciences, Tehran, Iran.

References

1. EPA, Office of air quality, Planning & Standards, Section 112: *Hazardous Air Pollutants List.* 1990.
2. Ministry of environment and forests, East Arjun Nagar, Delhi –110032, Central Pollution Control Board: *PARIVESH hazardous air pollutants.* 2009.
3. Pollution control department, bangkok, Air quality and noise management bureau: *Developement of environmental and emission standards of volatile organic compounds (VOCs) in Thailand.* 2009.
4. Subrahmanyam C, Renken A, Kiwi-Minsker L: **Novel catalytic non-thermal plasma reactor for the abatement of VOCs.** *Chem Eng J* 2007, **134:**78–83.
5. Subrahmanyam C, Renken A, Kiwi-Minsker L: **Catalytic abatement of volatile organic compounds assisted by non-thermal plasma: Part II. Optimized catalytic electrode and operating conditions.** *Appl Catal B-Environ* 2006, **65:**157–162.
6. Kim H, Ogata A, Futamura S: **Complete Oxidation of Volatile Organic Compounds (VOCs) Using Plasma-Driven Catalysis and Oxygen Plasma.** *I J PEST* 2007, **1:**46–51.
7. Agnihotri S, Cal MP, Prien J: **Destruction of 1, 1, 1-trichloroethane using dielectric barrier discharge nonthermal plasma.** *J Environ Eng* 2004, **130:**349–355.
8. An HQ, Huu TP, Van TL, Cormier JM, Khacef A: **Application of atmospheric non thermal plasma-catalysis hybrid system for air pollution control: Toluene removal,** ***Catal.*** *Today* 2011, **176:**474–477.
9. Oda T, Takahashi T, Yamaji K: **TCE decomposition by the nonthermal plasma process concerning ozone effect.** *IEEE T Ind Appl* 2004, **40:**1249–1256.
10. Oda T, Takahashi T, Kohzuma S: **Decomposition of dilute trichloroethylene by using non-thermal plasma processing-frequency and catalyst effect.** In *Industry Applications Conference. Thirty-Third IAS Annual Meeting.* 1998:1871–1876.
11. Mok Y, Lee SB, Oh JH, Ra KS, Sung BH: **Abatement of trichloromethane by using nonthermal plasma reactors.** *Plasma Chem Plasma Process* 2008, **28:**663–676.
12. Magureanu M, Mandache N, Parvulescu V, Subrahmanyam C, Renken A, Kiwi-Minsker L: **Improved performance of non-thermal plasma reactor during decomposition of trichloroethylene: Optimization of the reactor geometry and introduction of catalytic electrode.** *Appl Catal B-Environ* 2007, **74:**270–277.
13. Zhu T, Li J, Jin Y, Liang Y, Ma G: **Gaseous phase benzene decomposition by non-thermal plasma coupled with nano titania catalyst.** *Int J Environ Sci Tech* 2009, **6:**141–148.
14. Wang D, Namihira T, Akiyama H: *Pulsed Discharge Plasma for Pollution Control.* 2010.
15. Kim HH: **Nonthermal Plasma Processing for Air-Pollution Control: A Historical Review, Current Issues, and Future Prospects.** *Plasma Process Polym* 2004, **1:**91–110.
16. Taghvaei H, Shirazi MM, Hooshmand N, Rahimpour MR, Jahanmiri A: **Experimental investigation of hydrogen production through heavy naphtha cracking in pulsed DBD reactor.** *Appl Energy* 2012, **98:**3–10.
17. Jahanmiri A, Rahimpour MR, Mohamadzadeh Shirazi M, Hooshmand N, Taghvaei H: **Naphtha cracking through a pulsed DBD plasma reactor: Effect of applied voltage, pulse repetition frequency and electrode material.** *Chem Eng J* 2012, **191:**416–425.
18. Taghvaei H, Jahanmiri A, Rahimpour MR, Shirazi MM, Hooshmand N: **Hydrogen production through plasma cracking of hydrocarbons: Effect of carrier gas and hydrocarbon type.** *Chem Eng J* 2013, **226:**384–392.
19. Rahimpour MR, Jahanmiri A, Mohamadzadeh Shirazi M, Hooshmand N, Taghvaei H: **Combination of non-thermal plasma and heterogeneous catalysis for methane and hexadecane co-cracking: Effect of voltage and catalyst configuration.** *Chem Eng J* 2013, **219:**245–253.
20. Chen HL, Lee HM, Chen SH, Chang MB, Yu SJ, Li SN: **Removal of volatile organic compounds by single-stage and two-stage plasma catalysis systems: a review of the performance enhancement mechanisms, current status, and suitable applications.** *Environ Sci Technol* 2009, **43:**2216–2227.
21. Durme JV, Dewulf J, Leys C, Langenhove HV: **Combining non-thermal plasma with heterogeneous catalysis in waste gas treatment: A review.** *Appl Catal B-Environ* 2008, **78:**324–333.
22. Mo J, Zhang Y, Xu Q, Lamson JJ, Zhao R: **Photocatalytic purification of volatile organic compounds in indoor air: A literature review.** *Atmos Environ* 2009, **43:**2229–2246.
23. Indarto A, Choi JW, Lee H, Song HK: **Treatment of CCl4 and CHCl3 emission in a gliding-arc plasma.** *Plasma Devices Oper* 2006, **14:**1–14.
24. Főglein KA, Szabó PT, Babievskaya IZ, Szépvölgyi J: **Comparative study on the decomposition of chloroform in thermal and cold plasma.** *Plasma Chem Plasma Process* 2005, **25:**289–302.
25. Krawczyk K, Ulejczyk B, Song HK, Lamenta A, Paluch B: **Schmidt-Szałowski K:Plasma-catalytic reactor for decomposition of chlorinated hydrocarbons.** *Plasma Chem Plasma Process* 2009, **29:**27–41.
26. Ojala S, Pitkäaho S, Laitinen T, Koivikko NN, Brahmi R, Gaálová J, Matejova L, Kucherov A, Päivärinta S, Hirschmann C: **Catalysis in VOC Abatement.** *Top Catal* 2011, **54:**1224–1256.
27. Hu Y, Yuan C: **Low-temperature preparation of photocatalytic TiO_2 thin films on polymer substrates by direct deposition from anatase sol.** *J Mater Sci Technol* 2006, **22:**239–244.
28. Xu J, Ao Y, Fu D, Yuan C: **Synthesis of fluorine-doped titania-coated activated carbon under low temperature with high photocatalytic activity under visible light.** *J Phys Chem Solids* 2008, **69:**2366–2370.
29. Linga BVM, Reddy E, Subrahmanyam C: **Production of hydrogen from hydrogen sulfide assisted by dielectric barrier discharge.** *Int J Hydrogen Energ* 2012, **37:**2204–2209.
30. Jahanmiri A, Shirazia M, Hooshmanda N, Taghvaeia H: **Naphtha cracking through a pulsed DBD plasma reactor: Effect of applied voltage, pulse repetition frequency and electrode material.** *Chem Eng J* 2012, **191:**416–425.
31. Kogelschatz U: **Filamentary, patterned, and diffuse barrier discharges.** *IEEE T Plasma Sci* 2002, **30:**1400–1408.
32. Oda T, Kuramochi H, Ono R: **Trichloroethylene decomposition by the nonthermal plasma Combined with manganese-dioxide supported alumina.** *Int J PEST* 2008, **2:**50–55.
33. Francke KP, Miessner H, Rudolph R: **Cleaning of air streams from organic pollutants by plasma–catalytic oxidation.** *Plasma Chem Plasma Process* 2000, **20:**393–403.
34. Iijima S, Nakamura M, Yokoi A, Kubota M, Huang L, Matsuda H: **Decomposition of dichloromethane and in situ alkali absorption of resulting halogenated products by a packed-bed non-thermal plasma reactor.** *J Mater Cycles Waste Manage* 2011, **13:**206–212.
35. Urashima K, Chang JS: **Removal of volatile organic compounds from air streams and industrial flue gases by non-thermal plasma technology.** *IEEE Trans Dielectr Electr Insul* 2000, **7**(5):602–614.

36. Munter R: **Advanced oxidation processes–current status and prospects.** *Proc Estonian Acad Sci Chem* 2001, **50**(2):59–80.
37. Zhu T, Li J, Jin YQ, Liang Y, Ma G: **Decomposition of benzene by non-thermal plasma processing: Photocatalyst and ozone effect.** *Int J Environ Sci Technol* 2008, **5**(3):375–384.
38. Kang CS, You YJ, Kim KJ, Kim TH, Ahn SJ, Chung KH, Park NC, Kimura S, Ahn HG: **Selective catalytic reduction of NOx with propene over double wash-coat monolith catalysts.** *Catal Today* 2006, **111**:229–235.
39. Shelef M: **Selective catalytic reduction of NOx with N-free reductants.** *Chem Review* 1995, **95**:209–225.
40. Twigg MV: **Roles of catalytic oxidation in control of vehicle exhaust emissions.** *Catal Today* 2006, **117**:407–418.
41. Magureanu M, Mandache N, Parvulescu V: **Chlorinated organic compounds decomposition in a dielectric barrier discharge.** *Plasma Chem Plasma Process* 2007, **27**:679–690.
42. Vandenbroucke A, Vanderstricht A, Dinh MTN, Giraudon JM, Morent R, Geyter ND, Lamonier JF, Leys C: **Non-thermal plasma abatement of trichloroethylene with DC corona discharges.** In *19th International conference on Modelling, Monitoring and Management of Air Pollution; WIT Press*; 2011:147.
43. Karuppiah J, Subrahmanyam C: **The catalytic effect of MnOx and CoOx on the decomposition of nitrobenzene in a non-thermal plasma reactor.** *Chem Eng J* 2012, **180**:39–45.
44. Indarto A, Choi JW, Lee H, Song HK: **Decomposition of greenhouse gases by plasma.** *Environ Chem Lett* 2008, **6**:215–222.
45. Schmidt-Szałowski K, Krawczyk K, Sentek J, Ulejczyk B, Górska A, Młotek M: **Hybrid plasma-catalytic systems for converting substances of high stability, greenhouse gases and VOC.** *Chem Eng Res Des* 2011, **89**:2643–2651.
46. Lee WJ, Chen CY, Lin WC, Wang YT, Chin CJ: **Phosgene formation from the decomposition of 1, 1-C2H2Cl2 contained gas in an RF plasma reactor.** *J haz mat* 1996, **48**:51–67.
47. Einaga H: **Benzene oxidation with ozone over supported Manganese oxide catalysts: effect of catalyst support and reaction conditions.** *J Haz Mat* 2009, **164**:1236–1241.
48. Vandenbroucke A, Morent R, De Geyter N, Leys C: **Decomposition of Trichloroethylene with Plasma-catalysis: A review.** *J Adv Oxid Technol* 2011, **14**:165–173.
49. González-Velasco JR, Aranzabal A, López-Fonseca R, Ferret R, González-Marcos JA: **Enhancement of the catalytic oxidation of hydrogen-lean chlorinated VOCs in the presence of hydrogen-supplying compounds.** *Appl Catal B* 2000, **24**(1):33–43.

Response surface modeling of lead (II) removal by graphene oxide-Fe_3O_4 nanocomposite using central composite design

Mohammad Khazaei[1], Simin Nasseri[1,2*], Mohammad Reza Ganjali[3,4], Mehdi Khoobi[5], Ramin Nabizadeh[1], Amir Hossein Mahvi[1,2,6], Shahrokh Nazmara[1] and Elham Gholibegloo[7]

Abstract

Background: Magnetic graphene oxide (Fe_3O_4@SiO_2-GO) nanocomposite was fabricated through a facile process and its application as an excellent adsorbent for lead (II) removal was also demonstrated by applying response surface methodology (RSM).

Methods: Fe_3O_4@SiO_2-GO nanocomposite was synthesized and characterized properly. The effects of four independent variables, initial pH of solution (3.5–8.5), nanocomposite dosage (1–60 mg L^{-1}), contact time (2–30 min), and initial lead (II) ion concentration (0.5–5 mg L^{-1}) on the lead (II) removal efficiency were investigated and the process was optimized using RSM. Using central composite design (CCD), 44 experiments were carried out and the process response was modeled using a quadratic equation as function of the variables.

Results: The optimum values of the variables were found to be 6.9, 30.5 mg L^{-1}, 16 min, and 2.49 mg L^{-1} for pH, adsorbent dosage, contact time, and lead (II) initial concentration, respectively. The amount of adsorbed lead (II) after 16 min was recorded as high as 505.81 mg g^{-1} for 90 mg L^{-1} initial lead (II) ion concentration. The Sips isotherm was found to provide a good fit with the adsorption data ($K_S = 256$ L mg^{-1}, $n_S = 0.57$, $q_m = 598.4$ mg g^{-1}, and $R^2 = 0.984$). The mean free energy E_{ads} was 9.901 kJ/mol which confirmed the chemisorption mechanism. The kinetic study determined an appropriate compliance of experimental data with the double exponential kinetic model ($R^2 = 0.982$).

Conclusions: Quadratic and reduced models were examined to correlate the variables with the removal efficiency of Fe_3O_4@SiO_2-GO. According to the analysis of variance, the most influential factors were identified as pH and contact time. At the optimum condition, the adsorption yield was achieved up to nearly 100 %.

Keywords: Graphene oxide, Adsorption, Lead (II), Optimization, Central composite design

Background

Effluents containing Lead and other toxic metals (II) are increasingly discharged into the water supplies due to the expansion of industries [1]. The maximum levels lower than 15 ppb for lead (II) in drinking waters has been mandated by many environmental agencies and national standard organizations [2–4]. The strict limitations on discharging effluents contained lead (II) to the natural water bodies are attributed to the lead (II) potential health effects on children and adults [3].

Many processes such as precipitation, membrane filtration, adsorption, and ion exchange have been applied to remove lead (II) and other toxic metals from the industrial effluents [5]. Only a few methods such as using functionalized adsorbents and membrane technologies can be adopted to capture low concentrations around 1 mg L^{-1}, which is commonly occurred in drinking water sources [6]. Although, adsorption processes are

* Correspondence: khazaei@muq.ac.ir
[1]Department of Environmental Health Engineering, School of Public Health, Tehran University of Medical Sciences, Tehran, Iran
[2]Center for Water Quality Research, Institute for Environmental Research, Tehran University of Medical Sciences, Tehran, Iran
Full list of author information is available at the end of the article

useful in removal low concentrations of metal ions from aqueous solutions, but there are two main limitations regarding to the use of them; 1. low adsorption capacity [7, 8], and 2. difficult separation of adsorbent from treated water after the end of adsorption process [9–11].

Graphene oxide is an emerging carbon-based nonmaterial that has revealed the promising adsorptive properties [12, 13]. Graphene oxide (GO) creates a highly stable aqueous dispersion which prepares an excellent situation for effective contacts with target contaminants without needing to vigorous mechanical mixing [14]. The GO flakes have high specific surface area ranging from 600 to 3500 m^2 g^{-1} [15, 16]. The dispersibility property of GO is attributed to the plenty of hydrophilic functional groups on the GO flakes [15]. The GO flake surface contains different functional groups including epoxide and hydroxide, whereas, the edge of flakes are mainly contained a hedge of carboxylic groups [14].

Using magnetic agents like Fe_3O_4 has been considered as a way to separate the GO nanosheets from aqueous solution when the adsorption process is finished [17, 18]. Some methods employed for the adding of Fe_3O_4 on the GO surface are generally led to form reduced GO (rGO) [19, 20]. Because of the elimination of functional groups during the reduction process, rGO represents weak dispersity [14]. Hence, preserving the GO dispersibility in the aqueous solution as well as adding the magnetic property for separation purposes is under consideration.

Few literatures were reported applying non reduced Fe_3O_4/GO for the adsorption purposes [17, 21, 22]. Among them, some synthesis approaches have relied on the formation of covalent bonds between the GO sheets and Fe_3O_4 nanoparticles [17, 22] which has more stability than those methods based on physical attraction [21].

This research aimed to fabricate the covalent bond Fe_3O_4@SiO_2-GO nanocomposite as a highly dispersible and easy separatable adsorbent for the elimination of lead (II) from aqueous solution. Other purpose of the study was determining the optimal operational condition using response surface methodology (RSM) to achieve satisfactory lead (II) removal. The conventional optimization method, which altered one variable at a time by keeping the other variables constant, is a time consuming and costly approach that can not consider the interactive effects between variables. RSM technique is an empirical statistical approach used to evaluate the relationship between a set of controlled experimental variables and observed results. It can be applied to optimize and identify the performance of adsorption process. Minimum experimental runs are achievable by using RSM. Applying RSM reduces the experiment runs and the reagents consumption. It also facilitates the execution of experiments necessary for the construction of the response surface.

Methods

Materials

Graphite powder (particle size < 20 μm), tetraethyl orthosilicate (TEOS), (3-aminopropyl) triethoxysilane (APTES), n- hydroxysuccinimide (NHS) and 1- ethyl-3-(3-dimethyl aminopropyl) carbodiimide (EDC.HCl) were purchased from Sigma- Aldrich, Ltd. Co. All other chemicals such as sodium nitrate ($NaNO_3$), potassium permanganate ($KMnO_4$), sulfuric acid (H_2SO_4), hydrochloric acid (HCl), hydrogen peroxide aqueous solution (H_2O_2), iron chloride hexahydrate ($FeCl_3$, 6 H_2O), and iron chloride tetrahydrate ($FeCl_2$, 4 H_2O) were of reagent grade and used without further purification.

Preparation of graphene oxide (GO)

Graphene oxide was synthesized from the graphite powder by the modified Hummers et al. method [23]. Briefly, 2.0 g of graphite powder and 2.0 g of $NaNO_3$ were mixed with 92 mL of H_2SO_4 (98 %) in a flask and stirred in an ice bath vigorously for 0.5 h, and then 12.0 g of $KMnO_4$ was added to the above solution slowly. After stirring for 0.5 h, the ice bath was removed and the solution was stirred in a water bath at 35 °C for 6 h. After that, 160 mL of the DI water was added slowly to the flask. Then, the obtained mixture was stirred at 90^{0}Cfor 2 h. Afterward 400 mL of DI water was added and followed by addition of 12 mL of H_2O_2 (30 %), Upon which the color of mixture turned to bright yellow. The obtained suspension was washed with 1:10 HCl solution (150 mL) and DI water several times to remove metal ions [24]. The resultant dispersion was sonicated at 130 KHz for 2 h and centrifuged to obtain exfoliated graphene oxide [25].

Preparation of Fe_3O_4@SiO_2-NH_2

The Fe_3O_4 magnetic nanoparticles were synthesized using a coprecipitation method [26]. For the synthesis of Fe_3O_4@SiO_2- NH_2, 1.0 g of the obtained Fe_3O_4MNPs was dispersed in a mixture of 40 mL ethanol and 10 mL of DI water using an ultrasonic water bath. After that, o.5 mL TEOS and 2 mL $NH_3.H_2O$ (25 %) were added, and the mixture was stirred at 50 °C for 6 h. The solid product was collected by an external magnetic field, washed with ethanol and dried under vacuum. In the next step, 1 g of the obtained Fe_3O_4@SiO_2 was dispersed in 25 mL dried toluene and treated with addition of 1 mL APTES [27]. The mixture was refluxed for 24 h under nitrogen atmosphere. The product was washed with ethanol and then dried to obtain Fe_3O_4@SiO_2-NH_2 [28].

Preparation of Fe_3O_4@SiO_2-GO

The condensation reaction between amine groups of Fe_3O_4@SiO_2-NH_2 and carboxyl groups of GO was performed [28]. Typically, 0.2 g GO was dispersed in 50 mL DI water containing of 0.1 g NHS and 0.2 g EDC.HCl by ultrasonication for 2 h. Subsequently, 0.5 g $Fe_3O_4@SiO_2$- $NH_2$was added to the above mixture and stirred for 12 h at room temperature. The solid product was collected and washed with DI water and ethanol by magnetic separation and then dried under vacuum [17, 29]. Figure 1 shows a schematic view of the synthesis process.

To confirm the stability of nanocomposite, concentration of Iron after the adsorption process was measured. As shown in Tables 2, and 3, the leaching of Iron into the aqueous solution after contact times was negligible.

Characterization

The SEM images were taken with Hitachi- S4160 scanning microscope (Tokyo, Japan) to survey the morphological pattern and surface structural aspects of GO and $Fe_3O_4@SiO_2$-GO nanocomposite. A Nanoscope V multimode atomic force microscope (Veeco Instruments, USA) were used to perform AFM measurements. The AFM images were taken from samples which prepared by deposition a dispersed GO/methanol solution (70 mg mL^{-1}) onto a mica surface and allowing them to dry in air [25]. The images were taken under ambient condition by adjusting the instrument on the tapping mode.

Batch adsorption experiments

Using a thermostatic shaker, batch experiments were conducted in 100 mL Erlenmeyer flasks to study the removal of lead (II) on the $Fe_3O_4@SiO_2$-GO nanocomposite. The different volumes contained known quantities of as-dispersed $Fe_3O_4@SiO_2$-GO nanocomposite were added to 20 mL solution having predominated concentrations of Pb^{2+}. All solutions underwent constant mixing at the 300 rpm for different contact times determined by the experimental design. After ending the adsorption process, the nanocomposite was eliminated from the aqueous solution by a magnet. The equation (1) was applied to determine the removal efficiency of lead (II):

$$R(\%) = \frac{(C_0 - C_e)}{C_0} \times 100 \quad (1)$$

Where, R *(%)* is the removal efficiency, C_0 and C_t are the concentrations (as mg L^{-1}) of lead (II) at 0 and t minutes after the contact time, respectively.

The equilibrium adsorption capacity was also obtained as equation (2):

$$q_e = \frac{(C_0 - C_e)}{x_{ads}} \times 1000 \quad (2)$$

Where, q_e is the equilibrium capacity (mg g^{-1}), x_{ads} is the nanocomposite concentration in aqueous solution (mg L^{-1}), and 1000 is converting factor (mg g^{-1}).

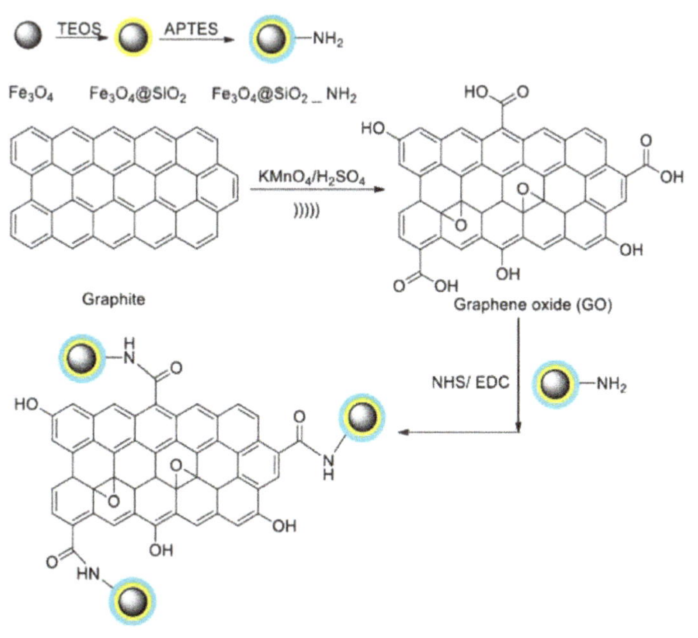

Fig. 1 Schematic of the chemical path to the synthesis of $Fe_3O_4@SiO_2$-GO nanocomposite. (TEOS: tetraethylorthosilicate, APTES: 3 aminopropyltriethoxysilane)

Lead (II) measurements in the aqueous solution were performed by using a Spectro Arcos ICP-optical emission spectrometer (SPECTRO Analytical Instruments, Kleve, Germany) based on radial plasma observation. The Spectro Arcos has a Paschen–Runge mount which equipped with 32 linear CCD detectors. The CCD detectors supply the ability of simultaneous monitoring of line intensities at wavelengths between 130 and 770 nm.

Isotherm and kinetic constants were obtained using the Solver "add-in" with Microsoft Excel spreadsheet program [30] according to the nonlinear forms of the equations.

Experimental design

Central composite design (CCD) was used to investigate the lead (II) removal. The RSM was employed to evaluate the combined effects of pH (X_1), GO-Fe_3O_4 dose (X_2), contact time (X_3), and initial lead (II) concentration (X_4) on the adsorption process. The experimental conditions of independent variables, which were derived from CCD, are summarized in Table 1. The lead (II) removal efficiency (Y) were served as output responses. Applying two blocks, one cube block and one star block, total 44 experiments were carried out, consisting of 20 center points, $2^4 = 16$ design point, and $2 \times 4 = 8$ axial points.

The details of 44 experiments are presented in Table 2. The chosen independent factors applied in the study were coded based on Eq. (3):

$$x_i = \frac{(X_i - X_0)}{\Delta X} \tag{3}$$

Where, x_i is a dimensionless coded value of the *ith* independent variable, X_0 is the center point value of X_i and ΔX is the step change value. A quadratic (second order) model as shown in Eq. (4) was applied to approximate the interaction between the response (Y) and four independent variables:

$$Y = b_0 + \sum_{i=1}^{k} b_i X_i + \sum_{i=1}^{k} b_{ii} X_i^2 + \sum_{i=1}^{k-1} \sum_{j=2}^{k} b_{ij} X_i X_j + c \tag{4}$$

Where, Y represents the dependent variable (lead (II) removal efficiency), b_0 is a constant value, b_i, b_{ii}, and b_{ij} refer to the regression coefficient for linear, second order, and interactive effects, respectively, Xi, and Xj are the independent variables, c denotes the error of prediction.

The above mentioned CCD analysis plus to the statistical analysis, such as ANOVA, F-test, and t-test were obtained using R software (version 3.0.3: 2014-03-06).

Table 1 The original and coded levels of independent variables

Original factors	Coded levels				
	-α	−1	0	+1	+α
pH X_1	3.5	4.75	6	7.25	8.5
Fe_3O_4@SiO_2-GO -X_2 (mg/L)	1	15.75	30.5	46.25	60
Time-X_3 (min)	2	9	16	23	30
Initial Pb^{2+} Concentration-X_4 (ppm)	0.5	1.625	2.75	3.87	5

Results and discussion

Characterization of GO-Fe_3O_4 nanocomposite

As shown in Fig. 2, a UV- visible spectrum obtained for the GO aqueous dispersion (orange line) displays a plasmon peak at 231 nm which is related to the $\pi \rightarrow \pi^*$ transitions due to the aromatic $C-C$ bonds. Also, a hump can be detected around 300 nm approving the $n \rightarrow \pi^*$ transitions of $C=O$ bonds [31, 32]. Gradually adding the lead (II) aqueous ions into the GO dispersion resulted in producing a growing humpy pattern around 300 nm which can be attributed to the affinity between lead (II) and $C=O$ bonds relating to the carboxylic groups in the GO structure [33].

Fabricated Fe_3O_4@SiO_2-GO was characterized with different techniques. Figure 3 shows the field emission SEM images of GO and Fe_3O_4@SiO_2-GO. Figure 3a illustrated the fluffy nature of GO layers which turned to agglomerated morphology after the formation of covalent bonds with Fe_3O_4@SiO_2-NH2 and producing Fe_3O_4@SiO_2-GO (Fig. 3b). The magnetic properties of the prepared nanocomposite were characterized using vibration sample magnetization (VSM). Figure 4 shows the magnetization curve patterns of Fe_3O_4, Fe_3O_4@-SiO_2-NH_2, and Fe_3O_4@SiO_2-GO. As inferred from Fig. 4, the maximum saturation magnetizations of Fe_3O_4, Fe_3O_4@SiO_2-NH_2, and Fe_3O_4@SiO_2-GO were 60.2, 43.8, and 22.3 emu g^{-1}, respectively.

The VSM curves (Fig. 4) shows that, the magnetic power of Fe_3O_4 nanoparticles were dropped into the one third of original state which was due to both the SiO_2-NH_2 coverage and the GO covalent bonds. But, the remaining 22.3 emu g^{-1} of saturation magnetization can still be considered as a powerful magnetic field to separate the nanocomposite from the aqueous solution, as shown in the Fig. 4d. Also, the coercivity and remanence were not observed after removing the magnetic field. From Fig. 4d, the yellow brown color of the GO dispersion revealed that the oxygenation of the graphene nanosheets has been effectively occurred during the synthesis [16, 34]. After 3 months from the GO preparation, there is no any visible sign of sedimentation which shows long-term dispersibility of GO in water.

The AFM image of GO nanosheets is illustrated in Fig. 5a. Also, Fig. 5b shows the distribution of GO obtaining 210 nanosheets found in a certain area of the mica surface which confirms preparing a well distributed

Table 2 Observed and predicted values for the quadratic model (T = 298 K)[a]

Run no.	Observed values (%)	Predicted values (%)	Residual	Run no.	Observed values	Predicted values	Residual
1	53.433	57.917	−4.484	23	98.579	100.000	−1.421
2	98.904	67.699	31.205	24	90.133	83.418	6.715
3	95.230	96.303	−1.074	25	80.601	85.100	−4.500
4	95.600	23.773	71.826	26	98.995	100.000	−1.005
5	95.317	94.748	0.570	27	99.263	95.067	4.196
6	95.375	94.747	0.628	28	94.576	94.739	−0.163
7	95.626	94.757	0.869	29	94.923	94.742	0.182
8	94.884	94.749	0.135	30	89.334	88.112	1.222
9	98.796	94.709	4.087	31	98.009	100.000	−1.991
10	92.002	94.739	−2.737	32	41.095	49.543	−8.448
11	87.971	87.427	0.544	33	93.478	94.836	−1.359
12	56.850	61.083	−4.234	34	95.341	94.742	0.599
13	98.432	66.637	31.796	35	94.931	94.798	0.133
14	99.493	91.859	7.634	36	96.083	99.816	−3.733
15	94.866	94.770	0.096	37	99.695	93.757	5.938
16	99.589	54.557	45.031	38	86.848	85.821	1.026
17	95.032	94.750	0.281	39	95.115	94.757	0.359
18	95.019	94.759	0.260	40	94.402	94.747	−0.345
19	92.438	84.665	7.773	41	94.495	98.033	−3.537
20	92.624	84.440	8.184	42	95.071	94.947	0.124
21	93.237	83.804	9.433	43	95.290	94.968	0.322
22	95.020	94.797	0.223	44	99.006	100.000	−0.994

[a]The average concentration of Iron (measured by ICP-OES) after ending contact times for 44 adsorption runs: 4.32 ± 1.01 ppb

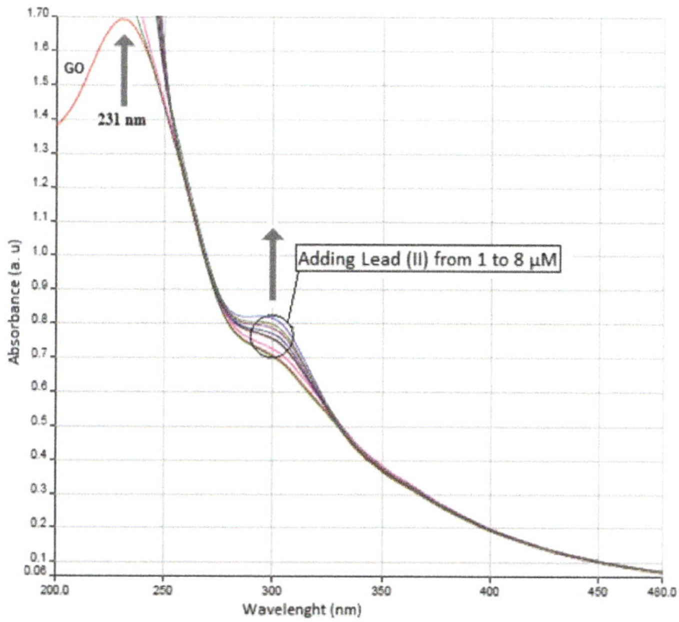

Fig. 2 UV-visible spectra for GO dispersion in water before (*Orange line*) and after adding the different concentrations of Lead (II). Lead (II) initial concentration = 1 μM, pH = 6.8, T = 298 K

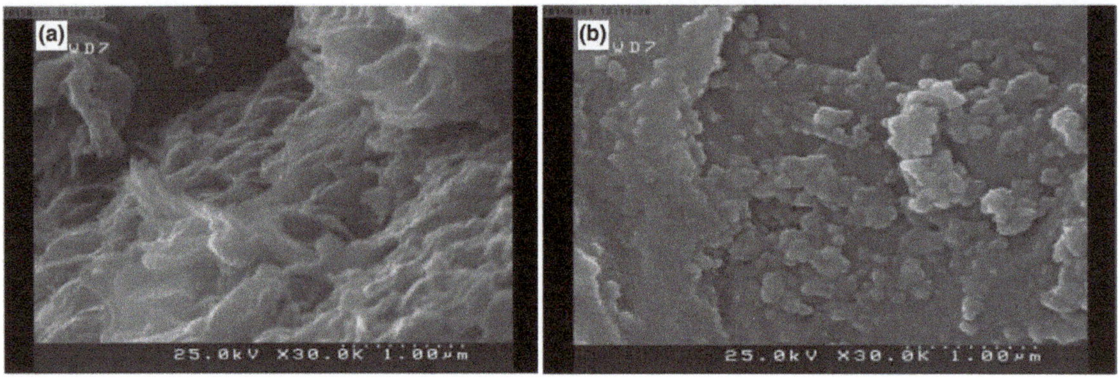

Fig. 3 Typical FE-SEM of GO (**a**), and $Fe_3O_4@SiO_2$-GO (**b**)

dispersion. As shown in Fig. 5b, the average thickness measured was 2.74 nm revealed producing few layered (1 and 2 layers) GO [35].

As shown in Fig. 5c, the thickness of a random GO sheet measured using the height profile (Line 1) in the AFM image, is about 0.75 nm. This sub-nanometer thickness confirms producing the GO monolayer [14].

Figure 6 shows the FT-IR spectra obtained for GO, Fe_3O_4, and $Fe_3O_4@SiO_2$-GO materials. Figure 6a depicts the characteristic features illustrated in the FT-IR spectrum for GO which are contained the adsorption bands attributed to the C-O stretching at 1055 cm^{-1}, the C–OH stretching at 1226 cm^{-1}, and the C-O carbonyl stretching at 1733 cm^{1} [36–38]. Furthermore, the O-H hydroxide stretching vibrations appear at 3419 cm^{-1}. Also, the adsorbed water molecules stretching at 1621 cm^{-1}, although it may feature due to the skeletal vibrations of un-oxidized graphitic remnants [39, 40].

As can be seen from Fig. 6b, the spectrum of the Fe_3O_4 shows the Fe-O stretching vibration at 591 cm^{-1}, and an intense OH band around 3400 cm^{-1}. The OH band is attributed to the stretching vibrations of Fe-OH groups attached on the Fe_3O_4 surface and also can be

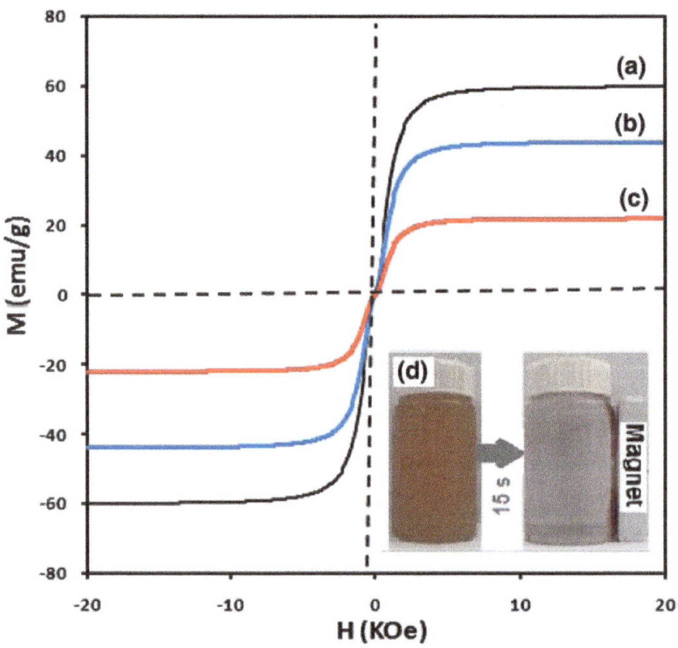

Fig. 4 Magnetic hysteresis loops of Fe_3O_4 (**a**), $Fe_3O_4@SiO_2-NH_2$ (**b**), and $Fe_3O_4@SiO_2$-GO (**c**). Photographic image of 1.4 mg mL^{-3} $Fe_3O_4@SiO_2$-GO dispersions in water before (*left image*) and after (*right image*) exposing to the external magnetic field for 15 s (**d**)

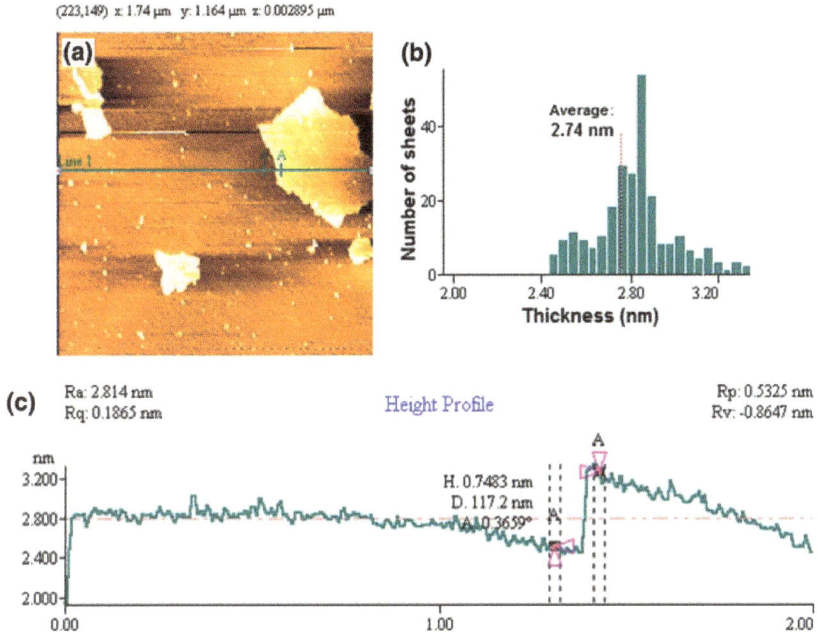

Fig. 5 Tapered mode AFM topography scan. Exfoliated graphene oxide deposited on a freshly cleaved mica surface (**a**). Histogram of platelet thicknesses from images of 210 platelets (the mean thickness is 2.74 nm) (**b**). Height profile through the green line (*Line 1*) presented in (**a**). Cross-section A-A through the sheet shown in (**a**) exhibiting a height minimum of 0.748 nm (**c**)

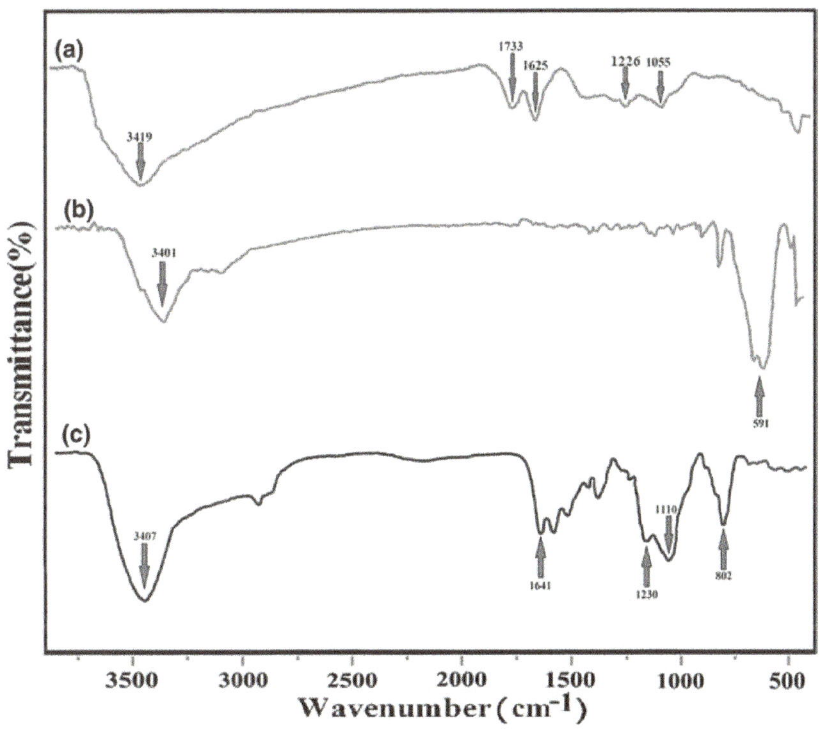

Fig. 6 FT-IR spectra of GO (**a**), Fe_3O_4 (**b**), and Fe_3O_4@SiO_2-GO (**c**)

assigned to the remaining water that was not eliminated from the surface of the Fe_3O_4 nanoparticles [41].

As depicted in Fig. 6c, the peak at 3401 cm^{-1} of Fig. 5c attributed to the $-NH_2$ vibration. Comparing Fig. 6c with Fig. 6a, the peak at 1733 cm^{-1} was almost disappeared, and a new broad peak was emerged at 1641 cm-1 corresponding to C = O characteristic stretching band of the amide group. The stretching band of the amide C–N peak appears at 1230 cm^{-1} [42]. Meanwhile, as shown in Fig. 6c, the peaks at 802 and 1110 cm^{-1} were obviously observed due to the Si–O vibrations. From these findings, it is recommended that APTES functionalized Fe_3O_4 was covalently bonded to GO through the amide linkage [22].

Response surface methodology model analysis

Predicted values for lead (II) removal efficiencies (%) applying quadratic model and reduced quadratic model were represented in Tables 2 and 3, respectively. The statistical significance of models was depicted in Tables 4 and 5 which represent the analysis of variance (ANOVA) for the quadratic model and reduced quadratic model, respectively.

The reduced quadratic model was applied by omitting the variables assigned to the P-values more than 0.05 in the quadratic model [43].

The values of the determination coefficient (multiple R^2) shown in Tables 4 and 5 indicated that 87.9 and 86.3 % of the variability in the response could be explained by the quadratic and reduced quadratic models, respectively.

If there have been various terms in the model and also the sample size has not been very large, the adjusted correlation coefficient (adjusted R^2) may represent values considerably smaller than the multiple correlation coefficients (Multiple R^2) [44]. In this experiment, the adjusted correlation coefficient value (adjusted $R^2 = 0.836$) are also noticeable to support the high significance of the models and approves a satisfactory adjustment for the reduced quadratic model to the experimental data [45–47].

The values of the determination coefficient (multiple R^2) shown in Tables 4 and 5 indicated that 87.9 and 86.3 % of the variability in the response could be explained by the quadratic and reduced quadratic models, respectively.

Table 3 Observed and predicted values for the reduced cubic model (T = 298 K)[a]

Run no.	Observed values (%)	Predicted values (%)	Residual	Run no.	Observed values	Predicted values	Residual
1	53.433	59.426	−5.994	23	98.579	100.000	−1.421
2	98.904	68.393	30.511	24	90.133	83.437	6.696
3	95.230	96.805	−1.575	25	80.601	86.087	−5.486
4	95.600	25.705	69.894	26	98.995	100.000	−1.005
5	95.317	94.994	0.323	27	99.263	95.744	3.519
6	95.375	94.994	0.381	28	94.576	94.994	−0.418
7	95.626	94.994	0.632	29	94.923	94.994	−0.070
8	94.884	94.994	−0.110	30	89.334	89.160	0.175
9	98.796	93.827	4.969	31	98.009	94.994	3.015
10	92.002	94.994	−2.992	32	41.095	50.054	−8.959
11	87.971	86.087	1.884	33	93.478	94.994	−1.516
12	56.850	59.426	−2.577	34	95.341	94.994	0.347
13	98.432	66.406	32.026	35	94.931	94.994	−0.063
14	99.493	93.430	6.063	36	96.083	100.000	−3.917
15	94.866	94.994	−0.128	37	99.695	93.715	5.980
16	99.589	56.162	43.426	38	86.848	88.655	−1.807
17	95.032	94.994	0.038	39	95.115	94.994	0.122
18	95.019	94.994	0.025	40	94.402	94.994	−0.591
19	92.438	84.254	8.184	41	94.495	100.000	−5.505
20	92.624	84.254	8.370	42	95.071	94.994	0.077
21	93.237	83.437	9.800	43	95.290	94.994	0.296
22	95.020	94.994	0.026	44	99.006	94.994	4.012

[a]The average concentration of Iron (measured by ICP-OES) after ending contact times for 44 adsorption runs: 2.44 ± 0.12 ppb

Table 4 Analysis of variance (ANOVA) for the quadratic model

Model formula in rsm (X_1,X_2,X_3,X_4)	DF	Sum of squares	Mean square	F-value	Probability (P)
First-order response	4	3307.4	826.85	31.7283	<0.0001
Two-way interactions	6	999.2	166.53	6.3903	0.0002
Pure quadratic response	4	1173.2	293.30	11.2546	<0.0001
Residuals	29	755.7	26.06	-	-
Lack of fit	28	750.5	26.80	5.1449	

Multiple $R^2 = 0.879$; Adjusted $R^2 = 0.820$; Lack of fit: 0.337

As revealed from Tables 4 and 5, the "lack of fit (LOF)" values were 0.337 and 0.355 for the quadratic and reduced quadratic models, respectively. The insignificant values of LOF (>0.05) and the significant *P*-values for both models prove that applying models is eligible to interpret the lead (II) removal process and also, the reduced model is the better choice because of the higher adjusted R^2 (0.836) and the higher value obtained for LOF (0.355) [43, 46].

Table 6 represents the regression analysis obtained from the reduced quadratic model. As shown, the significant of each coefficient was determined by *P*-value. Also, Values of "Prob > |t|" less than 0.05 in Table 6 indicate that all the model terms are significant. The bigger amounts of the t-values beside the smaller amounts of P-values show the more significant of the corresponding coefficients [46]. Based on the t- and *P* –value results, pH and time can be considered as the substantial effective factors on the lead (II) adsorption. The effect of each model term, also, can be observed from the coefficient estimate values represented in Table 6.

Contour plots depicted in Fig. 7 are the graphical illustrations of the regression analysis (Table 6) which represent the simultaneous effects of adsorbent-pH (a), time-pH (b), and time-adsorbent (c) on lead (II) removal efficiency as the response factor. As noted above, the interaction effects of pH (X_1) and Fe_3O_4@-SiO_2-GO dose (X_2) on the lead (II) removal is shown in Fig. 7a. The contact time and lead (II) initial concentration were fixed constant at 16 min and 2.49 mg/L, respectively. As shown, the lead (II) removal increased with increasing the Fe_3O_4@SiO_2-GO dosage. The maximum lead (II) removal was obtained in the range of pH from 6.5 to 8.5. In that range, the lead (II) removal was independent from the adsorbent dosage. In the pH values between 3–6.5, almost a direct relationship between pH and lead (II) removal was observed.

The effects of pH (X_1) and contact time (X_3) on lead (II) removal are shown in Fig. 7b. The adsorbent dose and lead (II) initial concentration were fixed constant at 30.5 mg/L and 2.49 mg/L, respectively. It is inferred from Fig. 7b that around the neutral pH, the lead (II) removal process was almost completed during the contact time up to 10 min. But for pH values less than 4, after the contact time more than 30 min, the removal efficiency near 70 % was achieved.

The effects of Fe_3O_4@SiO_2-GO dosage (X_2) and contact time (X_3) on lead (II) removal can be observed in Fig. 7c. The pH and lead (II) initial concentration were fixed constant at 6 and 2.49 mg/L, respectively. Figure 7b shows that, for the adsorbent doses more than 40 mg/L, regardless the contact time, the lead (II) removal efficiency revealed the levels permanently beyond 95 %.

Lead (II) removal showed to be very sensitive to changes in the pH both in low and high adsorbent dose. The removal capacity of Fe_3O_4@SiO_2-GO nanocomposite was rapidly increased when the pH increased from 3.5 to 8.5; as it was also reported by Madadrang [15]. pH influences both the surface charges of the functional groups on the surface of graphene oxide and also the species of lead ion in the aqueous solution [48].

Table 5 Analysis of variance (ANOVA) for the reduced quadratic model

Model term	DF	Sum of squares	Mean square	F-value	Probability (P)
pH	1	2859.39	2859.39	120.547	<0.0001
Adsorbent	1	204.08	204.08	8.6037	0.0058
Time	1	241.06	241.06	10.162	<0.0003
pH^2	1	1165.24	1165.24	49.124	<0.0001
pH × Adsorbent	1	200.98	200.98	8.4728	<0.01
pH × Time	1	219.01	219.01	9.2330	<0.005
Adsorbent × Time	1	491.94	491.94	20.739	<0.0001
Residuals	36	853.93	23.72	-	-

Multiple $R^2 = 0.863$; Adjusted $R^2 = 0.836$; Lack of fit: 0.355

Table 6 Regression analysis for the reduced quadratic model

Model term	Coefficient estimate	Std. error	t value	Pr (>|t|)	*P*-value
Intercept	−205.76106	27.09	−7.59	5.5×10^{-9}	<0.001
pH	65.73077	7.051	9.32	3.9×10^{-11}	<0.001
Adsorbent dosage	2.21028	0.444	4.98	1.6×10^{-5}	<0.001
Time	4.62763	0.920	5.03	1.3×10^{-5}	<0.001
pH^2	−3.69755	0.527	−7.01	3.20×10^{-3}	<0.001
pH x Adsorbent	−0.19222	0.066	−2.90	6.1×10^{-9}	<0.01
pH x Time	−0.42283	0.139	−3.04	4.4×10^{-3}	<0.01
Adsorbent x Time	−0.05370	0.012	−4.50	5.8×10^{-5}	<0.001

Increasing the protonation of functional groups on graphene oxide surface would be happen at acidic conditions and electropositivity of Fe_3O_4@SiO_2-GO surface would retard the adsorption rate, and finally, the removal efficiency of lead (II) can be reduced [18]. As inferred from Fig. 7a-b, when pH is less than 5, the lead (II) removal efficiency was weak. However, the adsorption of lead (II) was enhanced with the increasing pH from 5 to 8.5. Normally, the adsorption capacities of metal ions for most carbon based nanomaterials would increase with increases in the pH value. In this case, lead (II) can be adsorbed onto the graphene oxide surface by reacting lead (II) with - COOH and - OH groups [15, 49].

As shown in the contour plot exhibited in Fig. 7c, regardless the adsorbent dose, more than 75 % of lead (II) adsorption was achieved during the contact time less than 10 min and the adsorption process was completely done after passing twenty minutes. These findings revealed that the fast adsorption rate of the lead (II) can be attributed to the high affinity of lead (II) ions to the hydroxide (-OH), epoxide (-O-) and carboxylic (-COOH) groups on the GO nanosheets [15, 50, 51].

The optimum values of pH, adsorbent dose, and contact time determined by applying the reduced quadratic model were 6.9, 30.49 mg/L, and 16.01 min, respectively. The optimum concentration of initial lead (II) was not obtained from the reduced quadratic model because it was omitted from the model. But the results of quadratic model suggested 2.49 mg L^{-1} as the optimum value. Further studies such as isotherm and kinetic experiments were investigated according to the abovementioned optimum values obtained from the model.

Adsorption isotherms

In order to investigate the adsorption equilibrium of lead (II), isotherm models consisting of Langmuir (Eq. 5), Freundlich (Eq. 6), and Sips (Eq. 7) were applied. The original forms (nonlinear) of models can be expressed as follows:

$$q_e = \frac{q_m K_L C_e}{1 + K_L C_e} \tag{5}$$

$$q_e = K_f C_e^{1/n_F} \tag{6}$$

$$q_e = \frac{q_m(K_S C_e)^{n_S}}{1+ \ (K_S C_e)^{n_S}} \tag{7}$$

Where, q_e is the amount of lead (II) adsorbed on the absorbent at equilibrium (mg g^{-1}), C_e describes the equilibrium lead (II) concentration (mg L^{-1}), K_L is the Langmuir adsorption constant (L mg^{-1}) and q_m denotes the maximum adsorption capacity attributeing to the complete monolayer coverage of the adsorbent (mg g^{-1}). K_F is the Freundlich constant related to the maximum sorption capacity (mg g^{-1}), also, n_F is the Frendlich constant related to the heterogeneity factor. K_S (L g^{-1}) is the affinity constant and n_S denotes the surface heterogeneity. If n_S value is equal to the unity, the Sips isotherm is turned to the Langmuir isotherm, and consequently, the homogeneous adsorption can be modeled. Also, any deviation of n_S value from the unity (more than or less than unity) predicts the heterogeneous surface [52, 53].

The adsorption mechanism can be expressed by applying Dubinin–Radushkevich isotherm (Eq.8) which is based on the potential theory and assumes a Gaussian energy distribution.

$$q_e = q_m \exp\left(-B_{DR}\epsilon^2\right) \tag{8}$$

Where, ε is the Polanyi potential given by:

$$\epsilon = RTln\left(1 + \frac{1}{C_e}\right) \tag{9}$$

The B_{DR} constant (mol^2/J^2) is related to the mean free energy E_{ads} of the adsorption per molecule when it is transferred to the surface from infinity of the bulk phase.

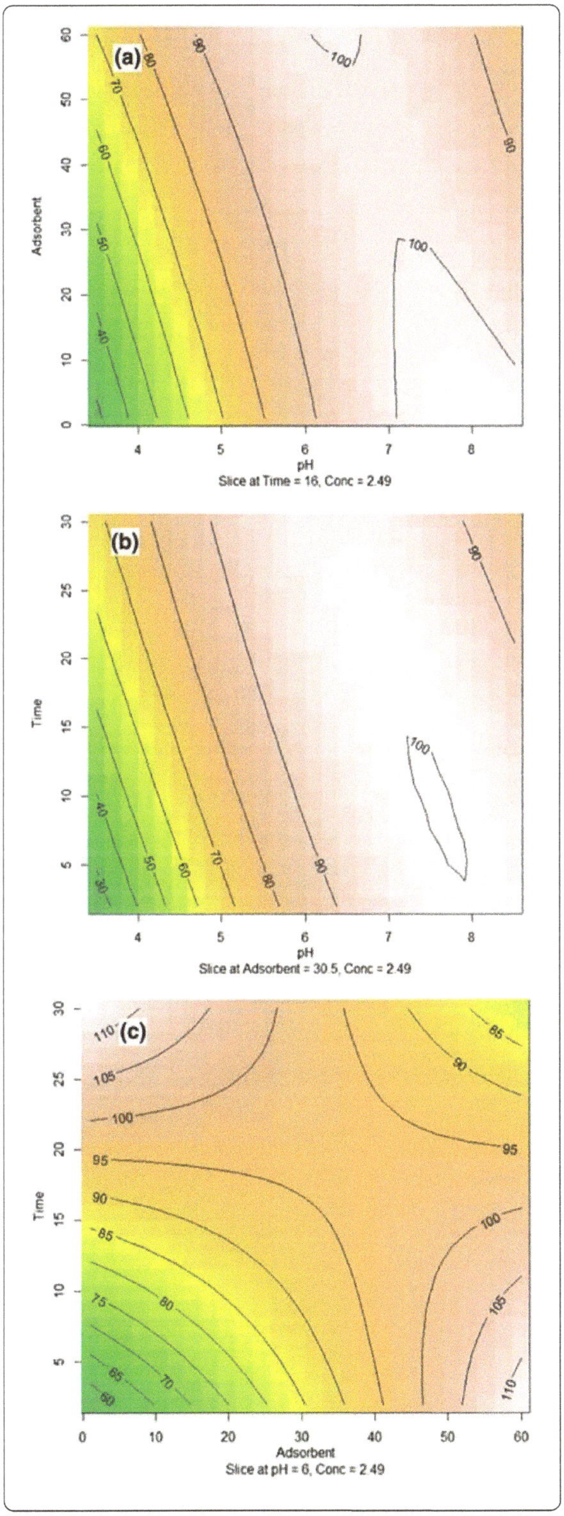

Fig. 7 Contour plots for the effect of factors on the lead (II) removal. Adsorbent dose (mg L^{-1}) and adsorption pH (**a**), contact time (min) and adsorption pH (**b**), adsorption time (min) and adsorbent dose (mg L^{-1}) (**c**)

$$E_{ads} = \frac{1}{\sqrt{2B_{DR}}} \tag{10}$$

Plotting the isotherm models versus the experimental results are depicted in Fig. 8a. The parameters of isotherm models can be observed in Fig. 8b. These parameters were determined according to the nonlinear regression by plotting q_e versus C_e assisted by Solver Add-Ins MS Excel [30].

As shown in Fig. 8b, the Sips isotherm model represents the higher correlation coefficient ($R^2 = 0.984$) comparing with the Langmuir ($R^2 = 0.964$) and Freundlich ($R^2 = 0.952$) models.

The Sips model includes three parameters and has the capability to apply for both the homogeneous and heterogeneous systems [54]. The Sips model (Eq. 5) integrates parameters from both the Langmuir and the Freundlich isotherm. The heterogeneous surface of adsorbent can be considered if the deviation of n_S value from the unity be occurred [53, 55]. However, the Sips isotherm moves toward a constant level at high concentrations whereas a pattern of Freundlich model can be observed at low concentrations [55].

According to the experimental data, the maximum adsorption uptake (q_m) was 505.8 mg g^{-1} which indicates the adsorption capacity higher than those reported by studies applying magnetic GO as lead (II) adsorbent [56] and is comparable with the studies using pristine GO [15, 49, 57]. The maximum adsorption uptake (q_m) obtained from Sips isotherm model was found to be 598.4 mg g^{-1} which was more than the values achieved both from the Langmuir model and the experimental data ($q_{m.Langmuir} = 497.8$ mg g^{-1}, $q_{m,exp} = 505.8$ mg g^{-1}). This indicates that the Sips model overestimates the q_m value which can be due to the heterogeneity characteristic considered in the Sips model. As shown in Fig. 8b, the deviation of n_S value from the unity ($n_S = 0.57$) as well as the n_F value more than unity ($n_F = 4.28$) can be assigned to the crosslinking effects beside the amount of functionalities such as -COOH and -OH on the adsorbent surface (see FTIR-spectra in Fig. 6). The isotherm curves were L-shaped, which shows the high affinity of surface groups towards lead (II) ions both at low and high concentrations [55]. As revealed from Fig. 8b, the mean free energy E_{ads} was 9.901 Kj/mol which seems to be the evidence of predomination the chemisorption mechanism [58].

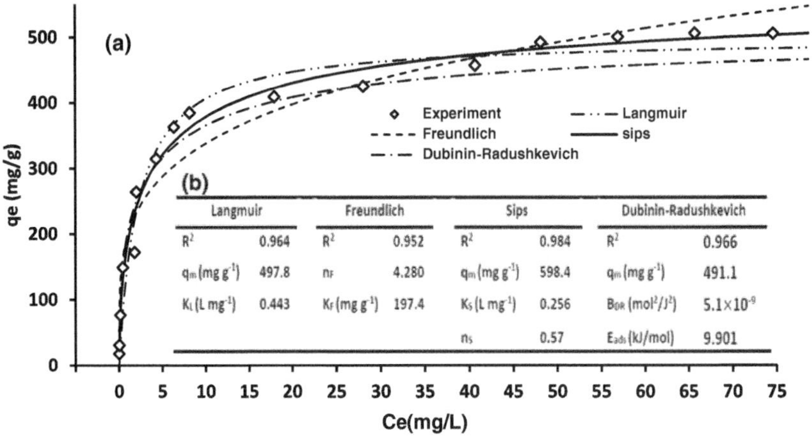

Langmuir		Freundlich		Sips		Dubinin-Radushkevich	
R^2	0.964	R^2	0.952	R^2	0.984	R^2	0.966
$q_m (mg\ g^{-1})$	497.8	n_F	4.280	$q_m (mg\ g^{-1})$	598.4	$q_m (mg\ g^{-1})$	491.1
$K_L (L\ mg^{-1})$	0.443	$K_F (mg\ g^{-1})$	197.4	$K_S (L\ mg^{-1})$	0.256	$B_{DR} (mol^2/J^2)$	5.1×10^{-9}
				n_S	0.57	$E_{ads} (kJ/mol)$	9.901

Fig. 8 Fitting results of different isotherms for lead (II) adsorption by Fe_3O_4@APTES -GO (**a**), and parameters obtained for the isotherm models (**b**). $q_{m,exp}$: 505.8, Adsorbent Dose: 30.5 mg L^{-1}, pH: 6, $C_{0,Lead(II)}$: 0.5–90 mg L^{-1}, time : 16 min

Adsorption kinetics

The experimental data were fitted with the original (nonlinear) forms of Lagergren-first-order (Eq. 11), pseudo-second-order (Eq. 12), and Double-exponential kinetic (Eq. 13) equations.

$$q_t = q_e(1-exp\ (-k_1 t)) \quad (11)$$

$$q_t = \frac{K_2 q_e^2 t}{1 + q_e k_2 t} \quad (12)$$

$$q_t = q_e - \frac{D_1}{x_{ads}} \exp(-k_{D_1} t) - \frac{D_2}{x_{ads}} \exp(-k_{D_2} t) \quad (13)$$

Where, q_t and q_e are the sorption capacity (mg g^{-1}) at time t and at the equilibrium time, respectively. k_1 and k_2 are the pseudo-first-order and pseudo-second-order rate constants, respectively. D_1 and D_2 (mg L^{-1}) are the rapid and slow steps, K_{D1} and K_{D2} (min^{-1}) are constants controlling the mechanism of slow and rapid phases, respectively. x_{ads} is the adsorbent dosage (g L^{-1}).

Figure 9a presents the nonlinear curves attributed to the kinetic models by applying equations 11, 12, and 13. Also, the kinetic parameters of lead (II) removal were illustrated in Fig. 9b.

According to the regression coefficient values of kinetic models, it was found that the double exponential kinetic model ($R^2 = 0.982$) obtains a better description to predict the kinetic data of lead (II) than both pseudo-first-order and pseudo-second-order models.

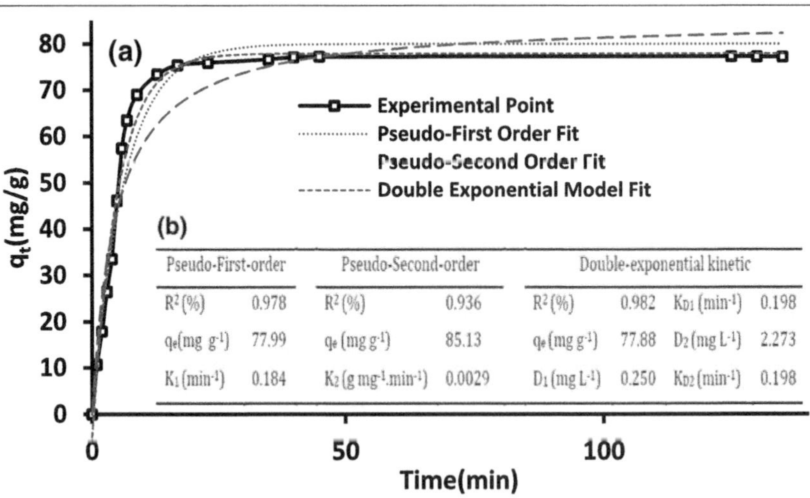

Pseudo-First-order		Pseudo-Second-order		Double-exponential kinetic			
R^2(%)	0.978	R^2(%)	0.936	R^2(%)	0.982	K_{D1} (min^{-1})	0.198
q_e(mg g^{-1})	77.99	q_e (mg g^{-1})	85.13	q_e (mg g^{-1})	77.88	D_2 (mg L^{-1})	2.273
K_1 (min^{-1})	0.184	K_2 (g $mg^{-1}.min^{-1}$)	0.0029	D_1 (mg L^{-1})	0.250	K_{D2} (min^{-1})	0.198

Fig. 9 Fitting results of different kinetic models for lead (II) adsorption by Fe_3O_4@APTES -GO (**a**), and parameters obtained from the kinetic models (**b**). Adsorbent Dose: 30.5 mg L^{-1}, pH: 6, $C_{0,Lead(II)}$: 2.36 mg L^{-1}

The values of constant parameters of double-exponential kinetic model revealed that the both external diffusion and internal diffusion have substantial effects on the lead (II) sorption using $Fe_3O_4@SiO_2$-GO nanocomposite [50].

Conclusions

Magnetic $Fe_3O_4@SiO_2$-GO nanocomposite was synthesized and applied to elimination the lead (II) from aqueous solution. Due to the high loading capacity of GO for metal ions, $Fe_3O_4@SiO_2$-GO revealed excellent performance in treatment the lead (II) contaminated waters. The removal process was found to be quick and facile, and the lead (II) adsorption process was almost completed up to 10 min contact time.

Main advantages of $Fe_3O_4@SiO_2$-GO nanocomposite include quick separation performed by using an external magnetic field and the noticeable lead (II) removal capacity (506 mg g^{-1}).

A central composite design (CCD) was applied to investigate the effects of four adsorption variables, namely pH, adsorbent dose, contact time, and initial lead ion concentration on the removal efficiency of lead (II).

Both the quadratic and reduced quadratic models were applied to correlate the variables to the response values. Results from the analysis of response surfaces indicated that pH, time, and the adsorbent dose were found to have significant effects on the removal efficiency of lead (II). The optimization of process was performed and the experimental values were found to be agreed satisfactorily with the predicted values.

The adsorption isotherms and kinetics were also investigated. Equilibrium adsorption data had best fit by the Sips isotherm model and chemisorption mechanism was predominated. Kinetic studies indicated that the double-exponential kinetic model is the preferred model to explain the equilibrium adsorption over the time.

Competing interests
The authors declare that they have no competing interests.

Authors' contributions
MK and SN have participated in all stages of the study (design of the study, conducting the experiment, analyzing of data and manuscript preparation). MRG and MK participated in graphene oxide synthesis and characterization. RN carried out technical RSM analysis of data. AHM participated in the intellectual helping in different stages of the study. SN performed data collection and carried out technical analysis. EG participated in fabrication and characterization of magnetic graphene oxide. All authors read and approved the final manuscript.

Acknowledgements
This research was part of a PhD dissertation of the first author and has been financially supported by a grant (NO, 28232-27-01-94) from Tehran University of Medical Sciences, Tehran, Iran. The authors would like to express their thanks to the Department of Environmental Health Engineering, School of Public Health, Tehran University of Medical Sciences for their collaboration.

Author details
[1]Department of Environmental Health Engineering, School of Public Health, Tehran University of Medical Sciences, Tehran, Iran. [2]Center for Water Quality Research, Institute for Environmental Research, Tehran University of Medical Sciences, Tehran, Iran. [3]Center of Excellence in Electrochemistry, Faculty of Chemistry, University of Tehran, Tehran, Iran. [4]Biosensor Research Center, Endocrinology & Metabolism Molecular-Cellular Sciences Institute, Tehran University of Medical Sciences, Tehran, Iran. [5]Department of Medicinal Chemistry, Faculty of Pharmacy and Pharmaceutical Sciences Research Center, Tehran University of Medical Sciences, Tehran 14176, Iran. [6]Center for Solid Waste Research, Institute for Environmental Research, Tehran University of Medical Sciences, Tehran, Iran. [7]Department of Chemistry, Faculty of Science, University of Zanjan, Zanjan, Iran.

References
1. Yang X, Xu J, Tang X, Liu H, Tian D. A novel electrochemical DNAzyme sensor for the amplified detection of Pb^{2+} ions. Chem Commun. 2010; 46(18):3107–9.
2. ISIRI. Drinking water physical and chemical specifications. Iran: Institute of Standards and Industrial Research; 2014.
3. EPA. Drinking water contaminants. National Primary Drinking Water Regulations 2015 [cited 2015 9/13/2015]; Available from: http://www.epa.gov/safewater/contaminants/index.html, 1/30/2010.
4. Ju X-J, Zhang S-B, Zhou M-Y, Xie R, Yang L, Chu L-Y. Novel heavy-metal adsorption material: ion-recognition P(NIPAM-co-BCAm) hydrogels for removal of lead(II) ions. J Hazard Mater. 2009;167(1–3):114–8.
5. Li Y-H, Di Z, Ding J, Wu D, Luan Z, Zhu Y. Adsorption thermodynamic, kinetic and desorption studies of Pb^{2+} on carbon nanotubes. Water Res. 2005;39(4):605–9.
6. Turan M, Mart U, Yüksel B, Çelik MS. Lead removal in fixed-bed columns by zeolite and sepiolite. Chemosphere. 2005;60(10):1487–92.
7. Mahvi A, Gholami F, Nazmara S. Cadmium biosorption from wastewater by Ulmus leaves and their ash. Eur J Sci Res. 2008;23(2):197–203.
8. Maleki A, Mahvi AH, Zazouli MA, Izanloo H, Barati AH. Aqueous cadmium removal by adsorption on barley hull and barley hull ash. Asian J Chem. 2011;23(3):1373–6.
9. Sekar M, Sakthi V, Rengaraj S. Kinetics and equilibrium adsorption study of lead(II) onto activated carbon prepared from coconut shell. J Colloid Interface Sci. 2004;279(2):307–13.
10. Sprynskyy M, Buszewski B, Terzyk AP, Namie nik J. Study of the selection mechanism of heavy metal (Pb^{2+}, Cu^{2+}, Ni^{2+}, and Cd^{2+}) adsorption on clinoptilolite. J Colloid Interface Sci. 2006;304(1):21–8.
11. Ho YS, McKay G. The kinetics of sorption of divalent metal ions onto sphagnum moss peat. Water Res. 2000;34(3):735–42.
12. Rezaee R, Nasseri S, Mahvi A, Nabizadeh R, Mousavi S, Rashidi A, et al. Fabrication and characterization of a polysulfone-graphene oxide nanocomposite membrane for arsenate rejection from water. J Environ Health Sci Eng. 2015;13(1):1–11.
13. Norouzi P, Larijani B, Ganjali M. Ochratoxin A sensor based on nanocomposite hybrid film of ionic liquid-graphene nano-sheets using coulometric FFT cyclic voltammetry. Int J Electrochem Sci. 2012;7:7313–24.
14. Dreyer DR, Park S, Bielawski CW, Ruoff RS. The chemistry of graphene oxide. Chem Soc Rev. 2010;39(1):228–40.
15. Madadrang CJ, Kim HY, Gao G, Wang N, Zhu J, Feng H, et al. Adsorption behavior of EDTA-graphene oxide for Pb (II) removal. ACS Appl Mater Interfaces. 2012;4(3):1186–93.
16. Stankovich S, Dikin DA, Dommett GH, Kohlhaas KM, Zimney EJ, Stach EA, et al. Graphene-based composite materials. Nature. 2006;442(7100):282–6.
17. Chen F, Yan F, Chen Q, Wang Y, Han L, Chen Z, et al. Fabrication of $Fe_3O_4@SiO_2@TiO_2$ nanoparticles supported by graphene oxide sheets for the repeated adsorption and photocatalytic degradation of rhodamine B under UV irradiation. Dalton Trans. 2014;43(36):13537–44.
18. Cui L, Wang Y, Gao L, Hu L, Yan L, Wei Q, et al. EDTA functionalized magnetic graphene oxide for removal of Pb(II), Hg(II) and Cu(II) in water treatment: Adsorption mechanism and separation property. Chem Eng J. 2015;281:1–10.
19. Alvand M, Shemirani F. Preconcentration of trace cadmium ion using magnetic graphene nanoparticles as an efficient adsorbent. Microchim Acta. 2014;181(1–2):181–8.
20. Teo PS, Lim HN, Huang NM, Chia CH, Harrison I. Room temperature in situ chemical synthesis of Fe_3O_4/graphene. Ceram Int. 2012;38(8):6411–6.

21. Liu Q, Shi J, Cheng M, Li G, Cao D, Jiang G. Preparation of graphene-encapsulated magnetic microspheres for protein/peptide enrichment and MALDI-TOF MS analysis. Chem Commun. 2012;48(13):1874–6.
22. Li Y, Wang X-Y, Jiang X-P, Ye J-J, Zhang Y-W, Zhang X-Y. Fabrication of graphene oxide decorated with Fe_3O_4@SiO_2 for immobilization of cellulase. J Nanoparticle Res. 2015;17(1):1–12.
23. Hummers Jr WS, Offeman RE. Preparation of graphitic oxide. J Am Chem Soc. 1958;80(6):1339–9.
24. Marcano DC, Kosynkin DV, Berlin JM, Sinitskii A, Sun Z, Slesarev A, et al. Improved synthesis of graphene oxide. ACS Nano. 2010;4(8):4806–14.
25. Cote LJ, Kim F, Huang J. Langmuir – Blodgett assembly of graphite oxide single layers. J Am Chem Soc. 2008;131(3):1043–9.
26. Hamadi H, Gholami M, Khoobi M. Polyethyleneimine-modified super paramagnetic Fe_3O_4 nanoparticles: an efficient, reusable and water tolerance nanocatalyst. 2011.
27. Tartaj P, Serna CJ. Synthesis of monodisperse superparamagnetic Fe/Silica nanospherical composites. J Am Chem Soc. 2003;125(51):15754–5.
28. He F, Fan J, Ma D, Zhang L, Leung C, Chan HL. The attachment of Fe_3O_4 nanoparticles to graphene oxide by covalent bonding. Carbon. 2010;48(11): 3139–44.
29. Wang W, Ma R, Wu Q, Wang C, Wang Z. Magnetic microsphere-confined graphene for the extraction of polycyclic aromatic hydrocarbons from environmental water samples coupled with high performance liquid chromatography–fluorescence analysis. J Chromatogr A. 2013;1293:20–7.
30. Hossain MA, Ngo HH, Guo W. Introductory of Microsoft Excel SOLVER function-spreadsheet method for isotherm and kinetics modelling of metals biosorption in water and wastewater. J Water Sustain. 2013;3(4):223–37.
31. Paredes JI, Villar-Rodil S, Solís-Fernández P, Martínez-Alonso A, Tascón JMD. Atomic force and scanning tunneling microscopy imaging of graphene nanosheets derived from graphite oxide. Langmuir. 2009;25(10):5957–68.
32. Maiti R, Manna S, Midya A, Ray SK. Broadband photoresponse and rectification of novel graphene oxide/n-Si heterojunctions. Opt Express. 2013;21(22):26034–43.
33. Yang D, Velamakanni A, Bozoklu G, Park S, Stoller M, Piner RD, et al. Chemical analysis of graphene oxide films after heat and chemical treatments by X-ray photoelectron and Micro-Raman spectroscopy. Carbon. 2009;47(1):145–52.
34. Li D, Muller MB, Gilje S, Kaner RB, Wallace GG. Processable aqueous dispersions of graphene nanosheets. Nat Nano. 2008;3(2):101–5.
35. Zhao G, Li J, Ren X, Chen C, Wang X. Few-layered graphene oxide nanosheets as superior sorbents for heavy metal ion pollution management. Environ Sci Technol. 2011;45(24):10454–62.
36. Titelman GI, Gelman V, Bron S, Khalfin RL, Cohen Y, Bianco-Peled H. Characteristics and microstructure of aqueous colloidal dispersions of graphite oxide. Carbon. 2005;43(3):641–9.
37. Stankovich S, Piner RD, Nguyen ST, Ruoff RS. Synthesis and exfoliation of isocyanate-treated graphene oxide nanoplatelets. Carbon. 2006;44(15):3342–7.
38. Abkenar SD, Khoobi M, Tarasi R, Hosseini M, Shafiee A, Ganjali MR. Fast removal of methylene blue from aqueous solution using magnetic-modified Fe_3 O_4 nanoparticles. J Environ Eng. 2014;141(1):04014049.
39. Cataldo F. Structural analogies and differences between graphite oxide and C60 and C70 polymeric oxides (Fullerene Ozopolymers). Fullerenes Nanotubes Carbon Nanostruct. 2003;11(1):1–13.
40. Sun X, Liu Z, Welsher K, Robinson JT, Goodwin A, Zaric S, et al. Nano-graphene oxide for cellular imaging and drug delivery. Nano Res. 2008;1(3): 203–12.
41. Yang X, Wang Y, Huang X, Ma Y, Huang Y, Yang R, et al. Multi-functionalized graphene oxide based anticancer drug-carrier with dual-targeting function and pH-sensitivity. J Mater Chem. 2011;21(10):3448–54.
42. Xu Y, Liu Z, Zhang X, Wang Y, Tian J, Huang Y, et al. A graphene hybrid material covalently functionalized with porphyrin: synthesis and optical limiting property. Adv Mater. 2009;21(12):1275–9.
43. Lenth RV. Response-Surface Methods in R, using rsm. J Stat Soft. 2009;32(7): 1–17.
44. Myers RH, Montgomery DC, Anderson-Cook CM. Response surface methodology: process and product optimization using designed experiments. vol. 705:2009. Hoboken, New Jersey: John Wiley & Sons.
45. Zhu H, Fu Y, Jiang R, Yao J, Xiao L, Zeng G. Optimization of copper(II) adsorption onto novel magnetic calcium alginate/maghemite hydrogel beads using response surface methodology. Ind Eng Chem Res. 2014;53(10): 4059–66.
46. Turkyilmaz H, Kartal T, Yildiz SY. Optimization of lead adsorption of mordenite by response surface methodology: characterization and modification. J Environ Health Sci Eng. 2014;12(1):5.
47. Amini M, Younesi H, Bahramifar N. Statistical modeling and optimization of the cadmium biosorption process in an aqueous solution using Aspergillus niger. Colloids Surf A Physicochem Eng Asp. 2009;337(1):67–73.
48. Luo S, Xu X, Zhou G, Liu C, Tang Y, Liu Y. Amino siloxane oligomer-linked graphene oxide as an efficient adsorbent for removal of Pb(II) from wastewater. J Hazard Mater. 2014;274:145–55.
49. Zhao G, Ren X, Gao X, Tan X, Li J, Chen C, et al. Removal of Pb (II) ions from aqueous solutions on few-layered graphene oxide nanosheets. Dalton Trans. 2011;40(41):10945–52.
50. Hadi Najafabadi H, Irani M, Roshanfekr Rad L, Heydari Haratameh A, Haririan I. Removal of Cu^{2+}, Pb^{2+} and Cr^{6+} from aqueous solutions using a chitosan/graphene oxide composite nanofibrous adsorbent. RSC Adv. 2015;5(21): 16532–9.
51. Wu W, Yang Y, Zhou H, Ye T, Huang Z, Liu R, et al. Highly efficient removal of Cu (II) from aqueous solution by using graphene oxide. Water Air Soil Pollut. 2013;224(1):1–8.
52. Repo E, Warchol JK, Kurniawan TA, Sillanpää MET. Adsorption of Co(II) and Ni(II) by EDTA- and/or DTPA-modified chitosan: kinetic and equilibrium modeling. Chem Eng J. 2010;161(1–2):73–82.
53. Guo L, Li G, Liu J, Yin P, Li Q. Adsorption of aniline on cross-linked starch sulfate from aqueous solution. Ind Eng Chem Res. 2009;48(23):10657–63.
54. Repo E, Warchoł JK, Bhatnagar A, Sillanpää M. Heavy metals adsorption by novel EDTA-modified chitosan–silica hybrid materials. J Colloid Interface Sci. 2011;358(1):261–7.
55. Repo E. EDTA-and DTPA-functionalized silica gel and chitosan adsorbents for the removal of heavy metals from aqueous solutions. 2011. Lappeenranta University of Technology Laboratory of Green Chemistry.
56. Ma Y, La P, Lei W, Lu C, Du X. Adsorption of Hg(II) from aqueous solution using amino-functionalized graphite nanosheets decorated with Fe3O4 nanoparticles. Desalin Water Treat. 2015;57:1–9. doi:10.1080/19443994.2014.998292.
57. Yang Y, Xie Y, Pang L, Li M, Song X, Wen J, et al. Preparation of reduced graphene oxide/poly (acrylamide) nanocomposite and its adsorption of Pb (II) and methylene blue. Langmuir. 2013;29(34):10727–36.
58. Kakavandi B, Kalantary RR, Jafari AJ, Nasseri S, Ameri A, Esrafili A, et al. Pb (II) adsorption onto a magnetic composite of activated carbon and superparamagnetic Fe3O4 nanoparticles: experimental and modeling study. Clean Soil Air Water. 2015;43:1157–66. doi:10.1002/clen.201400568.

18

Sawdust waste as a low-cost support-substrate for laccases production and adsorbent for azo dyes decolorization

Dalel Daâssi[1,2], Hela Zouari-Mechichi[1], Fakher Frikha[3], Susana Rodríguez-Couto[4,5], Moncef Nasri[1] and Tahar Mechichi[1*]

Abstract

Background: Laccases are multicopper oxidases with high potential for environmental and industrial applications. Low-cost laccase production could be achieved by solid state fermentation on agro-industrial by-products.

Methods: A number of agro-industrial solid wastes were tested as support-substrate for laccase production by *Coriolopsis gallica* under solid-state fermentation (SSF) conditions. Response surface methodology (RSM) was used to optimize the medium composition for laccase production. Initial screening by Plackett-Burman design was performed to select the major variables out of 20 tow medium components fellowing this Central composite design (CCD) was employed to optimize the level of the selected variables.

Results: Sawdust waste was shown to be the best support-substrate for laccase production by the *C. gallica*. Peptone as source of organic nitrogen, Cd^{2+} as laccase inducer and liquid/solid (L/S) ratio were found to have significant effects on laccase production. Operating at optimum concentrations of the most significant variables (peptone, 4.5 g L^{-1}, L/S ratio, 5.0 and Cd^{+2} 1.0 mM) extracellular laccase activity was enhanced from 1480 U L^{-1} (60.5 U g^{-1}), to 4880 U L^{-1} (200 U g^{-1}) which meant a 3.2-fold increase in laccase activity. On the other hand, sawdust waste was studied as a low cost adsorbent to remove the azo dyes Reactive Black 5 (RB5) and Acid Orange 51 (AO51). Decolorization percentages around 67 and 75 % were obtained in 24 h for RB5 and AO51, respectively.

Conclusion: When used as a support substrate, sawdust yielded the highest laccase production which was increased 3.2 times using RMS optimization.

Keywords: SSF, Sawdust, *C. gallica*, Optimization, Decolorization

Background

Laccases (p-diphenol: dioxygen oxidoreductases; EC 1.10.3.2) are particularly abundant in white-rot fungi, which are the only organisms able to degrade the whole wood components [1]. Most studies on laccase production by white-rot fungi have been performed in liquid cultures, which do not reflect the natural living conditions of such fungi (wood). In solid-state cultures, white *Coriolopsis* is assumed to be one of the most efficient lignin degraders -rot fungi grow under conditions close to their natural habitat. This may allow them producing certain enzymes and metabolites, which usually would not be produced or would only be produced at a low yield in submerged fermentation (SmF) conditions [2]. Agricultural and food wastes could be used as support-substrates to produce bulk chemicals and products with high commercial value like organic acids, proteins, alcohol and enzymes [3] by microorganisms. Furthermore, the utilization of these compounds helps in solving the pollution caused by their disposal [4].

Fungal growth in SSF is different from fungal growth in SmF because of different surface phenomena, moisture content and chemical composition of the support-substrate [5]. SSF provides a better oxygen circulation; it is a static process without mechanical energy

* Correspondence: tahar.mechichi@enis.rnu.tn
[1]Laboratory of Enzyme Engineering and Microbiology, Ecole Nationale d'Ingénieurs de Sfax, University of Sfax, Route de Soukra Km 4.5, BP 1173, Sfax 3038, Tunisia
Full list of author information is available at the end of the article

consumption and reproduces the natural living conditions of the white-rot fungi [4]. SSF constitutes an interesting alternative for fungal cultivation since the metabolites so produced are more concentrated, purification procedures are less costly, less wastewater is formed, product recovery is easier, bacterial contamination is lessened and is a simple process [6].

Two types of SSF systems can be differentiated depending on the nature of the solid support used. The first one involves cultivation on an inert support (synthetic material) [7] whereas, the second and most commonly-used system involves cultivation on a natural support (organic material) [8]. Many studies reported the exploitation of SSF to give an extra value to agro-industrial residues [9, 10] and different reactors for SSF were described [11].

In SSF, the selection of a suitable solid support-substrate is a critical factor. Ligninolytic enzymes have been successfully produced by SSF using various agro-industrial wastes such as banana waste [12], potato peelings [13], barley bran [14], wheat bran [8] and kiwi fruit [13]. In addition, the composition of the production medium is a key parameter in optimizing SSF processes because nutritional factors, such as the nature and concentration of carbon and nitrogen source and trace metals, can influence the growth and production of metabolites. Researchers are encouraged to apply statistical experimental approaches, e.g. Plackett-Burman (PB) design and response surface methodology (RSM), which provide a great amount of information based on only a small number of experiments [15].

It is very interesting to find new ways of producing laccase with higher activities at lower cost due to the enormous potential that this enzyme offers for the development of efficient biotechnological applications. Such applications include the detoxification of industrial effluents, mostly from textile-dyeing industry, which is considered as the most polluting one amongst all industrial sectors [16]. Effluents discharged from dyeing industries are highly colored and represents a serious concern worldwide since they contain different kinds of synthetic dyes. The use of dyes has generated much concern due to their toxic effects, since they have been reported to cause carcinogenesis, mutagenesis, chromosomal fractures, teratogenecity and respiratory toxicity [17].

Biosorption (adsorption) by lignocellulosic materials may be an alternative method for removing dyes from effluents. Several studies have shown the biosorption potential of different lignocellulosic materials [18, 19]. Because dye adsorbed lignocellulosics create another source of pollution, adsorption of dyes onto lignocellulosic materials does not completely solve this problem. In light of this situation, a two-step method combining biosorption and SSF may be an alternative approach and effective solution. The combination of these two methods, biosorption and biodecolorization by SSF, has potential to be a suitable process for dye removal and laccase production. Sawdust is an abundant by-product of the wood industry that is either used as cooking fuel or as packing material. Sawdust is easily available in the countryside at zero or negligible cost [20]. It contains various organic compounds (lignin, cellulose and hemicellulose) with polyphenolic groups that might be useful for binding dyes through different mechanisms [21, 22].

The aims of this study were: (a) to assess the potential of selected agro-wastes for laccase production by the white-rot fungus *C. gallica* under SSF conditions, (b) to optimize the laccase production by *C. gallica* under SSF conditions operating with sawdust waste as support-substrate using CCD and (c) to test the ability of the ligninolytic complex secreted in SSF conditions for azo dyes biodecolorization.

Methods

Chemicals

All chemicals were of certified reagent analytical grade. The following azo dyes were used: Reactive Black 5 (RB5) and Acid Orange 51 (AO51). They were purchased from Sigma-Aldrich (St. Louis, MO, USA). The characteristics of the dyes are summarized in Table 1. Stock dye solutions (0.1 % *w/v* in water) were stored in the dark at room at room temperature.

Support-substrates

Tip of palm ($3 \times 3 \times 2$ mm^3), oatmeal, wheat bran, straw ($3 \times 3 \times 2$ mm^3), filer paper (size $2 \times 2 \times 1$ mm^3), sawdust ($3 \times 2 \times 2$ mm^3), orange peelings (size $5 \times 5 \times 2$ mm^3), melon peelings (size $5 \times 5 \times 2$ mm^3), wood ($2 \times 3 \times 2$ mm^3) and olive leaves ($4 \times 2 \times 2$ mm^3) were used in this study as support-substrate under SSF conditions for laccase production by *C. gallica.*

Prior to use, the peelings of orange and melon were pre-treated as follows: they were first soaked for 1 h in 30 mL of 0.1 M KOH (10 g of fresh peelings) to neutralize organic acids [23]. Then, they were thoroughly washed with distilled water and dried at 30 °C for 2 days. The peelings were autoclaved at 120 °C for 1 h. The other support-substrates were used in dry state.

Fungal strain, media and culture conditions

The fungal isolate used in this study was *C. gallica.* The isolate is maintained in the culture collection of our laboratory in the Ecole Nationale d'Ingénieurs de Sfax (Tunisia). For short-term conservation, the isolate was cultured on 2 % malt extract and 1.5 % agar in Petri dishes at 30 °C for 4 days and stored at 4 °C until used.

C. gallica. was cultured in 250-mL Erlenmeyer flasks containing 5.0 g of the substrates. These substrates were

Table 1 Characteristics of the azo dyes used

Dye	CI[a] number	λ_{max} (nm)	Chemical structure
Reactive Black 5 (RB5)	20505	597	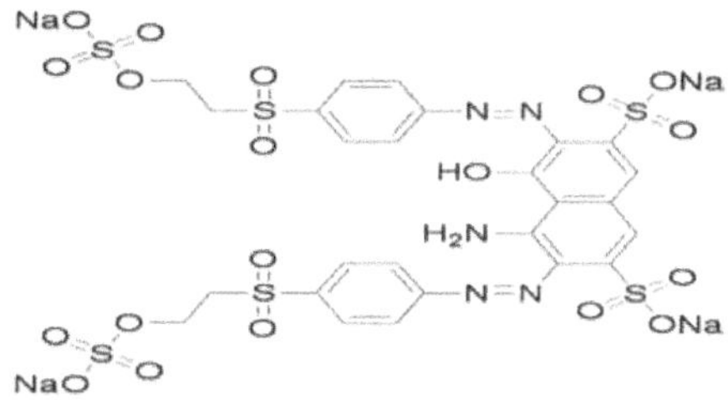
Acid Orange 51 (AO51)	26550	450	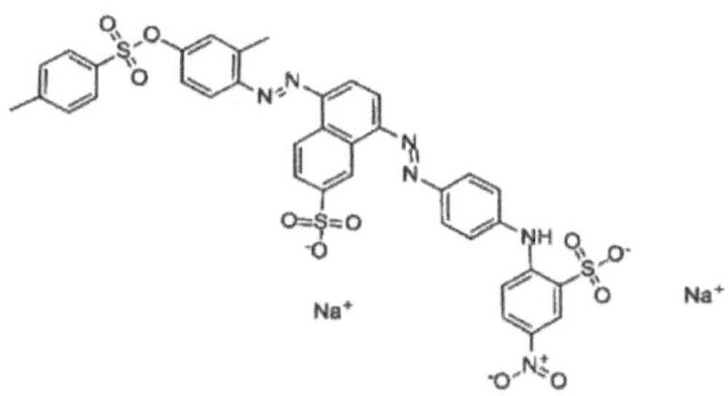

[a]*CI* color index

hydrated with 15 mL of 50 mM acetate buffer (pH 5.0). Inoculation was carried out directly in the Erlenmeyer flasks. Three plugs (diameter, 3 mm), from a 5-day growing fungus on malt extract agar (MEA) per Erlenmeyer were used as inoculum. The cultures were supplemented with laccase-inducing compounds (solution sterilized separately 60 mM) at the beginning of the cultivation. The Erlenmeyer flasks were incubated statically for 10 days in complete darkness at 30 °C.

Laccase activity determination

Laccase activity was measured by monitoring the increase in absorbance at 469 nm ($\varepsilon_{469nm} = 27{,}500\ M^{-1}\ cm^{-1}$) of a reaction mixture containing 10 mM 2,6-dimethoxyphenol in 100 mM acetate buffer, pH 5.0 [24]. Enzymatic reactions were carried out at room temperature (22–25 °C). One unit of enzyme activity was defined as the amount of enzyme oxidizing 1 µmol of substrate per min. The activities were expressed in U L^{-1}.

Plackett-Burmann design

Several parameters in the culture medium can affect laccase production. In order to identify these parameters, different components of the culture medium were evaluated using the PB experimental design [25]. The total number of trials to be carried out according to Plackett-Burmann is k + 1, where k is the number of variables. Each variable is represented at two levels, high and low which are denoted by "+" and "–", respectively; and also by five central points. The effect of each variable on each response was determined by subtracting the average response of the low level from that of the high level. Table 2 illustrates the factors under investigation as well as the levels of each factor used in the experimental design. Design expert, version 7.0 (STAT-EASE Inc., Minneapolis, USA) was used to analyze the experimental PB design. In our experiments, the variables with confidence levels above 95 % were considered as influencing laccase production significantly.

Response surface methodology

RSM was used to optimize the screened components that enhanced laccase production using the CCD [26]. Basically this optimization process involves three major steps: performing the statistically designed experiments, estimating the coefficients in a mathematical model and predicting the response and checking the adequacy of the model. Using the mathematical model, the levels of the variables giving maximum response can then be calculated. Each factor in the design was studied at five different levels ($-\alpha$, -1, 0, $+1$, $+\alpha$).

A set of 20 experiments was performed. All the variables were taken at a central-coded value considered as zero. The minimum and maximum ranges of variables investigated and the full experimental plan with respect to their values in actual and coded form is listed in Table 3. Upon completion of experiment, the laccase production was taken as dependent variable or response

Table 2 Range of different variables studied in the Plackett-Burmann design

Factors				levels		
Variables		Units	Variable code	Low (−)	Central point (0)	High (+)
Carbon sources (F1)	Glucose	g L^{-1}	X1	0	10	20
	Maltose	g L^{-1}	X2	0	10	20
	Saccharose	g L^{-1}	X3	0	10	20
	Starch	g L^{-1}	X4	0	10	20
Nitrogen sources (F2)	Casein Peptone	g L^{-1}	X5	0	10	20
	NH_4SO_4	g L^{-1}	X6	0	2.5	5
	KNO_3	g L^{-1}	X7	0	2.5	5
	Urea	g L^{-1}	X8	0	2.5	5
Phosphate (F3)	KH_2PO_4	g L^{-1}	X9	0	0.025	0.05
MgSO4 (F4)	$MgSO_4$	g L^{-1}	X10	0	0.25	0.5
Inductors (F5)	$CuSO_4$	mM	X11	0	0.5	1
	Ethanol	mL L^{-1}	X12	0	15	30
	Cd^{2+}	mM	X13	0	0.5	1
	$MnSO_4$	mM	X14	0	0.5	1
	Ferulic Acid	mM	X15	0	0.5	1
	Vanilllic acid	mM	X16	0	0.5	1
Buffer (F6)	Acetate-Na	mM	X17	0	10	20
	Citrate-Na	mM	X18	0	10	20
	Tartrate-Na	mM	X19	0	10	20
pH (F7)	pH		X20	3	4	5
Inoculum nombre (F8)	Inoculum	5 mm	X21	4	6	8
Liquid/solid ratio (F9)	L/S ratio		X22	1.5	4.75	8

(Y). The independent variables are coded for statistical calculation according to the following Eq. (1):

$$Xi = (xi - x0)/xi \quad (1)$$

Where Xi is the dimension less coded value of the independent variable xi, xi is the real value of that independent variable, x0 is the real value of that independent variable xi at the center point, △xi is the step change. The role of each variable, their interactions, and statistical analysis to obtain predicted yields is explained by applying the following quadratic Eq. (2):

Table 3 The range and the levels of the variables

Factor	Variable	Unit	Range and level of actual and coded values				
			−α	−1	0	1	α
peptone	A	g L^{-1}	0.688	2	4.5	7	8.311
Cd	B	mM	0.237	0.5	1	1.5	1.762
L/S	C	-	3.475	4	5	6	6.524

$$Y = \beta_0 + \sum \beta_i X_i + \sum \beta_{ij} X_i X_j + \sum \beta_{ii} X_i^2 \quad (2)$$

Where Y is predicted response, Xi and Xj are the levels of the independent variables.

Statistical analysis of the model was performed to evaluate the analysis of variance (ANOVA). Statistical significance of the model equation was determined by Fisher's test value, and the proportion of variance explained by the model was given by the multiple coefficient of determination, R squared (R^2) value. For each variable, the quadratic models were represented as contour plots (3D) and response surface curves were generated. Design expert, version 7.0 (STAT-EASE Inc., Minneapolis, USA) was used in this investigation.

Decolorization batch experiments of dyes-adsorbed sawdust

Batch decolorization experiments of azo dyes were performed after 10 days of fungal cultivation, as described in the SSF, sampling and extraction studies sub-section. Each decolorization cycle consisted of the addition of 2 mL of the azo dye (50 mg L^{-1}, final concentration) to the cultures. A new cycle was initiated after 24 h when no further change in the dye decolorization was detected. The experiments were performed in three-replicates and reported values are representative of three experiments.

A biotic control (without dye) and an abiotic control (without fungus) were conducted in parallel.

Samples were taken at the beginning of the process and at determined intervals, centrifuged (10,000 × g, 5 min) using a microcentrifuge (MSE Micro Centaur) and the residual dye concentration was spectrophotometrically measured from 500 to 700 nm and calculated by measuring the area under the plot. This approach takes into account the conversion of the dye molecules to other compounds absorbing at different wavelengths and then, the ratio of the area under the visible spectrum is always equal or lower than the ratio of the absorbances at the peak. The absorbances were corrected by subtracting the absorbance of culture without dye. The physical adsorption of the dye to the support was evaluated. Dye decolorization was expressed in terms of percentage according to sani et al. [27]. Biological decolorization was determined by subtracting the decolorization due to the physical adsorption of the dye to the support from the total decolorization.

Results and discussion

Selection of the support-substrate

Firstly, a series of experiments were carried out to select the best support-substrate for laccase production by *C. gallica* under SSF conditions. All the tested support-substrates facilitated the attachment of the fungus to them whereas their content in lignin, cellulose, hemicelluloses and sugars provided the required nutrients for fungal growth.

The profile of laccase production obtained on a particular cultivation day (10 days) using various support-substrates by *C. gallica* under SSF conditions is given in Fig. 1. The first sign of growth was seen on the 2nd or 3rd cultivation day. Laccase activity depended on the type of industrial solid waste used. There was a rapid increase in laccase activity in both sawdust and filter paper cultures during the first 10 days of fermentation with maximum laccase activities of 1480 U L^{-1} for the former and 1300 U L^{-1} for the latter on day 12.

Plackett-Burmann design

PB design was used to identify which variables had significant effects on laccase production by *C. gallica.* under SSF conditions using sawdust as support-substrate.

As shown in Table 2, 9 factors including 22 medium components were screened in PB experiments. The medium components screened consisted of different carbon and nitrogen sources, KH_2PO_4, $MgSO_4$, inducers of laccase activity, buffers, pH, inoculum size and liquid/solid (L/S) ratio. The upper and the lower limits of each variable were chosen to encompass the range in literature and to reflect what was done in practice after a preliminary investigation of the limits.

Figure 2 shows the effects of the variables on the response and significant levels. Confidence levels were accepted only when these were above 95 % ($p < 0.05$). Based on the statistical analysis, the factors having the greatest impacts on the production of laccase by *C. gallica.* under SSF conditions using sawdust as a support-substrate were identified as X5 (casein peptone), X8 (urea), X13 (Cd^{2+}) and X22 (L/S ratio). These components could be ranked as ratio L/S > Cd^{2+} > casein peptone > urea. The negative

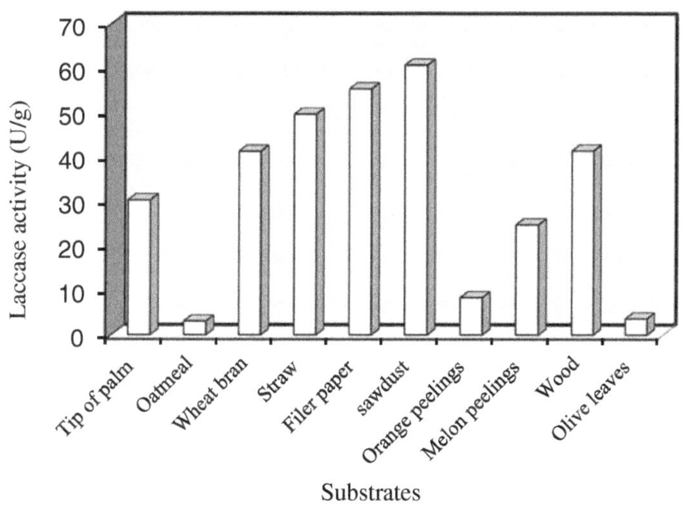

Fig. 1 Effect of different support-substrates on laccase production by *C. gallica* under solid-state fermentation (SSF) conditions (10 days)

Term	Estimated coefficients coded	Plotting the estimated	Standard deviation	Rapport t	Prob.>ltl
Constante	2100,3013		113,7519	18,46	<,0001
X1	-121,0976		110,3606	-1,10	0,3010
X2	-144,5142		112,1667	-1,29	0,2297
X3	-193,1171		115,6943	-1,67	0,1294
X4	-47,01615		120,4349	-0,39	0,7053
X5	481,25562		112,8365	4,27	0,0021
X6	-18,4735		111,5737	-0,17	0,8722
X7	32,028984		114,4011	0,28	0,7858
X8	-556,5186		126,8678	-4,39	0,0018
X9	132,86741		115,8334	1,15	0,2809
X10	222,19139		123,8311	1,79	0,1063
X11	-55,6713		118,3635	-0,47	0,6493
X12	37,058636		115,6943	0,32	0,7560
X13	491,51112		127,2733	3,86	0,0038
X14	-200,9592		118,3635	-1,70	0,1238
X15	-74,45382		112,1035	-0,66	0,5232
X16	117,48762		120,7927	0,97	0,3561
X17	16,480621		112,8365	0,15	0,8871
X18	91,978974		127,2733	0,72	0,4882
X19	146,98236		198,4603	0,74	0,4778
X20	194,29027		110,3606	1,76	0,1122
X21	-50,29473		110,3606	-0,46	0,6594
X22[-1]	-1962,144		148,7214	-13,19	<,0001
X22[0]	2667,7827		188,6833	14,14	<,0001
X22[1]	-705,6385		149,8432	-4,71	0,0011

Fig. 2 Effects of variables in Plackett-Burman design on laccase production by *C. gallica* under solid-state fermentation (SSF) conditions operating with sawdust as support-substrate

influence of urea was significant set at their high levels. Effects of the X5, X13 and X22 were all positive since laccase production increased with increasing concentrations.

In SSF, the concept of water availability or water solvent is vital because it determines the metabolism of microorganisms on solid matrices [28]. In this study humidity environment (L/S) was the most important factor influencing the production of laccase. Indeed, the production of laccase was much higher for a L/S ratio of 4.75 than for one of 1.5. Similar results were described by Rosales et al. [29].

Cd^{2+} (X13) had an acute effect on laccase activity. Thus, an increase of laccase activity was observed in cultures for samples containing high levels of Cd^{+2} (1 mM). This phenomenon was already reported by Baldrian and Gabriel [30], who showed that the activities of endo-1,4-β-glucanase, 1,4-β-glucosidase and laccase from *Pleurotus ostreatus* highly increased in the presence of Cd^{+2} at 2 mM (18.5 fold increase of laccase activity).

The source of organic nitrogen employed had an important effect on laccase synthesis. Thus, when using casein peptone (X5) maximal laccase activities were obtained. Laccase production was higher in the absence of glucose (X1) than with 20 g L^{-1} of glucose. Such negative effect of glucose on the production of laccase has been already described [31]. Therefore this factor was fixed at its lowest level. $MgSO_4$ (X10), KH_2PO_4 (X9), pH (X20), inoculum size (X21) and the nature of the buffer (sodium acetate (X17), tartrate (X18) or citrate (X19)) had a positive effect on the production of laccase but was not statistically significant as shown in Fig. 2.

All these remarks are summarized in Table 4. As a result, true values of the variables (excluding the three significant variables giving positive effect) in the medium were determined as follows : glucose as carbon source, 5.0 g L^{-1}; $MgSO_4 \cdot 7H2O$, 0.25 g L^{-1}; KH_2PO_4, 0.025 g L $^{-1}$; inoculum number, 6.0 plugs; sodium acetate as buffer, 25 mM, pH 5.0. The levels of three significant factors (casein peptone (X5), Cd^{2+} (X13) and L/S ratio (X22)) were determined from the optimization of operating conditions for the production of laccase.

Response surface methodology

RSM was used to optimize the nutrient medium for the production of laccase by *C. gallica* using the CCD. The

Table 4 CCD matrix of three variables with experimental values of laccase production

	Factor 1	Factor 2	Factor 3	Response R1	
Run	A:peptone	B:Cd	C:L/S	Experimental value	Predicted value
1	2.00	0.50	4.00	1778.00	1355.47
2	7.00	0.50	4.00	1490.90	1624.97
3	2.00	1.50	4.00	1036.36	788.91
4	7.00	1.50	4.00	3272.72	3179.23
5	2.00	0.50	6.00	1254.54	969.45
6	7.00	0.50	6.00	1709.09	1577.96
7	2.00	1.50	6.00	936.36	423.72
8	7.00	1.50	6.00	3109.09	3153.05
9	0.69	1.00	5.00	1036.36	1828.13
10	8.31	1.00	5.00	4254.54	4114.21
11	4.50	0.24	5.00	1045.45	1336.75
12	4.50	1.76	5.00	1745.45	2105.58
13	4.50	1.00	3.48	1990.90	2232.83
14	4.50	1.00	6.52	1509.09	1918.60
15	4.50	1.00	5.00	4327.30	4396.37
16	4.50	1.00	5.00	4600.00	4396.37
17	4.50	1.00	5.00	4327.30	4396.37
18	4.50	1.00	5.00	4745.45	4396.37
19	4.50	1.00	5.00	4763.64	4396.37
20	4.50	1.00	5.00	4054.54	4396.37

responses of the CCD design were fitted with a second-order polynomial Eq. (2). Except for the linear term A ($p < 0.05$) and the quadratic term A2 ($p < 0.05$), none of the other linear, quadratic and interaction terms were statistically significant (Table 4). The overall second-order polynomial equations for laccase production in expressed in coded variables (3) and actual variables (4) are:

$$(Y) = +4396.37 + 749.71 * A + 252.13 * B - 103.05 * C + 530.21 * A * B + 84.75 * A * C + 5.21 * B * C - 613.11 * A2 - 1150.84 * B2 - 998.32 * C2 \quad (3)$$

$$(Y) = -25766,5 + 589,1 * \text{peptone} + 7750,2 * \text{Cd} + 9717,2 * \frac{L}{S} + 424,2 * \text{peptone} * \text{Cd} + 33,9 * \text{peptone} * \frac{L}{S} + 10,4 * \text{Cd} * \frac{L}{S} - 98,1 * \text{peptone}^2 - 4603,4 * \text{Cd}^2 - 998,3 * \frac{L^2}{S^2} \quad (4)$$

Where, Y is laccase activity (U L^{-1}); A is casein peptone (g L^{-1}); B is Cd^{2+} (g L^{-1}). The statistical significance of the model equation was evaluated by the F-test for analysis of variance (ANOVA), which showed that the regression was statistically significant at 99 % ($p < 0.05$) confidence level. The model F-value of 20.5 for laccase production implies that the model is statistically significant. There is only 0.01 % likelihood that large model F value could occur by chance. The value of p > F less than 0.05 indicates that the model terms are also significant. The R^2 value, being a measure of the goodness of fit of the model, indicated that the 95 % of the total variation was explained by the model. The adjusted R^2 value was 90 %. At the same time a relatively lower value of the coefficient of variation (CV = 17.47 %) indicates a better precision and reliability of the experiments carried out (Table 5).

The plot of predicted values versus experimental values in Fig. 3 also shows that all the predicted values of RSM model are located in close proximity to the experimental values. This supports the hypothesis that the model Eq. (2) is sufficient to describe the response of the experimental observations pertaining to laccase production. The Student's t distribution and corresponding values, along with parameter estimates are given in Table 5. The ANOVA results showed that among the 22 variables, tree had significant effects ($p < 0.05$): A (casein peptone), B (Cd^{2+}) and C (L/S ratio).

Table 5 Results of the regression analysis of the central composite design (CCD)

Source	Sum of Squares	Degrees of freedom	Mean Square	F-value	*P*-value Prob > F	Significance
Model	39501352.1	9	4389039.1	20.5	<0.0001	significant
Residual	2141646.9	10	214164.7			
Lack of Fit	1749316.7	5	349863.3	4.5	0.0633	not significant
Pure Error	392330.2	5	78466.0			
Cor Total	41642999.1	19				
R^2	0.95					

The relationships between culture medium variables and response can be better understood by examining the planned series of contour plots (Fig. 4a, b and c), which were generated from the predictive model described above. Three-dimensional response surface curves were plotted to study the interaction between the two factors selected and to determine the optimum concentration of each of them for maximum laccase productivity (R1) (Fig. 4). The coded model was used to generate three-dimensional diagrams and a contour plot of calculated response surface from the interaction between casein peptone (A) and Cd^{2+} (B), casein peptone (A) and L/S ratio (C), Cd^{2+} (B) and L/S ratio (C) (Fig. 4a, b and c, respectively) as a function of the six variables being at their constant levels. The shapes of contour plots indicate the nature and extent of the interactions. The prominent interactions of significant components are shown by the elliptical nature of the contour plot in Fig. 5. The optimal values of variables are obtained when moving along the major and minor axis of the ellipse and the response at the centre point yields maximum laccase production.

The main objective of the optimization was to determine the optimum values of variables for laccase activity

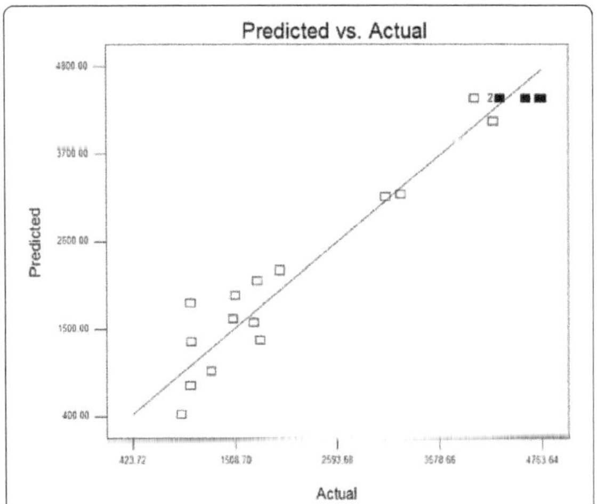

Fig. 3 Comparison between the observed values and the predicted values of (RSM) model: zero error is shown as a *thin line*

from the model obtained experimentally. From the response surface (Fig. 4) and perturbation plot (Fig. 5) it is obvious that casein peptone had a significant effect on laccase production compared to other variables. Figure 5 shows that the R1 response increases as the concentration of peptone from casein does. When the L/S ratio took values close to the center (4.75–5.0) and casein peptone took high concentrations (5.5 g L^{-1}), laccase activity reached 4163 U L^{-1}.

Cd^{2+} (C) had an acute effect on laccase activity. Figure 5c shows that the maximum laccase yield was 3992 U L^{-1} in the presence of Cd^{+2} at its central level (1 mM). However, a rapid decline in laccase productivity was observed at higher Cd^{2+} concentrations (1.25 mM). This positive effect of Cd^{2+} addition on the production of laccase was also reported by Baldrian and Gabriel [32] who found an 18.5-fold increase of laccase activity when $Cd(NO_3)_2$ (2 mM) was added to 12-day-old liquid cultures of *P. ostreatus*. In addition, Staszczak and Jarosz-Wilkołazka [33] reported that the treatment of 7-day-old mycelia with 10–200 μM Cd^{2+} resulted in considerably higher levels of laccase activity (three to five fold increase at 100 μM Cd^{2+}). These results strongly support the interpretation that the proteasome-mediated proteolytic pathway plays an important role in the regulation of *C. gallica.* laccase activity in response to Cd^{2+}.

The laccase activity was 4763 U L^{-1} in the optimized media with the three components at their central levels. Design Expert predicted the maximum laccase yield to be 4800 U L^{-1} in an optimized medium composed of Cd^{2+} (1 mM); casein peptone 4.5 g L^{-1}, L/S ratio (5.0), $MgSO_4$ (0.5 g L^{-1}, KH_2PO_4 0.05 g L^{-1}, inoculum size 6.0 plugs and 25 mM sodium acetate pH 5.0 as buffer. Laccase yield in the optimized medium was 4800 U L^{-1}, which is 3.2-fold higher than the laccase activity obtained in the initial medium (1480 U L^{-1}).

The model is significant and Lack of fit is not significant thus proving the validity. The good agreement between the predicted and the experimental results verified the validity of the model, and the improvement of laccase production also indicated that RSM was a powerful tool for determining the exact optimal values of the individual factors and the maximum response value.

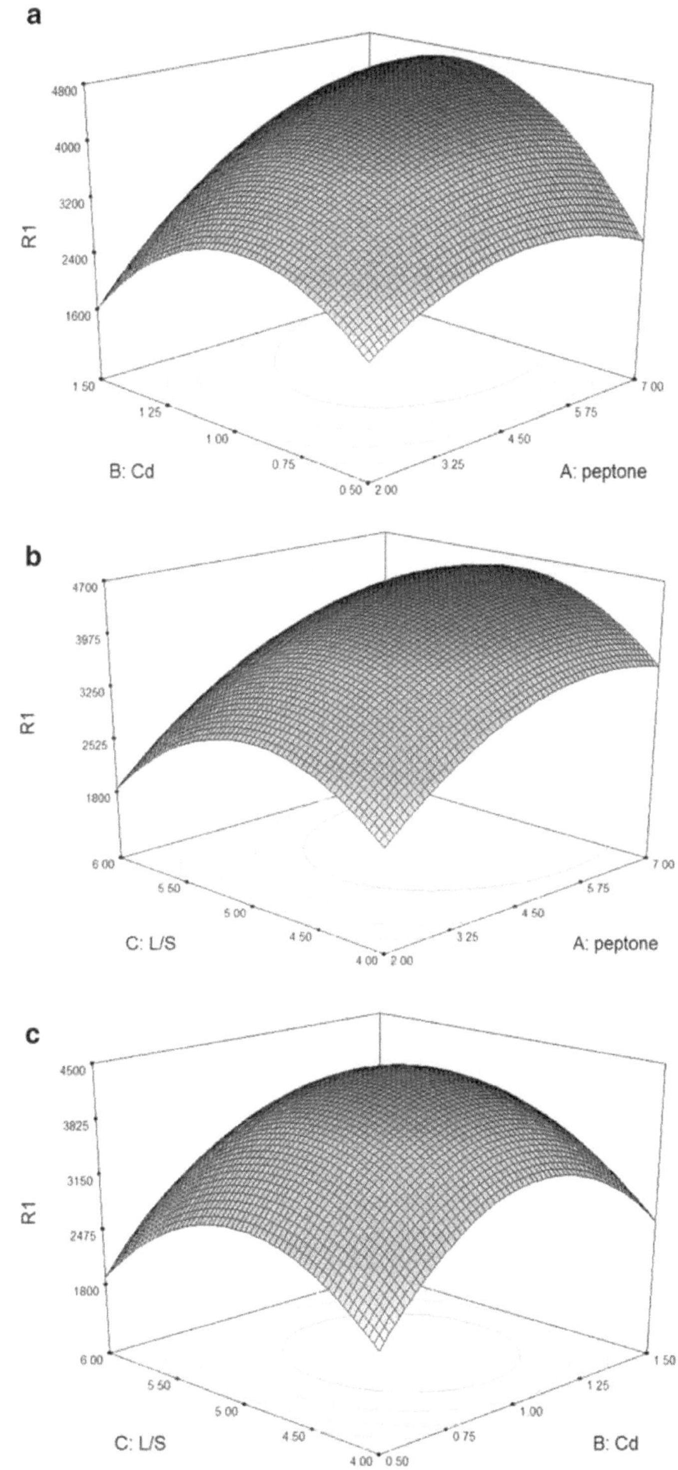

Fig. 4 Response surface and contour plots of laccase production by *C. gallica.* under solid-state fermentation (SSF) conditions operating with sawdust as support-substrate showing the effect of two variables (other variables were kept at zero in coded unit): significant interaction between (**a**): peptone (*A*) and Cd^{2+} (*B*); (**b**): peptone (*A*) and L/S ratio (*C*); (**c**): Cd^{2+} (*B*) and L/S ratio (*C*)

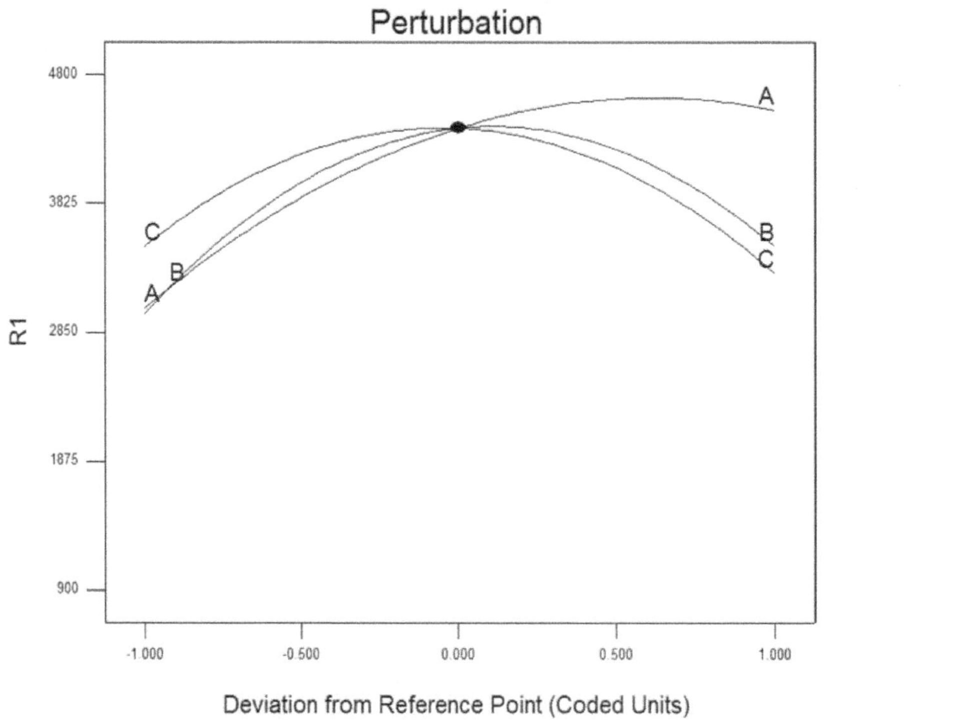

Fig. 5 Perturbation graph showing the effect of each independent variable on laccase production while keeping other variables at their respective mid-point levels. (*A*) Casein peptone, (*B*) Cd^{2+} and (*C*) L/S ratio

Batch decolorization experiments under SSF conditions

Adsorption techniques employing low-cost adsorbents are widely used to remove certain classes of chemical pollutants from water, especially those that are practically unaffected by conventional biological wastewater treatments. Sawdust, a relatively abundant and inexpensive material is currently being investigated as an adsorbent to remove contaminants from water such as: dyes, oil, toxic salts and heavy metals [34, 35].

To test the efficiency on dye removal of the above cultures, the decolorization of RB-5 and AO51 was studied. Both RB5 and AO51 belong to the class of azo compounds which are the most widely used in textile industries. This class characterizes by one or more nitrogen-nitrogen double bonds called azo groups in their chemical structure. These molecules are chemically stable and difficult to biodegrade. Several studies reported the toxicity of RB-5 [36] and AO51 [37].

Figure 6a and b show the decolorization percentage obtained for each batch. The decolorization obtained in the 1st and 2nd batch was higher than that attained in the 3rd batch for RB5 and AO51. This was likely due to the rapid adsorption of the dye onto both the fungal mycelium and the sawdust waste during the first decolorization stages as it was evidenced for the change in color of the fungal mycelium and the lignocellulosic waste (40.7 and 50.8 % adsorption percentages in the 1st batch for AO51 and RB5, respectively). Once the fungal mycelium and the sawdust waste were saturated with the dye, the decolorization was only due to the action of laccase enzymes. Decolorization percentages around 67–75 % were obtained in 24 h (1st batch) for RB5 and AO51, respectively.

As is observed in Fig. 6, the differences between the controls and SSF are significant in the 2nd batch specially AO51. In the case of RB-5 the 2nd batch shows a low variation between controls and SSF cultures compared to AO51. This suggests that the decolorization of RB-5 is realized essentially by physical adsorption of the dye to the sawdust waste during the decolorization stages. However, Biological decolorization determined by subtracting the decolorization due to the physical adsorption of the dye to the support from the total decolorization was low. SSF using sawdust can be a suitable process for RB-5 decolorization. Several studies reported that the azo dye RB-5 is difficult to biodegrade and needs a mediator redox in the case of enzymatic decolorization [36, 37].

Therefore, two mechanisms were involved in dye degradation by *C. gallica* cultures: biodegradation and

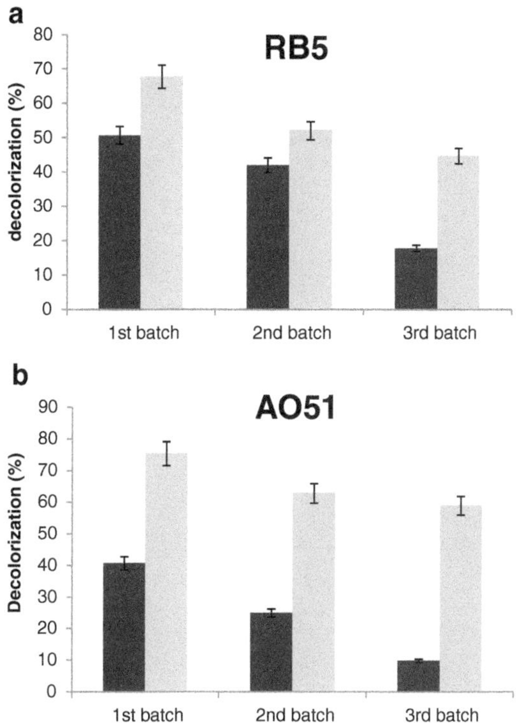

Fig. 6 Decolorization of the azo dyes (**a**) Reactive Black 5 (RB5) and (**b**) Acid Orange 51 (AO51) by *C. gallica* cultures grown on sawdust waste under solid-state fermentation conditions in three successive batches

adsorption. The determination of the amount of dye bound to the fungal mycelium was unfeasible, since it was impossible to remove the dye from it. This might be attributed to the physical-chemical property of sawdust used as support substrate in SSF.

A similar trend toward decolorization efficiency using rice bran as a substrate for the removal of textile dyestuff from wastewater decolorization of the adsorbed textile dyes from textile wastewater was reported by Kadam et al. [38]. It was also found that decolorization degrees between 49 and 94 % could be obtained under semi-solid-state fermentation of sunflower seed shells by *Trametes pubescens* [39].

Conclusions

Waste materials have little or no economic value and often present a disposal problem. Therefore, there is a need to valorize these low-cost by-products. So, their use as support-substrate for laccase production, add economic value and help in reducing the cost of waste disposal. The developed SSF process showed to be an effective system for sawdust waste upgrading by producing high laccase activity levels and removing azo dyes.

Competing interests

The authors declare that they have no competing interests.

Authors' contributions

DD performed laboratory experiments and wrote the first draft of the manuscript. HZM participated in conception and design of the experiments, FF participated in the analysis of data, SR-C participated in interpretation of data and revision of manuscript. TM and MN supervised the experimental work, coordinated tasks between authors and made final revision of the manuscript. All authors read and approved the final manuscript.

Acknowledgments

This project received funding from the Tunisian ministry of higher education and scientific research and the International Foundation for Science (IFS), under grant agreement no. F 4620-1.

Author details

[1]Laboratory of Enzyme Engineering and Microbiology, Ecole Nationale d'Ingénieurs de Sfax, University of Sfax, Route de Soukra Km 4.5, BP 1173, Sfax 3038, Tunisia. [2]Department of Biology, Faculty of Sciences and Arts, Khulais, University of Jeddah, Jeddah, Saudi Arabia. [3]Faculty of Sciences, University of Sfax, Route de Soukra Km 4,5, Sfax 3000, Tunisia. [4]CEIT, Unit of Environmental Engineering, Paseo Manuel de Lardizábal 15, 20018 San Sebastian, Spain. [5]IKERBASQUE, Basque Foundation for Science, Alameda de Urquijo 36, 48011 Bilbao, Spain.

References

1. Kahraman SS, Gurdal IH. Effect of synthetic and natural culture media on laccase production by white-rot fungi. Bioresource Technol. 2002;82:215–7.
2. Gonzales GV, Torres EF, Aguilar CN, Gomez SJR, Godinez GD, Augur C. Advantages of fungal enzyme production in solid-state over liquid fermentation systems. Biochem Eng J. 2003;13:157–67.
3. Martins ES, Silva D, Da Silva R, Gomes E. Solid-state production of thermostable pectinases from thermophilic *Thermoascus urantiacus*. Process Biochem. 2002;37:949–54.
4. Rodríguez-Couto S, Sanroman MA. Application of solid-state fermentation to food industry-a review. J Food Eng. 2005;22:211–9.
5. Eliasashvili V, Penninckx M, Kachlishvili E, Tsiklauri N, Metreveli E, Kharziani T, et al. *Lentinus edodes* and *Pleurotus* species lignocellulolytic enzymes activity in submerged and solid-state fermentation of lignocellulosic wastes of different composition. Bioresource Technol. 2008;99:457–62.
6. Pandey A, Soccol CR, Mitchell D. New developments in solid state fermentation. I. Bioprocesses and products. Process Biochem. 2000;35:1153–69.
7. Rodríguez-Couto S. A promising inert support for laccase production and decolouration of textile wastewater by the white-rot fungus *Trametes pubescesns*. J Hazard Mater. 2012;233–234:158–62.
8. Neifar M, Jaouani A, Ellouze-Ghorbel R, Ellouze-Chaabouni S, Penninckx M. Effect of culturing processes and copper addition on laccase production by the white-rot fungus *Fomes fomentarius* MUCL 35117. Lett Appl Microbiol. 2009;49:73–8.
9. Sharma RK, Arora DS. Production of lignocellulolytic enzymes and enhancement of in vitro digestibility during solid state fermentation of wheat straw by *Phlebia floridensis*. Bioresource Technol. 2010;3:9248–53.
10. Kumar NSM, Ramasamy R, Manonmani HK. Production and optimization of L- asparaginase from *Cladosporium sp.* using agricultural residues in solid state fermentation. Ind Crop Prod. 2013;43:150–8.
11. Singhania RR, Patel AK, Soccol CR, Pandey A. Recent advances in solid state fermentation. Biochem Eng J. 2009;44:13–8.
12. Reddy GV, Ravindra BP, Komaraiah P, Roy KRRM, Kothari IL. Utilization of banana waste for the production of lignolytic and cellulolytic enzymes by solid substrate fermentation using two *Pleurotus species* (*P. ostreatus* and *P. sajor-caju*). Process Biochem. 2003;38:1457–62.
13. Rosales E, Rodríguez-Couto S, Sanromán A. New uses of food waste: application to laccase production by *Trametes hirsute*. Biotechnol Lett. 2002;24:701–4.
14. Rodríguez-Couto S, Rosales E, Gundín M, Sanromán MÁ. Exploitation of a waste from the brewing industry for laccase production by two *Trametes* species. J Food Eng. 2004;64:423–8.

15. Bezerra MA, Santelli RE, Oliveira EP, Villar LS, Escaleira LA. Response surface methodology (RSM) as a tool for optimization in analytical chemistry. Talanta. 2008;76:965–77.
16. Rodríguez-Couto S. Exploitation of biological wastes for the production of value-added products under solid-state fermentation conditions. Biotechnol J. 2008;3:859–70.
17. Costan G, Bermingham N, Blaise C, Ferard JF. Potential ecotoxic effects probe (PEEP): a novel index to assess and compare the toxic potential of industrial effluents. Environ Toxic Water. 1993;8:115–40.
18. Wang X, Chen JP. Biosorption of Congo red from aqueous solution using wheat bran and rice bran: batch studies. Separ Sci Technol. 2009;44:1452–66.
19. Ozmen N, Yesilada O. Valorization and biodecolorization of dye adsorbed on lignocellulosics using white rot fungi. Bioresources. 2012;7:1656–65.
20. Garg VK, Amita M, Kumar R, Gupta R. Basic dye (methylene blue) removal from simulated wastewater by adsorption using Indian Rosewood sawdust: a timber industry waste. Dyes Pigments. 2004;63:243–50.
21. Ajmal M, Khan AH, Ahmad S, Ahmad A. Role of sawdust in the removal of copper (II) from industrial wastes. Water Res. 1998;32:3085–91.
22. Shukla A, Zhang YH, Dubey P, Margrave J, Shukla SS. The role of sawdust in the removal of unwanted materials from water. J Hazard Mater. 2002;95:137–52.
23. Stredansky M, Conti E. Xanthan production by solid state fermentation. Process Biochem. 1999;34:581–7.
24. Yaropolov AI, Skorobogatko OV, Vartanov SS, Varfolomeyev SD. Laccase-proprieties, catalytic mechanism, and applicability. Appl Biochem Biotechnol. 1994;49:257–80.
25. Plackett RL, Burmann JP. The design of optimum multifactorial experiments. Biometrika. 1946;33:305–25.
26. Montgomery DC. Design and analysis of experiments. 4th ed. New York, NY: Wiley; 1997.
27. Sani RK, Azmi W, Banerjee UC. Comparison of static and shake culture in the decolorization of textile dyes and dye effluents by *Phanerochaete chrysosporium*. Folia Microbiol. 1998;43:85–8.
28. Pérez-Guerra N, Torrado-Agrasar A, Lopez-Macias C, Pastrana L. Main characteristics and applications to denim washing. Process Biochem. 2003; 40:1673–8.
29. Rosales E, Rodríguez Couto S, Sanromán MÁ. Reutilisation of food processing wastes for production of relevant metabolites: application to laccase production by *Trametes hirsute*. J Food Eng. 2005;66:419–23.
30. Baldrian P, Gabriel J. Lignocellulose degradation by *Pleurotus ostreatus* in the presence of cadmium. FEMS Microbiol Lett. 2003;220:235–40.
31. Prasad KK, Mohan SV, Rao RS, Pati BR, Sarma PN. Laccase production by *Pleurotus ostreatus* 1804: Optimization of submerged culture conditions by Taguchi DOE methodology. Biochem Eng J. 2005;24:17–26.
32. Baldrian P, Gabriel J. Copper and cadmium increase laccase activity in *Pleurotus ostreatus*. FEMS Microbiol Lett. 2002;206:69–74.
33. Staszczak M, Jarosz-Wilkołazka A. Inhibition of the proteasome strongly affects cadmium stimulated laccase activity in *Trametes versicolor*. Biochimie. 2005;87:755–62.
34. Shukla SS, Yu LJ, Dorris KL, Shukla A. Removal of nickel from aqueous solutions by sawdust. J Hazard Mater B. 2005;121:243–6.
35. Mosayebzadeh RA. Removal of basic dye methylene blue from aqueous solutions using sawdust and sawdust coted with polypyrrole. J Iran Chem Soc. 2010;7:339–50.
36. Saratale RG, Saratale GD, Chang JS, Govindwar SP. Bacterial decolorization and degradation of azo dyes: a review. J Chin Inst Eng. 2011;42:138–57.
37. Daâssi D, Zouari-Mechichi H, Frikha F, Martinez MJ, Nasri M, Mechichi T. Decolorization of the azo dye Acid Orange 51 by laccase produced in solid culture of a newly isolated *Trametes trogii* strain. 3 Biotech. 2013;3:115–25.
38. Kadam AA, Telke AA, Jagtap SS, Govindwar SP. Decolorization of adsorbed textile dyes by developed consortium of *Pseudomonas sp. SUK1* and *Aspergillus ochraceus NCIM-1146* under solid state fermentation. J Hazard Mater. 2011;189:486–94.
39. Rodriguez-Couto S, Osma JF, Toca-Herrera JL. Removal of synthetic by an eco-friendly strategy. Eng Life Sci. 2009;9:116–23.

19

On-line micro column preconcentration system based on amino bimodal mesoporous silica nanoparticles as a novel adsorbent for removal and speciation of chromium (III, VI) in environmental samples

Hamid Shirkhanloo[1,2*], Aisan Khaligh[3], Farideh Golbabaei[4], Zargham Sadeghi[1*], Amir Vahid[2] and Alimorad Rashidi[2]

Abstract

Background: Chromium (VI) has toxic and carcinogenic effects. So, determination and speciation of chromium in environmental samples is very important in view of health hazards. In this study, solid phase extraction (SPE) based on bulky amine-functionalized bimodal mesoporous silica nanoparticles (NH_2-UVM-7) as a novel nanoadsorbent was applied for preconcentration and speciation of chromium (III, VI) in water samples.

Methods: UVM-7 was synthesized via atrane route and subsequently functionalized with amino silane via grafting method. In SPE procedure, polymer tubing as a micro-column was filled with NH_2-UVM-7 adsorbent. Preconcentration and speciation of Cr (III) and Cr (VI) ions with NH_2-UVM-7 were obtained in water samples due to the fact that only Cr (VI) ions can be complexed with-NH_2 groups at optimized pH. Finally, chromium concentration was determined by flame atomic absorption spectrometry (F-AAS).

Results: TEM, XRD, and SEM results confirmed the beneficial properties of NH_2-UVM-7 as the adsorbent for chromium extraction. Under the optimal conditions, linear calibration curve, detection limit and preconcentration factor were obtained 6–320 μg/ L, 1.2 μg/L and 66.7, respectively (RSD < 5 %). The efficiency of nanoadsorbent for preconcentration and extraction of Cr (VI) was 96 %, whereas it was less than 5 % for Cr (III).

Conclusions: The developed NH_2-UVM7-based SPE/F-AAS method has enough sensitively and simplicity for speciation and determination of Cr (VI) and Cr (III) ions in real water samples. Good recoveries, with low detection limits and good preconcentration factors are the main advantages of this procedure.

Keywords: Chromium, Speciation, Removal, Solid phase extraction, Amine-functionalized UVM-7, Flame atomic absorption spectrometry

Background

Heavy metals in industrial and municipal effluent water (IMEW) are important sources of water contamination. The contamination and quality of IMEW are its main concern especially in the regions with limited water resources The refinery effluents are one of the most important water pollution sources which can release a large quantity of heavy metals by crude oil-processing and petrochemical industries. In such region, heavy metals such as Ni, V, Pb, Hg, Cr and Co, etc. enter into the soil, water and plants and cause environmental pollutions and poison food chain [1–4]. So, in the viewing of health risk hazards, determination of heavy metals in environmental samples is very important [5–7].

The hexavalent chromium has a serious environmental pollution and threatens human health [8]. Chromium species exist mainly in two different oxidation states in

* Correspondence: hamidshirkhanloo@yahoo.ca; research@piho.org
[1]Occupational and Environmental Health Research Center (OEHRC), Iranian Petroleum Industry Health Research Institute (IPIHRI-PIHO), Tehran 1485733111, Iran
[2]Research Institute of Petroleum Industry (RIPI), Tehran 14665-1137, Iran
Full list of author information is available at the end of the article

the environment, Cr (III) and Cr (VI), which have contrasting physiological effects. The Cr (III) compounds play an important role in the metabolism of glucose and certain lipids [9, 10]. On the contrary, the Cr (VI) has toxic and carcinogenic effects and damage macromolecules, proteins and DNA [11]. The World Health Organization (WHO) states that 50 μg/L of Cr (VI) are considered to be too high as compared to its gen-toxicity [11–13]. Exposure may occur from natural or industrial sources of chromium. The general population is exposed to chromium by inhaling ambient air, ingesting food, and drinking water containing chromium. WHO has set a permissible limit of 0.05 mg/L for total chromium in drinking water [14]. Thus, the accurate determination of chromium ions has become increasingly necessary to study problems associated with environmental water pollution.

In order to provide a timely warning of chromium exposure, it is highly desirable to develop suitable procedures for chromium speciation. The most sensitive analysis techniques for determination of chromium species include ion chromatography inductively coupled plasma mass spectrometry (IC-ICP-MS) [15], luminescence quenching [16], stripping voltammetry [17], flame atomic absorption spectrometry (F-AAS) [18], neutron activation analysis (NAA) [19], inductively coupled plasma optical emission spectrometry (ICP-OES) [20], isotope-dilution mass spectrometry (ID-MS) [21], and electrothermal atomic absorption spectrometry (ET-AAS) [22, 23]. However, high instrumental and operational costs, low concentration levels of analytes, high levels of matrices, and high detection limits are common disadvantages of many of these methods. In order to simplify the analytical approaches, a separation/preconcentration step prior to analysis is required. Liquid-liquid extraction (LLE) [24, 25], homogeneous liquid-liquid extraction [26], solid phase extraction (SPE) [27, 28], liquid-phase microextraction (LPME) [29], and cloud point extraction (CPE) [30], etc., have been used for the preconcentration and/or separation of trace and ultra-trace amounts of chromium.

Among variety of methods, SPE is widely applied for the trace metal ions preconcentration because of its advantages including simplicity, minimal cost, rapidity, safety and ease of automation, lesser waste generation, lesser matrix effect, availability and easy recovery, high preconcentration efficiency, and easy adaptation of solid phase in a mini column coupled to a continuous flow preconcentration system [31]. In the SPE procedure, the choice of the appropriate sorbent is a critical factor to obtain full recovery and a high preconcentration factor. Many adsorbents such as activated carbons, nano sulfur, composite materials (CM), mesoporous silicate materials, and mesoporous silicate nanoparticles (MSN) have been successfully used for this purpose.

Since 1992, mesoporous silicate materials, especially MCM-41, have been received growing attention because of their unique properties such as high surface area and tunable pore size which facilitate the diffusion of large reactants and products inside the pores [32, 33]. These properties allow easy access of functional groups (R = OH, CN, S, NH_2) into the structure, which increases the adsorption capacity due to the combination of chemical and physical adsorption processes [34]. The mesoporous silicate nanoparticles (MSN) have higher surface area and therefore higher physical adsorption than mesoporous silicate materials [35]. The properties of MSN have been investigated by many research groups in many fields such as catalysis [35], separation [36], optic [37], biotechnology [38–40], and selective adsorbents. These nanomaterials are widely used as adsorbents for adsorption of heavy metal ions from aqueous solution in the field of water treatment [41, 42]. UVM-7 is an interesting material which can be considered as a nanometric version of the well-known MCM-41 material, and the most outstanding feature of this material is its peculiar architecture: a continuous network constructed from aggregates formed from connected mesoporous silicate nanoparticles in the range of meso/macropores, and so it has a bimodal pore system [43].

In this study, UVM-7 as bimodal mesoporous nanoparticle was synthesized and subsequently functionalized with amino silane via grafting method. The main purpose of the present research is to develop a novel analytical method for speciation and preconcentration of trace amounts of Cr (VI)/Cr (III) ions in water samples without the application of any chelating agents. The method is based on the combination of NH_2-UVM7-packed micro-column SPE and F-AAS detection method. To the best of our knowledge, no attempt has been made to apply NH_2-UVM-7 in SPE procedure for preconcentration of heavy metal ions, especially for speciation of Cr ions, in water samples. All main factors for the quantitative recoveries of Cr ions were investigated and optimized. The developed method was successfully applied for speciation and determination of analytes in real water samples. Also, the synthesized adsorbent can be used for removal of Cr (VI) ions from water samples.

Methods

Apparatus and materials

The determination of chromium ions was performed using spectra GBC flame atomic absorption spectrometer (F-AAS, GBC, Plus 932, Australia) under the conditions given by the manufacturer with air-acetylene flame and deuterium background correction. A Cr hollow cathode lamp operating at a current of 6 mA and a wavelength of 357.9 nm with a spectral bandwidth of 0.2 nm was used. The instrumental conditions were listed in Table 1. The pH values were measured with a Metrohm pH-meter (model 744, Herisau, Switzerland). A peristaltic pump (Lambda, Switzerland) was used in the SPE process.

All chemical compounds and reagents used for experiments and analysis were of analytical grade and purchased from Merck (Darmstadt, Germany). Cr (III) stock solution was prepared by dissolving of appropriate amount of Cr $(NO_3)_3.9H_2O$ (Merck,) as 1000 mg L^{-1} solution in 1 % HNO_3. Cr (VI) stock solution was prepared by dissolving of appropriate amount of $K_2Cr_2O_7$ (Merck) as 1000 mg L^{-1} solution in 1 % HCl. Standard and experimental solutions were prepared daily by dilution of the stock solution. The pH adjustments of samples were made using nitric acid (0.1 mol/L) for pH 1-2, and appropriate buffer solutions including sodium acetate (CH_3COONa/CH_3COOH, 1-2 mol/L) for pH 3-7, and ammonium chloride (NH_3/NH_4Cl, 0.2 mol/L) for pH 8-10. Deionized water obtained from a Millipore Continental Water System (Bedford, MA, USA) was used throughout this study. All the laboratory glassware and plastics were cleaned by soaking in 10 % (v/v) nitric acid for at least 24 h and then rinsed with deionized water prior to use.

Synthesis and functionalization of UVM-7

The general procedure for synthesis of UVM-7 is the atrane route, in which the presence of the polyalcohol is the key to balancing the hydrolysis and condensation reaction rates. In a typical synthesis, TEOS (tetraethyl ortho-silicate) was added to predetermine amounts of $TEAH_3$ (triethanolamine). The solution was heated up to 140 °C under vigorous stirring. After cooling down to 90 °C, CTAB (cetyltrimethylammonium bromide) was added to this solution. Hereafter, water was added slowly to the solution under stirring until a white suspension was obtained. This suspension was kept for 4 h at room temperature. The solid was filtered, washed with sufficient amounts of water and acetone and dried in an oven at 80 °C overnight. Thermocalcination of the as-synthesized UVM-7 was carried out under flow of air up to 550 °C for 6 h with a heating rate of 1 °C/min to remove both the surfactant and $TEAH_3$ from the as-synthesized UVM-7. The final molar composition of the reactants was 1.0 TEOS: 3.5 $TEAH_3$: 0.25 CTAB: 90 H_2O.

For the functionalization of calcined UVM-7 with amine groups, 1.2 g of triethoxysililpropylamine ($C_9H_{23}NO_3Si$) and 2 g of calcined UVM-7 were added to appropriate amount of toluene and refluxed for 24 h at 80 °C, followed by filtering and washing with proper amounts of ethanol and deionized water. The obtained bulky amine-functionalized UVM-7 was dried at 80 °C overnight.

Table 1 Instrumental conditions for chromium determination by F-AAS

Parameters	F-AAS
Wavelength	357.9 nm
Slit	0.2 nm
Lamp curent	6 mA
Injection mode	Manual
Volume Injection	2.2 mL/min
Mode	Integration
Fuel	Air-Acetylene

Characterization of adsorbent

X-ray diffraction (XRD) patterns were recorded on a Seifert TT 3000 diffractometer (Ahrensburg, Germany) using nickel filtered Cu-Kα radiation of wavelength 0.15405 nm. The textural properties of the sorbent including surface area, pore volume, and pore size distribution were determined by nitrogen adsorption–desorption isotherms at-196 °C using BELSORP-mini porosimeter (Bell Japan, Inc.). Prior to analysis the samples were degassed under vacuum at 300 °C for 4 h until a stable vacuum of 0.1 Pa was reached. The specific surface areas and pore volume of the sorbents were calculated by the Brunauer-Emmett-Teller (BET) and Barrett-Joyner-Halenda (BJH) methods, respectively. Scanning electron microscopy (SEM, Phillips, PW3710, Netherland) was used for surface image analysis of the sorbents. The morphology of sorbent was examined by transmission electron microscopy (TEM, CM30, Philips, Netherland). The elemental analyzer (CHNS/O, PerkinElmer, 2400 Series II, USA) was used for determination of elemental composition of sample. CHN instrument performs elemental ratio calculations of H/C, N/C, S/C or C/N.

General procedure

In SPE procedure, thin wall polymer tubing with outer diameter of 0.55 cm, inner diameter of 0.5 cm, length of 5 cm, and wall thickness of 0.05 cm filled by bulky nanoparticles of NH_2-UVM-7 was used as a preconcentration micro-column. An aliquot of the sample solution (100 mL) containing 20 μg/L of Cr (VI) and/or Cr (III) was adjusted to pH = 2 with nitric acid solution (0.1 N). The resulting sample solution was pumped through the NH_2-UVM-7 packed micro-column at a flow rate of 2.5 mL/min. The micro-column was then rinsed with 5 mL deionized water. Afterwards, the retained Cr (VI) ions were completely eluted from the solid phase with 1.5 mL of 0.3 mol/L NaOH solution. Finally, the concentration of Cr (VI) ions in the eluent was determined by F-AAS. The recovery was calculated by using Eq. 1, where C_i is the initial concentrations of analytes in solution phase, and C_f is the concentration of analytes determined by F-AAS after the SPE process. All the experimental data were the averages of triplicate determinations.

$$\text{Recovery}\,\% = \frac{(C_i\text{-}C_f)}{Ci} \times 100 \quad (1)$$

In the optimum pH conditions, Cr (VI) ions were complexed with amine groups of NH_2-UVM-7 and total chromium was calculated by oxidation of Cr (III) to Cr (VI) with H_2O_2 solution (1 mL, 0.2 M). Then, Cr (III) concentration of water sample was simply calculated by the difference between total chromium and Cr (VI) concentrations. A blank solution was also run under the same analytical conditions without adding any chromium ions. The NH_2-UVM-7 adsorbent was used freshly for blank experimental run. Moreover, the same procedure was repeated for unmodified UVM-7 sorbent. The extraction conditions were listed in Table 2.

Results

XRD analysis

XRD patterns of calcined UVM-7 and amine-grafted UVM-7 are shown in Fig. 1. There are three resolved diffraction peaks in XRD patterns of NH_2-UVM-7 and UVM-7, which can be indexed as the (100), (110), (200) and (210) reflections associated with hexagonal symmetry (d_{110} and d_{200} were overlapped with each other). However, these peaks are broad, which is the characteristic of mesoporous materials synthesized via atrane route. After the attachment of organic groups on the silica wall of UVM-7, the main three diffraction peaks are still clear which means that functionalization procedure did not had worth effect on the structural order of UVM-7.

Table 2 Extraction Conditions of proposed method for chromium speciation

Parameter	Value
Working pH	2
Amount of NH_2-UVM-7	0.12 g
Sample volume of SPE	100 mL
Volume of sample injection	1.5 mL
Linear range (method)	6-320 µg/L
Limit of detection (LOD)	1.2 µg/L
Preconcentration factor (PF)	66.7
Buffer concentration	0.03 mol/L
Volume of back-extraction solvent (NaOH)	1.5 mL
Concentration of back-extraction solvent (NaOH)	0.3 mol/L
Linear range (F-AAS)	0.4 - 15 mg/L
Correlation coefficient of F-AAS	$R^2 = 0.9956$

N_2 physisorption

The nitrogen adsorption-desorption isotherms of UVM-7 and NH_2-UVM-7 were determined and displayed in Fig. 2. The corresponding isotherm of both samples displays two distinct regions at medium and at high relative pressure which can be attributed to the presence of bimodal pore system. The first is related to the presence of small mesopores (IUPAC clacification), and the second is related to the large mesopores, respectively. The observation of these two distinct regions in both the samples, UVM-7 and NH_2-UVM-7, confirms that the UVM-7 bimodal pore system is remained almost intact after the functionalization with triethoxysililpropylamine. Textural properties of UVM-7 and NH2-UVM-7 were determined and presented in Table 3. The specific surface area (S_{BET}) of UVM-7 and NH_2-UVM-7 calculated from the linear part of the BET equation were 863 m^2/g and 626 m^2/g, respectively. Decreasing of BET surface area, pore volume, and pore diameter of NH_2-UVM-7 in comparison with initial UVM-7 is due to the grafting of aminosilane on silica walls. The unit cell parameter (a_0) and the average pore wall thickness (W_t) of the sorbents were calculated by the equations of $a_0 = 2.d_{100}/\sqrt{3}$ and $W_t = a_0 - (d_p/1.05)$, respectively, where d_p is the pore diameter of adsorbent and d_{100} is obtained from XRD diffractograms. As shown in Table 3, these two parameters are almost constant for both the sorbents.

Elemental analysis

Elemental analysis provides further evidence for the amount of amine functional groups grafteed on UVM-7. The yield of functionalization can be calculated using the elemental analysis results (the ratio of nitrogen content of the amine-functionalized UVM-7 divided by the amount of nitrogen of the triethoxysililpropylamine used for functionalization). The nitrogen content was 4.83 wt %. Moreover, by determining the nitrogen content of the remaining toluene it was found that about 99 % of the triethoxysililpropylamine was grafted on the UVM-7.

SEM imaging

The SEM was performed to illustrate the morphology and particle size distribution of the calcined NH_2-UVM-7. As shown in Fig. 3, NH_2-UVM-7 has a highly porous morphology and the mesoporous silica particles are in nanometer range (30 nm). Moreover, functionalization did not led to bulky silica nanoparticles.

TEM imaging

TEM image also illustrates pore structure of NH_2-UVM-7. As shown in Fig. 4, the mesopores are clearly visible in the silica nanoparticles and particle size of the samples is in

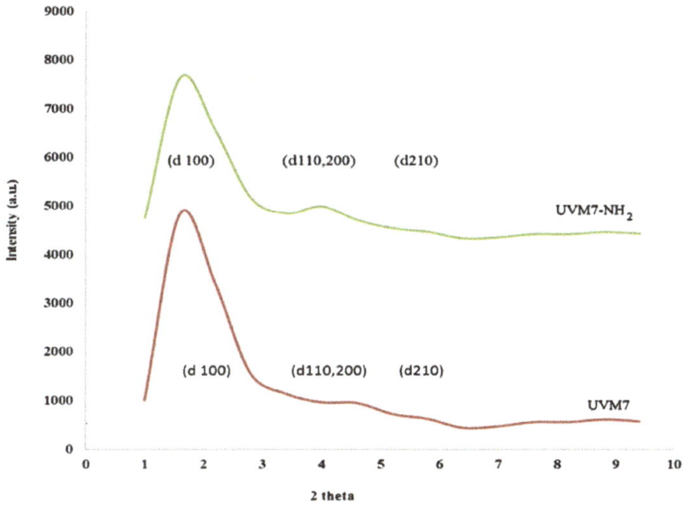

Fig. 1 Low angle XRD patterns of calcined NH_2-UVM-7 and UVM-7

nanometer range around 30 to 40 nm as those observed in SEM image.

Effect of pH, sample volume and amount of NH_2-UVM-7

In the SPE studies, the pH of the sample solution is an important parameter to obtain quantitative recoveries of metal ions, because it affects the surface charge of the adsorbent, the degree of ionization and speciation of the adsorbate. The influence of sample pH on speciation and recovery efficiency of Cr (VI)/Cr (III) ions by NH_2-UVM-7 was investigated at different pH values (1-10) by using buffered sample solutions containing Cr (III) and Cr (VI) ions, according to the general procedure. The complexation was strongly conditioned by the pH of solutions and subsequently affects extraction efficiency of the complex. As shown in Fig. 5, the highest extraction efficiency (>97 %) for Cr (VI) was achieved in the pH range of 1 -3.2, whereas the recovery values for Cr (III) were below 5 % in the same pH. Thus, the procedure was applied to speciation of Cr (VI)/Cr (III) ions at pH = 2. For higher pH values (pH > 3), the recovery percentages of Cr (VI) ions decreased with increase in pH.

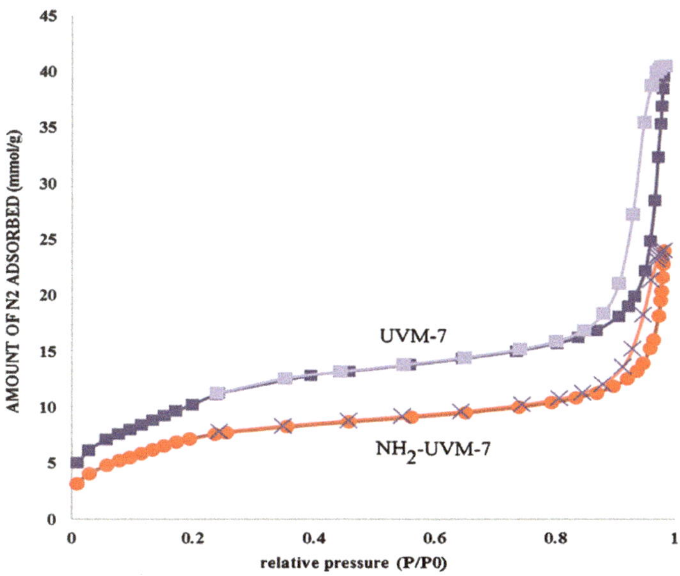

Fig. 2 Nitrogen physisorption isotherms of NH_2-UVM-7 and UVM-7

Table 3 Textural properties of UVM-7 and NH_2-UVM-7

Sample	$S^a_{BET}(m^2/g)$	$d^b_{sp}(nm)$	$d^c_{lp}(nm)$	$V^d_{sp}(cm^3/g)$	$V^e_{lp}(cm^3/g)$	$a^f(nm)$	W_t $^g(nm)$
UVM-7	863	2.67	52.2	0.42	0.84	5.59	2.92
NH_2-UVM-7	626	2.62	42.2	0.27	0.41	5.59	2.97

[a]BET specific surface area, [b]diameter of small pores, [c]diameter of large pores, [d]Volume of small pores, [e]Volume of large pores, [f]Unit cell parameter obtained from XRD diffractograms ($2d_{100}/\sqrt{3}$), [g]Wall thickness(nm) obtained by following equation: $W_t = a - (d_p/1.05)$

The extraction mechanism of Cr (VI) ions on the NH_2-UVM-7 may be based on the electrostatic attractions between metals ions and NH_2 groups of nanoadsorbent, which is highly dependent on solution pH. The NH_2 groups on the surface of the NH_2-UVM-7 can either be protonated ($-NH_3^+$) at low pH or be deprotonated (NH^-) at high pH. The variation in adsorption capacity of Cr (VI) at different pH values may be attributed to the affinities of NH_2-UVM-7 nanoadsorbent for the different anionic species of Cr (VI) existing at acidic pH conditions namely $HCrO_4^-$, CrO_4^{2-} and $Cr_2O_7^{2-}$. It is clear that negatively charged $HCrO_4^-$ and $Cr_2O_7^{2-}$ are easily adsorbed to the positively charged NH_3^+ at low pH values due to the electronic attraction. By using UVM-7 as the SPE adsorbent for preconcentration of Cr (IV) ions, it was observed that the extraction efficiencies were less than 5 % in the studied pH range. This is because the physical adsorption of Cr (VI) ions by unmodified UVM-7 is the main mechanism. So, the NH_2-UVM7 is favorite adsorbent for speciation and determination of Cr (VI)/Cr (III) ions in water samples by SPE method and can be used for on-line removal Cr (VI) in water samples at pH = 2.

Sample volume is one of the most important parameters of SPE procedure. The effect of aqueous sample volume on the recoveries of analyte ions was examined by passing different volumes (10-200 mL) of sample solution from the micro-column, according to the general procedure. The results were illustrated in Fig. 6. Quantitative recoveries of Cr (VI) ions were obtained using 10-100 mL of sample solution. At higher volumes, the recoveries were decreased. Therefore, 100 mL was selected as the optimum sample volume for further experiments of SPE. The preconcentration factor (PF) for preconcentration and extraction is calculated by the ratio of the highest sample volume for analyte (100 mL) and the lowest final eluent volume (1.5 mL). In the present study the possible preconcentration factor was 66.7.

The effect of the adsorbent dosage on the recoveries of Cr (VI) ions was investigated using various amounts of NH_2-UVM-7 in the range of 0.03–0.2 g (Fig. 7). It was observed that the extraction efficiency of the system was remarkably affected by NH_2-UVM-7 amount, and quantitative extraction was obtained using 0.1-0.2 g of NH_2-UVM-7. Therefore, in order to achieve a suitable preconcentration, 0.12 g of NH_2-UVM-7 was chosen as optimum leading to a final adsorbent.

Effect of matrix and various eluents

In this section, the interfering effect of various matrix ions, most probably present in the environmental samples, on the recoveries of Cr (VI) ions from NH_2-UVM-7 based SPE was examined. The procedure of SPE was performed using a 100 ml sample containing 100 μg/L of analyte and 1–2 mg/L of different concentration of matrix ions. The tolerate amounts of each ion were the concentration values tested that caused less than 5 % the absorbance alteration. As shown in Table 4, the ions

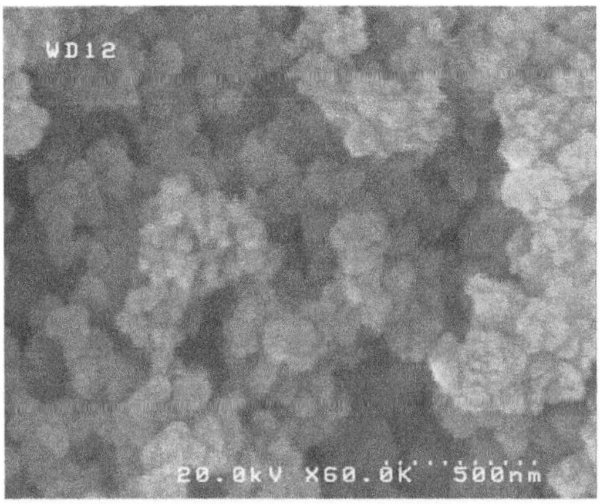

Fig. 3 SEM image of NH_2-UVM-7

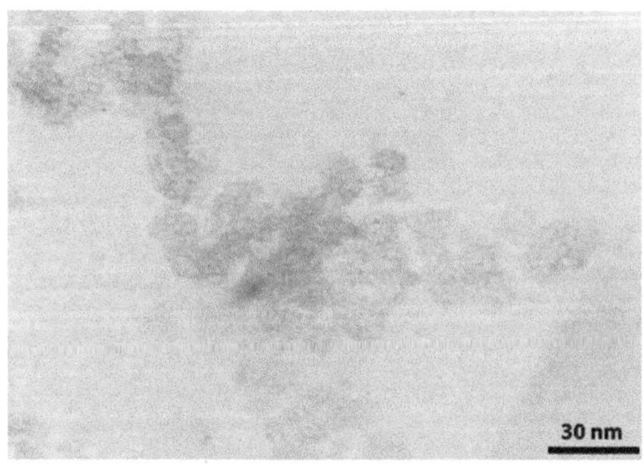

Fig. 4 TEM image of NH_2-UVM-7

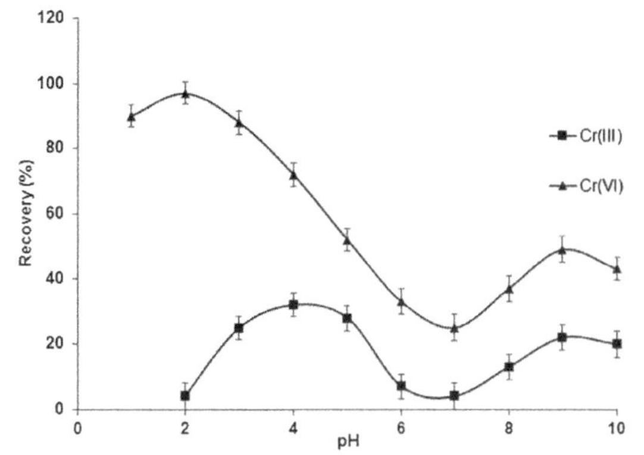

Fig. 5 The influence of solution pH on the recovery of Cr (**VI**) (▲) and Cr (**III**) (■) ions with NH_2-UVM-7 (▲). Conditions: sample volume 100 mL; adsorbent amount 0.12 g; eluent 1.5 mL of 0.3 mol/L NaOH; sample flow rate 2.5 mL/min

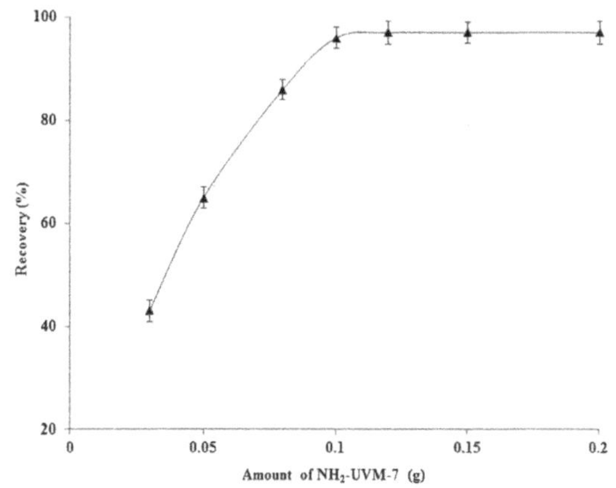

Fig. 7 The influence of amount of NH_2-UVM-7 on the recovery of Cr (**VI**) ions. Conditions: sample volume 100 mL; solution pH 2; eluent 1.5 mL of 0.3 mol/L NaOH; sample flow rate 2.5 mL/min

normally present in natural waters has no significant influence on the adsorption of Cr (VI) ions under the experimental conditions used.

The proposed method was based on back-extraction of Cr (VI) ions from NH_2-UVM-7 with a suitable basic elution solution. Increasing of the pH leads to dissociation and releasing of chromium ions into the aqueous phase. A volume of 1.5 mL of various eluents such as NaOH, NH_3, and EtOH (ethanol) with different concentration of 0.2-1 mol/L were tested as the eluent. The results showed that 1.5 mL of 0.3 mol/L NaOH quantitatively extracted chromium ions from the solid phase. At high concentration of NaOH, the recovery percentage was decreased (Fig. 8).

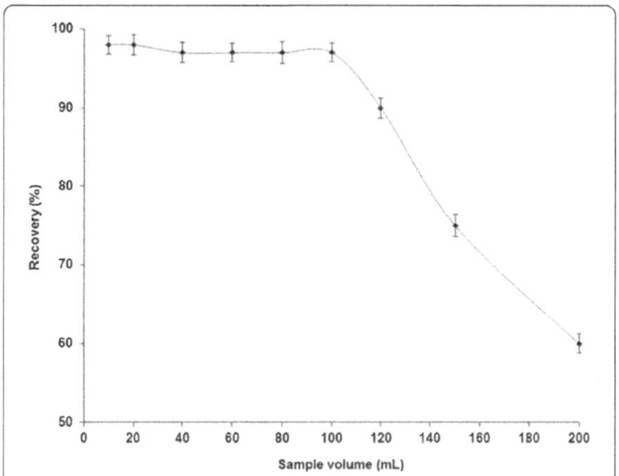

Fig. 6 The influence of sample volume on the recovery of Cr (**VI**) ions. Conditions: solution pH 2; adsorbent amount 0.12 g; eluent 1.5 mL of 0.3 mol/L NaOH; sample flow rate 2.5 mL/min

Method validation

The developed method was applied for speciation/preconcentration and determination of Cr (VI) and Cr (III) ions in different water samples including Tap and drinking water (Tehran, Iran), river water (Kan, Tehran, Iran), waste water (petrochemical factory, Tehran, Iran) and industrial water (Tehran, Iran). The spiked samples were prepared to demonstrate the accuracy and reliability of the method for determination of Cr (III) and Cr (VI). The remaining aliquots were spiked with increasing quantities of Cr (VI) and Cr (III) and analyzed by the developed SPE method. As it can be seen from Table 5, a good agreement was obtained between the added and measured analytes amount, which confirms the accuracy of the procedure and its independence from the matrix effects. The recovery of spiked samples is satisfactorily reasonable and was confirmed using addition method, which indicates the capability of the system in the determination of Cr (VI) and Cr (III) in water and biological samples. The validation of the presented procedure was also performed by the analysis of certified reference material, NIST SRM 1643e (Trace elements in water), from the National Institute of Standard and Technology (NIST, Gaithersburg, USA), for chromium values. The results found were in good agreement with the certified values of SRM (Table 6).

Adsorption capacity

The adsorption capacity of NH_2-UVM-7 was determined for Cr (VI) by using column technique. 100 mL of aqueous solutions containing 5-500 mg/L Cr (VI) at optimized pH were passed through a micro-column filled with 0.12 g of NH_2-UVM-7 at a flow rate of 0.5-5 ml/min. After Cr (VI) was eluted from the nanosorbent with 1.5 mL of NaOH (0.3 mol/L), the concentration of Cr

Table 4 The effect of matrix ions on chromium speciation and determination by proposed method

Ions	Maximum tolerance ratio (matrix ion conc./Cr conc.)
Ni^{2+}, Mg^{2+}, Ca^{2+}, Co^{2+}, Al^{3+}, K^+, Na^+, V^{3+}, Mn^{2+}, Fe^{3+}, Pb^{2+}, Zn^{2+}	2000
PO_4^{3-}, Cl^-, CO_3^{2-}, SO_4^{2-}, NO_3^-	1000

This work was performed using 100 mL of 100 μg/L Cr (VI) standard solution

(VI) in eluent was determined by F-ASS. In order to successfully represent the dynamic adsorptive behaviour, it is important to have a satisfactory description of the equation state between the two phases composing the adsorption system. In this study the Langmuir adsorption isotherm was employed for Cr (VI) adsorption by NH_2-UVM-7 adsorbent. The Langmuir model assumes uniform energies of adsorption onto the surface of NH_2-UVM-7. The Langmuir equation is defined as Eq. 2:

$$\frac{C_e}{q_e} = \frac{1}{bQ_{max}} + \frac{C_e}{Q_{max}} \tag{2}$$

Where C_e is the equilibrium concentration of metal ions in solution phase (mg/L) and q_e is the amount of metal ions adsorbed at equilibrium (mg/g), Q_{max} is maximum adsorption capacity (mg/g) on unit mass of adsorbent, and b is the Langmuir constant (L/mg), related to the free energy of adsorption. The Langmuir model provided a good fit throughout the concentration range. The applicability of the isotherm models and the high values of the correlation coefficients ($R^2 = 0.9958$) for Cr (VI) suggest favourable adsorption by NH_2-UVM7 at 45 °C. The value of Q_{max} in Langmuir plots was 192 mg/g for Cr (VI) ions at 45 °C. The values of Q_{max} and effective time for flow rate are depended on temperature of solution. According to the results, the maximum capacity of adsorbent in column condition due to the shorter contact time is 5 % less than batch system, which is apparently quite expected. The Langmuir isotherm plots at different temperatures and the value of model constants were shown in Fig. 9 and Table 7, respectively.

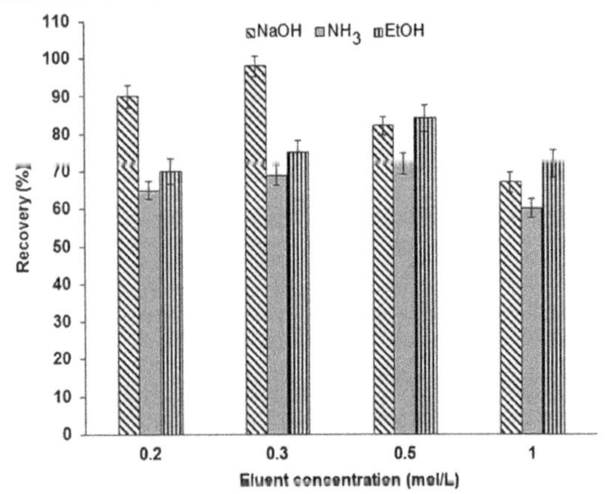

Fig. 8 Effect of different eluents on the recovery of Cr (VI) ions from NH_2-UVM-7 phase. Conditions: sample volume 100 mL; solution pH 2; adsorbent amount 0.12 g; sample flow rate 2.5 mL/min; eluent volume 1.5 mL

Discussion

The results showed that the quantitative recovery of Cr (VI) ions was obtained using 12 mg of NH_2-UVM-7 sorbent at pH = 2. At sample pH of 3.5-5, Cr (III) ions physically adsorbed on UVM-7 and NH_2-UVM-7 sorbents with recovery percentages of 33 % and 29 %, respectively. The NH_2 groups functionalized on UVM-7 were used for speciation of chromium ions at optimized pH, but they were decomposed by using strong acid or base. For back extraction of retained Cr (VI) from NH_2-UVM-7, the concentration of sodium hydroxide must be less than 0.5 mol/L. However, the pH value of the sample should be adjusted according to the chemistry of the compound of interest. It seems that, at the optimum pH the Cr (VI) ions are in the anionic form and so easily complexed with protonated amine groups (NH_3^+) of functionalized UVM-7. Therefore, by controlling pH and amount of sorbent, Cr (VI) ions can be removed from waters. So, the NH_2-UVM-7 packed micro-column SPE is a favorite method for speciation and determination of chromium ions in environmental samples, and also can be used for on-line removal of Cr (VI) in water samples at optimum pH of 2. Because of high surface area of nanosorbent (S/V) a very little amount of NH_2-UVM-7 (0.12 g) was used for removal of Cr (VI) in water sample with good adsorption capacity as 192 mg/g. Understanding the chemistry of the compound with analysis such as ionizability and hydrophobicity can be useful in designing appropriate conditions to obtain efficient extraction recovery. The results of this study showed that the sodium hydroxide solution (0.3 mol/L) was more efficient eluent for Cr (VI) back extraction from the sorbent (Fig. 8). The NaOH solution is organic free eluent and can prevent co-elution of organic compounds possibly present in the real samples. In the SPE, the volume required to elute the Cr (VI) from the nanosorbent, depends on the sorbent mass and strength of Cr (VI) retention by NH_2-UVM-7. In this study, the lowest satisfactory eluent volume is 1.5 mL, giving a suitable preconcentration factor of 66.7. Using this volume, efficient recovery of 97 % can be achieved. In optimized sample volume and sample flow rate less than 5 ml/min, Cr (VI) extraction is applicable with an efficient recovery. In this study sample flow rates up to 3 ml/min were applied with acceptable recovery of 97 %. Therefore, to be

Table 5 The reliability of proposed method for determination and speciation of Cr (III) and Cr (VI) in natural water samples

Sample	Added (μg/L)		Found (μg/L)[a]		Total Cr [a]	Recovery (%)	
	Cr^{3+}	Cr^{6+}	Cr^{3+}	Cr^{6+}		Cr^{3+}	Cr^{6+}
Tap water	—	—	22.8 ± 1.2	ND[b]	22.8 ± 1.2	—	—
	50	—	71. 5 ± 3.4	ND	71.5 ± 3.4	97.4	—
	—	20	23.1 ± 1.8	19.5 ± 1.1	42.6 ± 2.3	—	97.5
Drinking water	—	—	8.7 ± 0.4	11.2 ± 0.5	19.9 ± 0.7	—	—
	50	—	57.9 ± 2.8	10.8 ± 0.4	68.7 ± 3.2	98.4	—
	—	20	8.4 ± 0.3	30.5 ± 1.3	38.9 ± 1.6	—	96.5
Waste water [c]	—	—	94.6 ± 4.8	52.3 ± 3.1	146.9 ± 6.8	—	—
	50	—	145.4 ± 6.5	50.1 ± 2.7	195.5 ± 9.6	101.6	—
	—	50	93.3 ± 4.3	100.6 ± 5.4	193.9 ± 8.5	—	96.6
River	—	—	17.6 ± 0. 8	9.4 ± 0.3	27.0 ± 1.4	—	—
	10	—	27.3 ± 1.3	9.6 ± 0.4	36.9 ± 1.9	97.0	—
	—	20	17.9 ± 0.7	28.9 ± 1.6	46.8 ± 2.4	—	97.5
Industrial water	—	—	49.1 ± 2.2	125.3 ± 5.1	174.4 ± 9.1	—	—
	40	—	88.6 ± 4.2	122.7 ± 4.8	211.3 ± 9.8	98.8	—
	—	40	48.8 ± 2.2	163.8 ± 6.7	212.6 ± 11.2	—	96.3

[a]Mean of three determinations ± confidence interval (P = 0.95, n =5), [b]Not Detected, [c] from petrochemical factory

confident, the sample flow rate of 2.5 ml/min was selected, providing a reduced extraction time for as large as 100 mL sample volume. However, as the results shows, it would be possible to increase the sample flow rate even more as 4 mL/min without significant loss in the analyte recovery. In order to show the effect of possible matrix components on the developed method, the interfering effects of various matrix ions, most probably present in the environmental samples were examined (Table 4). The ions added to the samples are mostly present in the real water samples and can be used as closely related interferences present in matrices. The results clearly show the non-effectiveness of the all added components for each concentration on the recoveries obtained from developed method. Many sample preparation methods were used for metal extraction. Recently, liquid-liquid extraction and liquid-liquid microextraction (LLE, LLME) methods have been used for some heavy metals [44]. Although the LLME technique may be useful in some conditions, however the analyte extraction is too hard as such solutions are extremely difficult to be separated. Therefore, due to such problems, nowadays, there is a strong trend towards replacing LLE by SPE. Based on reported methods for optimizing of SPE [45, 46], authors generally have used 5 factors to optimize the method for environmental samples while, in this study, 8 parameters were screened. This allows that a robust and more reliable method is introduced for environmental monitoring of Cr (VI) and Cr (III) ions. Therefore, to make an advantage from this study compare to the other, further experiments of reproducibility of the method were carried out on spiked water samples to validate the possible use of the developed SPE for determination of Cr (VI) and Cr (III) ions. A comparison of the current method with the other reported methods was also given in Tables 8 and 9. It can be seen that the PF and LOD values of the present method, for determination of trace chromium ions, are

Table 6 Validation of proposed method for chromium determination by certified reference material (N = 5)

Bovine serum	Certified (μg/L)	Found[a] (μg/L)	Recovery (%)
NIST SRM 1643e	20.40 ± 0.24	19.48 ± 0.87	95.49 ± 0.44

[a]Mean value ± ts/√N, SRM 1643e consists of approximately 250 mL of acidified water in a polyethylene bottle

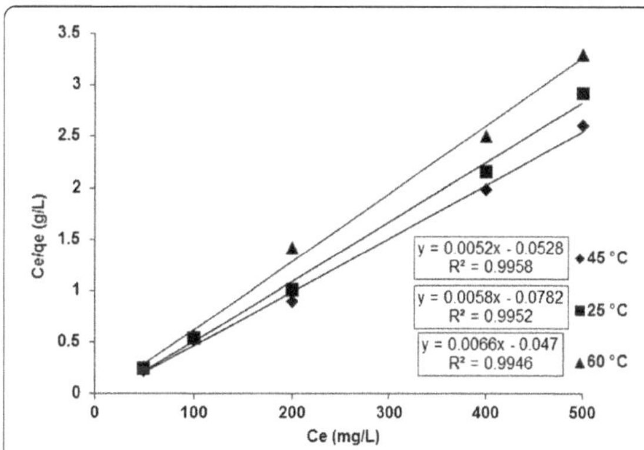

Fig. 9 Langmuir plot for chromium adsorption by NH_2-UVM-7 at different temperatures

Table 7 The Langmuir isotherm parameters for Cr (VI) adsorption by NH_2-UVM-7 at different temperatures

Temperature(°C)	Langmuir isotherm			
	Q_{max}(mg/g)	Max C_e/q_e	R^2	$t_{effective}$(min)
25	172.4	2.61	0.9952	100
45	192.3	2.92	0.9958	88
60	151.5	3.31	0.9946	83

better than, or comparable to that reported in the literature [47–56]. The limit of detection, preconcentration factor and adsorption capacity were 1.2 μg/L, 66.7, and 192 mg/g, respectively. Lower LOD values of some other works are related with higher sensitivity of the instrument used in these studies (Table 8). Also, the low sample volume (100 mL) caused to get relatively low preconcentration factor of 66.7. The adsorption of chromium ions on the most adsorbent used in SPE techniques requires formation of hydrophobic complexes using chelating agents [52–54]. However, in the developed method, NH_2-UVM-7 was investigated as a novel sorbent for the speciation and preconcentration of trace amounts of Cr (VI) and Cr (III) ions without application of any chelating agents. Hazer and Demir used SPE method based on Poly 1, 3-thiazol-2-yl methacrylamide-co-4-vinyl pyridine-co-divinylbenzene for the speciation analysis of chromium. The limit of detection, preconcentration factor and adsorption capacity were obtained as 2.4 μg/L, 30 and 80 mg/g, respectively [56]. Duran et al. used activated carbon from tea-industry wastes (TIWAC) for preconcentration and speciation of chromium without complexing agent, prior to determination by flame atomic absorption spectrometry [55]. The preconcentration factor and adsorption capacity for activated carbon were 50 and 61 mg/g, respectively. Soylak et al. studied on chromium speciation based on coprecipitation of Cr (III) by using praseodymium (III) hydroxide (Pr $(OH)_3$) precipitate and neodymium (III) Hydroxide. In their studies, the recovery extraction for Cr (VI), LOD and PF was lower than our developed method [57, 58]. Finally, the developed method based on the combination of NH_2-UVM-7 packed micro-column SPE and F-AAS detection method was successfully applied for speciation and determination of Cr (III)/Cr (VI) ions in real water samples. In addition, the NH_2-UVM-7 can be used for removal of Cr (VI) in water samples with high capacity and good repeatability.

Conclusions

The simple, fast, reliable, and economical technique for speciation and determination of trace amount of Cr (VI) and Cr (III) ions in real water samples was developed by combining the SPE technique based on NH_2-UVM-7 adsorbent with F-AAS detection method. The developed method allows us to obtain good recovery (>97 %), reproducibility, and good preconcentration factor (66.7) without using the chelating agent. In addition, the method was free of interference. Factors influencing the SPE method were optimized. The recovery efficiency of UVM-7 and NH_2-UVM-7 for Cr (VI) were found to be 5 % and 96 %, respectively, at pH =2. So, the extraction recoveries of Cr (VI) anion are depended on chemically adsorption by protonated amine group (NH_3^+) of NH_2-UVM-7. The developed SPE/F-AAS method based on NH_2-UVM-7 sorbent was successfully applied for speciation and determination of Cr (VI) and Cr (III) ions in real water samples. This method is comparable respect to powerful techniques as DLLME-ET-AAS (Table 8). The adsorption capacity of NH_2-UVM-7 for Cr (VI) ions is higher than that chelate modified SPE procedures reported in literature up to now (Table 9). The developed procedure has some advantages over other SPE methods in literature, such as low consumption of only 0.12 g NH_2-UVM-7 as adsorbent and also 1.5 mL of eluent per extraction, high sorption capacities, low detection limits, good preconcentration factor and good reusability (up to 15 cycles). The developed method can be used for removal of Cr (VI) in water samples at optimized pH. It is

Table 8 Comparison of the proposed SPE/F-AAS method with various reported procedures for determination of chromium in water samples

Detection method	Separation technique	PF[a]	LOD[b](μg/L)	Reference
ICP -MS	DLLME[c]	—	0.110	[48]
ET-AAS	SPE[d]	20	0.050	[49]
ET-AAS	BDES[e]	27	0.010	[50]
F-AAS	CPE[f]	58	0.180	[51]
CAdSV[a]	EDCS[g]	—	0.007	[47]
F-AAS	SPE[h]	66.7	1.2	This work

[a]Preconcentration factor, [b]Limit of detection, [c]Dispersive liquid- liquid micro extraction, [d]Solid phase extraction, [e]Bi-directional electrostacking, [f]Cloud point extraction, [g]Electro deposition on cell surface, [h]Nano solid phase extraction by NH_2-UVM-7

Table 9 Comparison of the proposed method with other SPE procedures for determination of chromium in water samples

SPE adsorbent	LOD[a] (μg/L)	PF[b]	Adsorption capacity (mg/g)	Reference
DPC-Poly C-18[c]	2.4	12	———	[52]
ENVI-18 DSK ™ disk	20	300	———	[53]
APDC/MWCNT[d]	0.96	100	9.5	[54]
TIWAC[e]	4.5	50	61.0	[55]
Polymer [f]	2.4	30	80.2	[56]
NH_2-UVM-7	1.2	66.7	192.0	This work

[a]Limit of detection, [b]Pre-concentration factor, [c]1,5-diphenylcarbohydrazide (DPC)-Polysorb C-18 beads, [d]Ammonium pyrrolidine dithiocarbamate (APDC)/ multi-walled carbon nanotubes, [e]Tea-industry waste activated carbon, [f]Poly (1,3-thiazol-2-yl methacrylamide-co-4-vinyl pyridine-co-divinylbenzene)

expected that the developed method could successfully be utilized for speciation, preconcentration, and determination of chromium ions in different environmental and biological samples.

Competing interests
The authors declare that they have no competing interests.

Authors' contributions
HSH, ZS and AKH participated in the design of the study, analysis, interpretation of data and helped to draft the manuscript. FG supervised the study in all steps and has been consulted by AV. Technical assistance has been provided by AMR. All authors read and approved the final manuscript.

Acknowledgements
The authors are thankful to the Iranian Petroleum Industry Health Research Institute (IPIHRI) and Research Institute of Petroleum Industry (RIPI), Tehran, Iran, for their support for this work. The authors are thankful to M.J. Kian and F. Eftekhar, S. H. Abbasi and A. M. Mortazavi for supporting this work.

Author details
[1]Occupational and Environmental Health Research Center (OEHRC), Iranian Petroleum Industry Health Research Institute (IPIHRI-PIHO), Tehran 1485733111, Iran.
[2]Research Institute of Petroleum Industry (RIPI), Tehran 14665-1137, Iran.
[3]Department of Chemistry, Semnan University, Semnan 35131-1911, Iran.
[4]Occupational Health Engineering Department, School of Public Health, Tehran University of Medical Sciences, Tehran 6446-14155, Iran.

References

1. Okoronkwo NE, Igwe GC, Onwuchekwa EC. Risk and health implications of polluted soils for crop production. African J Biotechnol. 2005;4:1521–4.
2. Dhankhar R, Chhikara S, Rana L, Sangwan S. Impact assessment of soils treated with refinery effluent. Eur J Soil Biol. 2009;45:459–65.
3. Atubi O. Effects of warri refinery effluents on water quality from the Iffie River, Delta State, Nigeria. American Rev Polit Econ. 2011;9:45–56.
4. Asgharipour MR, Sirousmehr AR. Comparison of three techniques for estimating phytotoxicity in municipal solid waste compost. Ann Biol Res. 2012;3:1094–101.
5. Duruibe JO, Ogwuegbu MOC, Egwurugwu JN. Toxicity, heavy metal pollution and human biotoxic effects. Int J Phy Sci. 2007;2:112–8.
6. U.S. Department of Health and Human Services: Chromium. National Institute for Occupational Safety and Health (NIOSH). Atlanta, GA: Centers for Disease Control (CDC), publication No: CDC-2005-149; 2007.
7. U.S. Department of Occupational Safety and Health. Toxic and hazardous substances. Atlanta, GA: Occupational safety and health standards, Occupational Safety and Health Administration (OSHA), Code of Federal Regulations: 29 CFR 1910.100; 2012.
8. U.S. Office of Water & Waste Management. Drinking water standards and health advisories. Washington, DC: Environmental Protection Agency (EPA), EPA Code: 820-R-11-002; 2011.
9. Katz SA, Salem S. The toxicity of chromium with respect to its chemical speciation: a review. J Appl Toxicol. 2006;13:217–24.
10. Kotas J, Stasicka Z. Chromium occurrence in the environment and methods of its speciation. Environ Pollut. 2000;107:263–83.
11. U.S. Department of Health and Human Services: toxicological profile for chromium. Public Health Service, Agency for Toxic Substances and Disease Registry (ATSDR), Publication No: ATSDR-HE-CS-2001-0005; 2000.
12. U.S. Department of Human Hazardous Exposure. Documentation of the Threshold Limit Values and Biological Exposure. Index 7th Ed. Atlanta, GA: American Conference of Governmental Industrial Hygienists (ACGIH); 2011.
13. National Health and Nutrition Examination Survey (NHNES). Chromium compounds. Atlanta, GA, USA: Centers for Disease Control; 2010.
14. International Program on Chemical Safety (IPCS): Chromium. Environmental Health Criteria 61. Switzerland: World Health Organization; 2003 [http://www.inchem.org/documents/ehc/ehc/ ehc61.htm]
15. Laborda F, Grriz M, Bolea E, Castillo J. Determination of total and soluble Cr (VI) in compost by ion chromatography-inductively coupled plasma mass spectrometry. Int J Environ An Ch. 2007;87:227–35.
16. Hosseini MS, Belador F. Cr (III) /Cr (VI) speciation determination of chromium in water samples by luminescence quenching of quercetin. J Hazard Mater. 2009;165:1062–7.
17. Jorge EO, Rocha MM, Fonseca ITE, Neto MMM. Studies on the stripping voltammetric determination and speciation of chromium at a rotating-disc bismuth film electrode. Talanta. 2010;81:556–64.
18. Kiran K, Kumar KS, Prasad B, Suvardhan K, Babu LR, Janardhanam K. Speciation determination of Cr (III) and Cr(VI) using preconcentration cloud point extraction with flame atomic absorption spectrometry. J Hazard Mater. 2008;150:582–6.
19. Chai ZF, Zhang ZY, Feng WY, Chen CY, Xu DD, Hou XL. Study of chemical speciation of trace elements by molecular activation analysis and other nuclear techniques. J Anal At Spectrom. 2004;19:26–33.
20. Suleiman JS, Hu B, Huang CZ. On-line speciation of Cr (III) and Cr (VI) using microcolumn packed with immobilized used green tea leaves (UGTLs) and determination by ICP-OES in environmental water samples. Atom Spec. 2007;28:234–40.
21. Rahman GMM, Kingston HMS, Towns TG, Vitale RJ, Clay KR. Determination of hexavalent chromium by using speciated isotope-dilution mass spectrometry after microwave speciated extraction of environmental and other solid materials. Anal Bioanal Chem. 2005;382:1111–20.
22. Burguera M, Burguera JL. On-line electrothermal atomic absorption spectrometry configurations, Atomic Spectroscopy. Spectrochim Acta B. 2007;62:884–96.
23. Olmedo P, Pla A, Hernandez AF, Lopez-Guarnido O, Rodrigo L, Gil F. Validation of a method to quantify chromium, cadmium, manganese, nickel and lead in human whole blood, urine, saliva and hair samples by electrothermal atomic absorption spectrometry. Anal Chim Acta. 2010;659:60–7.
24. Beni A, Karosi R, Posta J. Speciation of hexavalent chromium in waters by liquid–liquid extraction and GFAAS determination. Microchem J. 2007;85:103–8.
25. Shirkhanloo H, Khaligh A, Mousavi HZ, Eskandari MM, Miran-Beigi AA. Ultra-trace speciation and determination in blood samples by ionic liquid-based dispersive liquid–liquid microextraction. Chem papers. 2015;69:779–90.
26. Ebrahimzadeh H, Yamini Y, Kamare F, Shariati S. Homogeneous liquid–liquid extraction of trace amounts of mononitrotoluenes from waste water samples. Anal Chim Acta. 2007;594:93–100.
27. Li Z, Chang X, Hu Z, Huang X, Zou X, Wu Q, et al. Zincon-modified activated carbon for solid-phase extraction and preconcentration of trace lead and chromium from environmental samples. J Hazard Mater. 2009;166:133–7.
28. Narin I, Kars A, Soylak M. Novel solid phase extraction procedure on amberlite XAD-1180 for speciation of Cr (III), Cr (VI) and total chromium in environmental and pharmaceutical samples. J Hazard Mater. 2008;150:453–8.
29. Zeng C, Lin Y, Zhou N, Zheng J, Zhang W. Room temperature ionic liquids enhanced the speciation of Cr (VI) and Cr (III) by hollow fiber liquid phase microextraction combined with flame atomic absorption spectrometry. J Hazard Mater. 2012;237:365–70.
30. Liang P, Sang H. Speciation of chromium in water samples with cloud point extraction separation and preconcentration and determination by graphite furnace atomic absorption spectrometry. J Hazard Mater. 2008;154:1115–9.
31. Soliman EM, Saleh MB, Ahmed S. Alumina modified by dimethyl sulfoxide as a new selective solid phase extractor. Talanta. 2006;69:55–60.
32. Thielemann J, Girgsdies F, Schlogl R, Hess C. Pore structure and surface area of silica SBA-15, influence of washing and scale up. Beilstein J Nanotechnol. 2011;2:110–8.
33. Kokunešoski M, Gulicovski J, Matovic B, Logar M, Milonjic SK, Babic B. Synthesis and surface characterization of ordered mesoporous silica SBA-15. Mater Chem Phys. 2010;124:1248–52.
34. Lenin H, Carmen G, Julio L, Aurelio B, Ramon MM, Dolores M, et al. Bases for the synthesis of nanoparticulated silicas with bimodal hierarchical porosity. Solid State Sci. 2006;8:940–51.
35. Taguchi A, Schuth F. Ordered mesoporous materials in catalysis. Microp Mesop Mater. 2005;77:1–45.
36. Nakanishi K, Tanaka N. Sol-gel with phase separation, hierarchically porous materials optimized for high-performance liquid chromatography separations. Acc Chem Res. 2007;40:863–73.

37. Zanjanchi MA, Ebrahimian A, Alimohammadi Z. A spectroscopic study on the adsorption of cationic dyes into mesoporous AlMCM-41 materials. Optical Mater. 2007;29:794–800.
38. Lu J, Liong M, Zink JI, Tamanoi F. Mesoporous silica nanoparticles as a delivery system for hydrophobic anticancer drugs. Small. 2007;8:1341–6.
39. Slowing II, Trewyn BG, Lin VSY. Mesoporous silica nanoparticles for intracellular delivery of membrane-impermeable proteins. J Am Chem Soc. 2007;129:8845–9.
40. Torney F, Trewyn BG, Lin VSY. Mesoporous silica nanoparticles deliver DNA and chemicals into plants. Nature Nanotech. 2007;2:295–300.
41. Yang H, Xu R, Xue XM, Li FT, Li GT. Hybrid surfactant template mesoporous silica formed in ethanol and its application for heavy metal removal. J Hazard Mater. 2008;152:690–8.
42. Xue XM, Li FT. Removal of Cu (II) from aqueous solution by adsorption onto functionalized SBA-16 mesoporous silica. Microporous Mesoporous Mater. 2008;116:116–22.
43. El Haskouri J, Morales JM, Ortizde Zárate D, Fernández L, Latorre J, Guillem C, et al. Nanoparticulated silicas with bimodal porosity: chemical control of the pore sizes. Inorg Chem. 2008;47:8267–77.
44. Bouabdallah I, Zidane I. Liquid-liquid extraction of copper (II), cadmium (II), and lead (II) using tripodal N-donor pyrazole ligands. Arkivok. 2006;11:59–65.
45. Tuzen M, Narin I. Solid phase extraction system for atomic absorption spectrometric determination of some trace metals in environmental samples (XAD-4/PAN). Anal Lett. 2004;37:473–89.
46. Soylak M, Dogan M. Column preconcentration/separation and atomic absorption spectrometric determinations of some heavy metals in table salt samples using amberlite XAD-1180. Turk J Chem. 2003;27:235–42.
47. Bobrowski A, Mocak J, Dominik J, Pereira H, Knap W. Metrological characteristics and comparison of analytical methods for determination of chromium trace in water samples. Acta Chim Slov. 2004;51:77–93.
48. Ina R, Audrius P, Birut P, Evaldas N. Determination of Cr (VI) by dispersive liquid-liquid microextraction and dried-droplet laser ablation ICP-MS. Cur Anal Chem. 2010;6:310–5.
49. Xue A, Qian S, Huang G, Chen L. Separation and preconcentration of chromium speciation on chitosan and determination by graphite furnace atomic absorption spectrometry. J Anal At Spectrom. 2000;15:1513–5.
50. Yang L, He Y, Gan W, Li M, Qu Q, Lin X. Determination of Cr (VI) and Pb (II) in drinking water by electrokinetic flow analysis system and graphite furnace atomic absorption spectrometry. Talanta. 2001;55:271–9.
51. Agrawal YK, Sharma KR. Speciation, liquid–liquid extraction, sequential separation, preconcentration, transport and ICP-AES determination of Cr (III), Mo (VI) and W (VI) with calix-crown hydroxamic acid in high purity grade materials and environmental samples. Talanta. 2005;67:112–20.
52. Wang J, Xue B. Sequential injection analysis for Cr (VI) and Cr (III) with renewable surface reflection spectrophotometry. Anal Sci. 2006;22:1233–6.
53. Mohammadhosseini M, Tehrani MS, Ganjali MR. Preconcentration, determination and dpeciation of chromium(III) using solid phase extraction and flame atomic absorption spectrometry. J Chin Chem Soc. 2006;53:549–57.
54. Tuzen M, Soylak M. Multiwalled carbon nanotubes for speciation of chromium in environmental samples. J Hazard Mater. 2007;147:219–22.
55. Duran C, Ozdes D, Gundogdu A, Imamoglu M, Senturk HB. Tea-industry waste activated carbon, as a novel adsorbent, for separation, preconcentration and speciation of chromium. Anal Chim Acta. 2011;688:75–83.
56. Hazer O, Demir D. Speciation of chromium in water samples by solid-phase extraction on a new synthesized adsorbent. Anal Sci. 2013;29:729–34.
57. Soylak M, Aydin A. Speciation of Cr (III) and Cr (VI) in environmental samples by using coprecipitation with praseodymium(III) hydroxide and determination by flame atomic absorption spectrometry. J Iranian Chem Soc. 2012;9:263–7.
58. Soylak M, Kizil N. Neodymium (III) hydroxide coprecipitation-FAAS system for the speciation of chromium in natural waters. Atom Spect. 2013;34:216–20.

Mercury pollution for marine environment at Farwa Island, Libya

Adel A.S. Banana[1], R. M. S. Radin Mohamed[2] and A. A. S. Al-Gheethi[2,3*]

Abstract

Background: Farwa is an Island in Libya receives petrochemical wastes generated from General Company of Chemical Industries (GCCI) since more than 40 years.

Aim: The present work aimed to determine the concentrations of mercury (Hg^{+2}) in fish, marine plants and sediment collected from Farwa lagoon to evaluate effect of industrial wastewater from GCCI on the marine environment.

Methods: Hundred and twelve samples of fish, pearl oyster, cuttlefish sediments and marine plants were analyzed to determine Hg^{2+} concentration during the period from January to August 2014 by using Atomic Absorption Spectrometer (AAS).

Results: The highest concentration of Hg^{2+} was detected in *Pinctada radiata* (11.67 ± 3.30 μgg^{-1}) followed by *Serranus scriba* (6.37 ± 0.11 μg g^{-1}) and *Epinephelus marginatus* (6.19 ± 0.02 μg g^{-1}). About 75 % of marine plants contained the maximum contaminations during the summer season. In fish samples Hg^{2+} concentrations exceeded the levels provided by international standards.

Conclusions: The fish at Farwa lagoon is heavily contaminated with Hg^{2+} which may represent a source for mercury poisoning for human.

Keywords: Mercury, Fishes, Contamination, Farwa Island

Background

The increasing of industrial activities has led to increase the contamination of environment with several types of pollutants as due to discharge of industrial wastewater into the environment and aquatic system. petrochemicals factors is among various of industrials process which produce heavily contaminated wastewater. In the developed countries the wastewater are treated using advanced technologies such as reverse osmosis, nanotube carbon, adsorption process using different types of adsorbents as well as photo-degradation processes of degradable toxic compounds. Those technologies have high efficiency to remove most toxic substances from wastewater before final disposal into the environment. Others technologies such as multi-walled carbon nanotube/tungsten oxide (MWCNT/WO_3) and alumina nano-particles polyamide membrane still under investigation and they exhibited high efficiency for the removal and degrade various types of pollutants based on the lab scale experiments [1–7].

In the term of heavy metals contamination, the petrochemical industries represent one of the main sources for generation of these toxics into the environment. the adsorption process materials is the most common treatment process to remove heavy metals from wastewater. Recently, some authors focused on improvement this process to be high efficiency. Gupta et al. [8] has combined the magnetic properties of iron oxide with adsorption properties of carbon nanotubes to increase the removal of Cr^{2+} ions.

Heavy metals are groups of elements with high molecular weights that are not degraded when taken into the body; instead, they accumulate in specific body organs and cause illness. Heavy metals have the potential to disrupt the metabolism and biological activities of many proteins because it can oxidize the sulfhydryl groups [9]. Among several of heavy metals, mercury (Hg^{2+}) is the most toxic

* Correspondence: adelalghithi@gmail.com
[2]Faculty of Civil & Environment Engineering, UTHM, Parit Raja, Malaysia
[3]High Institute of health sciences, Sana'a, Yemen
Full list of author information is available at the end of the article

element for organisms [10–12]. Hg^{2+} is very toxic pollutant that contaminates fish around the world, therefore fish represent the main source of Hg^{2+} for human [13]. The studies indicated that mercury accumulation in the oceans correlates with the rising tide of mercury pollution. The most serious Hg^{2+} poisoning has been occurred due to consumption of Hg^{2+} contaminated fish and other seafood polluted by industrial wastewater [14]. However, information for mercury contamination of fishes and marine environment in Libya is unavailable; this might due to absence of academic research for more than 40 years. Therefore, the present work aimed to evaluate the concentrations of Hg^{2+} in fish, sea woods and sediments at Farwa Island, Libya that received petrochemical wastes generated from General Company of Chemical Industries (GCCI) for more than 40 years.

Methods

Study area

Farwa Island is located on the Mediterranean in West Zawya, Libya (33° 04' N, 1° 50' E to 33° 08' N and 11° 32' E) from Abu- Kamash east to the Tunisian border in the west (Fig. 1). It comprises Farwa lagoon that covering an area of 32 km^2 and is the largest lagoon on the Libyan coast. GCCI is located at Abu- Kamash chemical complex. GCCI was opened in 1970s and consist of 3 units that produce 104,000 tonnes/year Ethylene di-chloride, 60, 000 tonnes poly vinyl chloride (PVC), 50,000 tonnes caustic soda and 45,000 tonnes chlorine. In addition to sodium carbonate, sodium hypochlorite and HCl. GCCI has four dumping sites, two of them are located on the west while another two are located on the east.

Collection and analysis of samples

Hundred ninety two samples (in triplicate, 3 sample/ month) of fishes, oysters, cuttlefish, magnoliophyta plants and sediments were collected from marine environment around of Farwa Island, Libya during the period from January to August 2014. The marine organisms collected samples included ten types of fishes, only one type of oyster and one type of cuttlefish. These samples were collected using local fishermen. Magnoliophyta plant samples were collected from different location around Farwa Lagoon, Zone I (100 m), Zone II (1000 m) and Zone III (3000 m). These locations represent the distance between the sampling point and the factory and they were selected because its very close to GCCI and the possibility to heavy contamination with Hg^{2+} is high. The samples were transported inside ice box to the laboratory and kept in deep freezer at −20 °C until analysis.

Sample preparation and analysis were carried out according to Bernhard [15]. Liver, muscle, gill, heart, air sac and stomach-intestine were removed before the analysis [16]. Fish samples were homogenized in a blender. Magnoliophyta plants were cut out into small pieces (5 mm in diameter) and then homogenized in a blender. A weight of 10 g of homogenate for each of fish and magnoliophyta plants was digested according to APHA [17]. In briefly; five mL of HNO_3 (65 %) and 5 mL of H_2SO_4 were added into sample placed inside flask (100 mL). The mixture was heated on a hot plate (70–80 °C) for 30 min to the lowest volume (20 mL) before precipitation occurs. The digestion step was continued until light colored, clear solution was observed. The flask walls was washed with distilled water and filtered using Whatman, 125 mm Ø, filter papers (Cat No. 1001 England). The filtrate was

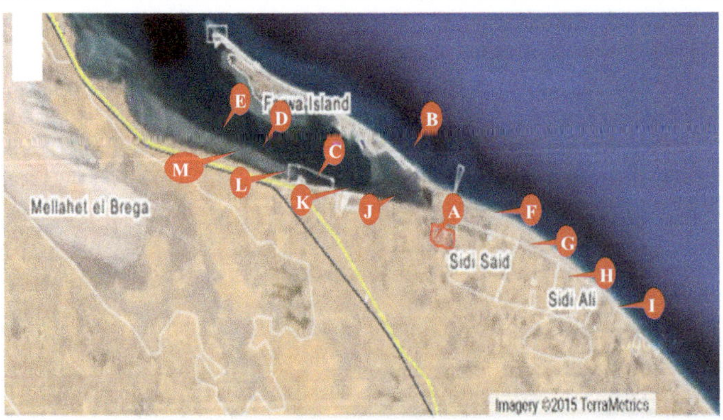

Fig. 1 Google map of study area, A) GCCI B) site of fish samples collection C) site of marine plant samples collection (100 m); D) site of marine plant samples collection (1000 m); E) site of marine plant samples collection (3000 m); F) site of sediment samples collection (100 m, W); G) site of sediment samples collection (500 m, W); H) site of sediment samples collection (1000 m, W); I) site of sediment samples collection (3000 m, W); J) site of sediment samples collection (100 m, E); K) site of sediment samples collection (500 m, E); L) site of sediment samples collection (1000 m, E); site of sediment samples collection (3000 m, E)

transported into a volumetric flask (100 mL) with 10 mL water and mixed thoroughly.

Sediment samples (1 kg) were collected by using grab sampler from eight sites located on the west and east of GCCI. Samples were transported to the laboratory and dried in oven at 50 °C. After that, sediment samples were powdered and passed through 160 μm sieve. The samples packed in paper bags and stored in deep freezer at −20 °C prior to analysis. The mercury was extracted from the samples with 10 mL HNO_3/HCl (1:3 v/v) by using a microwave digestion system as described above.

The Hg^{2+} concentrations in the digested samples were determined by an atomic absorption spectrophotometer (AAS) (Model P.E.A ANALYST 100, HGA-800 and MHS-10, Perkin Elmer, USA).

Table 1 ANOVA Analysis of Hg^{2+} concentrations in different fish samples during the period of study from January to August 2014

Sample		Sum of Squares	df	Mean Square	F	Sig.
Serranus scriba	Between groups	54.369	7	7.767	1257.814	.000
	Within groups	.099	16	.006		
	Total	54.468	23			
Oedalechilus labeo	Between groups	28.478	7	4.068	2697.193	.000
	Within groups	.024	16	.002		
	Total	28.502	23			
Diplodus vulgaris	Between groups	6.588	7	.941	1146.640	.000
	Within groups	.013	16	.001		
	Total	6.602	23			
Dicentrarchus labrax	Between groups	4.697	7	.671	712.616	.000
	Within groups	.015	16	.001		
	Total	4.712	23			
Lithognathus mormyrus	Between groups	70.353	7	10.050	2138.378	.000
	Within groups	.075	16	.005		
	Total	70.428	23			
Epinephelus marginatus	Between groups	99.308	7	14.187	16690.375	.000
	Within groups	.014	16	.001		
	Total	99.321	23			
Sarpa salpa	Between groups	11.577	7	1.654	301.838	.000
	Within groups	.088	16	.005		
	Total	11.664	23			
Sciaena umbra	Between groups	3.448	7	.493	467.260	.000
	Within groups	.017	16	.001		
	Total	3.465	23			
Pagrus pagrus	Between groups	3.373	7	.482	98.591	.000
	Within groups	.078	16	.005		
	Total	3.451	23			
Caranx crysos	Between groups	5.237	7	.748	949.947	.000
	Within groups	.013	16	.001		
	Total	5.249	23			
Pinctada radiata	Between groups	310.444	7	44.349	6809.846	.000
	Within groups	.104	16	.007		
	Total	310.548	23			
Sepia officinalis	Between groups	2.703	7	.386	639.161	.000
	Within groups	.010	16	.001		
	Total	2.713	23			

The concentrations of heavy metals was calculated ($\mu g\ g^{-1}$) using Eqs. (1)

$$MetalConcentration = A \times B/C$$

Where
A = concentrations of metals in digested solution $\mu g\ g^{-1}$
B = final volume of digested solution mL
C = sample size, gram

Data analysis
The data were not normally distributed, therefore, they were log transformed and subjected to parametric statistics. The differences in Hg^{2+} concentrations of samples investigated were tested by ANOVA. The statistical analyses was performed SPSS (version 11.5).

Results and discussion

The present study investigated the mercury contamination of marine environment included fishes, oysters, cuttlefish, magnoliophyta plants and sediments at Farwa Island, Libya that are received industrial wastewater generated from GCCI since 40 years ago. The concentration of mercury at this place has not reported before, thus the current work was conducted to evaluate the effect of petrochemical wastewater on the environment. The results revealed that the Hg^{2+} concentration differed significantly ($p < 0.05$) during the period of study (Table 1). These variables may be due to the climatic conditions of the area, winter season extends from November to March and is generally cold and rainy with unstable winds blowing from different directions which lead to cause dilution of Farwa lagoon, while summer season (May to September) is rather hot and dry [18]. The mean of Hg^{2+} concentrations in fish, oysters and cuttlefish samples collected during the period study are presented in Table 2. It can be noted that the Hg^{2+} concentrations ranged from 3.13 ± 1.5 $\mu g\ g^{-1}$ in *Serranus scriba* to 0.34 ± 0.33 $\mu g\ g^{-1}$ in *Sciaena umbra*. The distributions of Hg^{2+} concentrations for each species in the period from January to August 2014 are depicted in Fig. 2. It shown that the highest concentration of Hg^{2+} was detected in *Pinctada radiata* (11.67 ± 3.30 $\mu g g^{-1}$) in August, followed by *Serranus scriba* (6.37 ± 0.11 $\mu g\ g^{-1}$) in July and *Epinephelus marginatus* (6.19 ± 0.02 $\mu g\ g^{-1}$) in February. The *Serranus scriba* have high concentration of Hg^{2+} during the study period from January to July followed by *Epinephelus marginatus*, the average was 2.83 *vs.* 2.18 μg g-1. The lowest Hg^{2+} concentrations were detected in *Pagrus pagrus* (0.001 $\mu g\ g^{-1}$) and *Sciaena umbra* (0.01 $\mu g\ g^{-1}$). Both types contained the lowest average concentrations during the period of study (0.33 and 0.36 $\mu g\ g^{-1}$ respectively). *Lithognathus mormyrus* has the highest Hg (3.59 ± 0.19 $\mu g\ g^{-1}$) among the fish samples collected in April, whereas *Oedalechilus labeo* has the highest Hg (3.59 ± 0.01 $\mu g\ g^{-1}$) among the fish samples collected in May. In June, the highest Hg^{2+} was determined in *Lithognathus mormyrus* (4.97 ± 0.04 $\mu g\ g^{-1}$).

The analysis for association between Hg^{2+} concentrations in fish, oysters as well as cuttlefish samples and months indicated that the concentration of Hg^{2+} in *Serranus scriba, Dicentrarchus labrax, Sciaena umbra* and *Pinctada radiata* associated significantly ($p < 0.05$) to the seasons with R^2 0.64, 0.24, 0.21 and 0.34 respectively (Table 3). The Hg^{2+} concentrations in magnoliophyta plants are presented in Table 4. It can be noted that the maximum concentration was detected in the samples

Table 2 Hg^{2+} concentrations in Fishes collected from Farwa lagoon, Libya which received petrochemical wastes from General Company of Chemical Industries (GCCI), (±SD represent the standard division from the mean, $n = 24$ for each sample)

Sample No.	Family name	English name	Science name	Hg concentration ($\mu g\ g^{-1}$)
1	Serranidae	Painted comber	Serranus scriba	3.13 ± 1.5
2	Mugilidae	Boxlip Mullet	Oedalechilus labeo	1.4 ± 1.1
3	Sparidae	Common Two-Banded Seabream	Diplodus vulgaris	1.4 ± 0.53
4	Moronidae	European seabass	Dicentrarchus labrax	0.89 ± 0.45
5	Sparidae	Striped sea bream	Lithognathus mormyrus	1.5 ± 0.7
6	Serranidae	Dusky Grouper	Epinephelus marginatus	1.9 ± 2.0
7	Sparidae	Salema	Sarpa salpa	0.99 ± 0.71
8	Sciaenidae	sculpin	Sciaena umbra	0.34 ± 0.33
9	Dentex macrophthalmus	Red porgy	Pagrus pagrus	0.39 ± 0.38
10	Carangidae	blue runner	Caranx crysos	0.78 ± 0.48
11	Oyster	Rayed Pearl Oyster	Pinctada radiata	2.3 ± 3.6
12	Cuttlefish	common cuttlefish	Sepia officinalis	0.63 ± 0.34

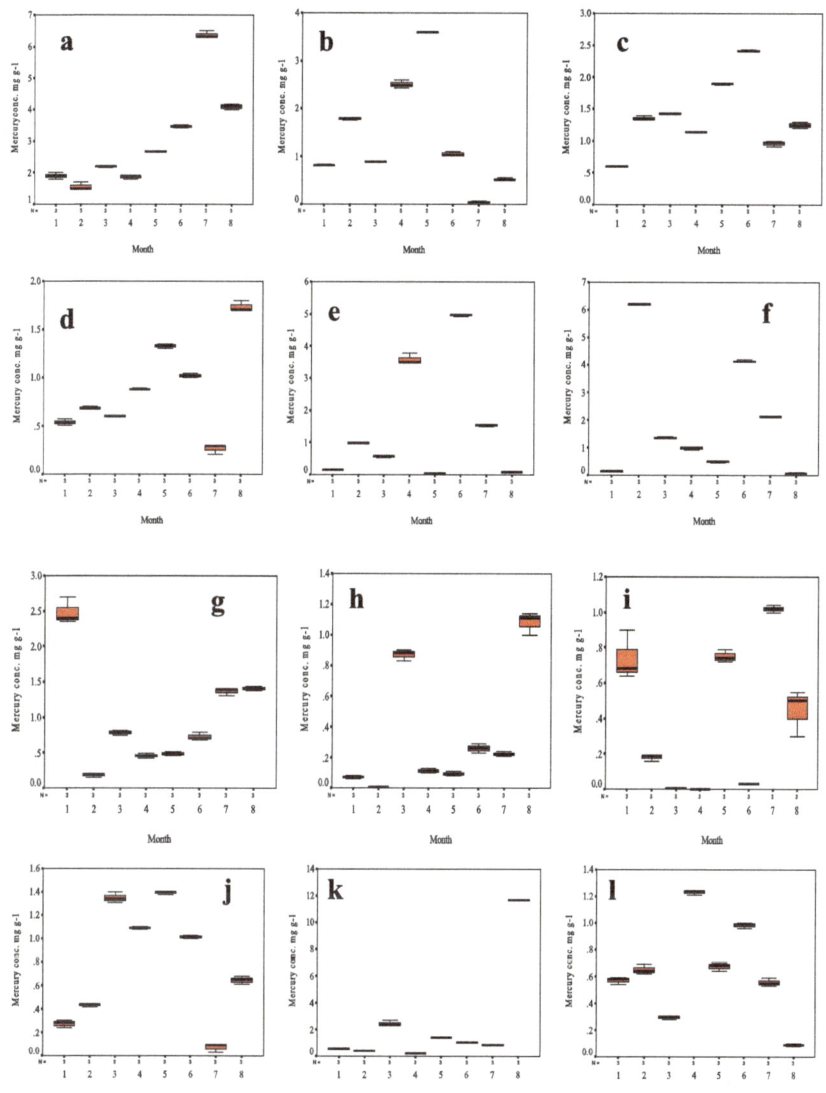

Fig. 2 Seasonal distribution of Hg^{2+} concentrations in fish, oysters and cuttlefish samples collected from Farwa lagoon, Libya; **a**) *Serranus scriba;* **b**) *Oedalechilus labeo,* **c**) *Diplodus vulgaris;* **d**) *Dicentrarchus labrax;* **e**) *Lithognathus mormyrus;* **f**) *Epinephelus marginatus;* **g**) *Sarpa salpa;* **h**) *Sciaena umbra;* **i**) *Pagrus pagrus;* **j**) *Caranx crysos;* **k**) *Pinctada radiate;* **l**) *Sepia officinalis*

collected from place near of GCCI (100 m). The highest concentrations were determined in samples collected during April, where, 2.33 ± 0.60, 1.44 ± 0.42 and 0.96 ± 0.12 μg g^{-1} were determined in samples collected from zone I, II and III respectively. The lowest Hg^{2+} was recorded in samples collected from zone III (0.02 ± 0.00 μg g^{-1}) during January. In comparison with the study conducted by Pergent-Martini [19] which was carried out on the mercury contamination in the *Posidonia oceanica* Collected from mediterranean sea. It can be noted that the Hg^{2+} concentrations in this study was quite high. There would be due to dispose of wastewater generated from GCCI into the sea without treatment process since 40 years ago.

The present study revealed that the concentrations of Hg^{2+} in all types of fish samples were more than the standards limits recommended by FDA and FAO-WHO [20, 21]. According to U.S. EPA [22], Hg^{2+} should be less than 0.3 μg g^{-1} wet fish muscle tissue for protection of human health. However, Zaza et al. [13] reported that

Table 3 Measures of association between Hg^{2+} concentrations in fish, *oysters as well as cuttlefish* samples and months

Sample*month	R	R Squared	Eta	Eta Squared	Significance (p value)
Serranus scriba	0.80	0.64	0.99	0.99	0.01
Oedalechilus labeo	−0.228	0.05	1.00	0.99	0.14
Diplodus vulgaris	0.327	0.11	0.99	0.99	0.06
Dicentrarchus labrax	0.493	0.24	0.99	0.99	0.01
Lithognathus mormyrus	0.191	0.04	0.99	0.99	0.18
Epinephelus marginatus	−0.173	0.03	1.00	1.00	0.21
Sarpa salpa	−0.068	0.01	0.99	0.99	0.38
Sciaena umbra	0.454	0.21	0.99	0.99	0.01
Pagrus pagrus	0.215	0.05	0.98	0.98	0.16
Caranx crysos	0.006	0.00	0.99	0.99	0.45
Pinctada radiata	0.587	0.34	1.00	1.00	0.01
Sepia officinalis	−0.188	0.04	0.99	0.99	0.19

the minimum level of Hg^{2+} is 0.5 μg g^{-1} for fish species. In the present study, the minimum concentration of Hg^{2+} was 1 μg g^{-1} in *Pagrus pagrus.* Fish consumption is one of the major factors of Hg^{2+} intake for humans [23, 24]. Hg^{2+} is very dangerous for pregnant woman because mercury is most harmful to developing foetuses, infants, and young children.

High Hg^{2+} concentration was detected in sediment samples collected from the West of GCCI than those collected from the East. However, both sites contain high concentration of Hg^{2+}. The Hg^{2+} concentration decreased significantly ($p < 0.05$) as the site distance from GCCI, the maximum Hg^{2+} was noted in sediment samples taken from the west (100 m from GCCI) where 11.14 ± 4.11 μg g^{-1} was recorded in April 2014 (Table 5). Among the sediment samples collected from the east, the samples taken in June contain 4.67 ± 1.62 μg Hg^{2+} g^{-1}. The pollution of environmental area around GCCI represent a serious problem due to that the surrounding areas are used for agricultural purpose such as for Grapes, olives and almonds. More than 1500 people are living around the GCCI.

Table 4 Hg^{2+} concentrations in magnoliophyta plant samples collected from different distance of GCCI at Farwa lagoon, Libya (±SD represent the standard division from the mean, $n = 3$ for each sample per month)

Sample/month	Hg^{2+} concentrations (μg g^{-1})		
	Zone I (100 m)	Zone II (1000 m)	Zone III (3000 m)
1	0.82 ± 0.20	0.93 ± 0.13	0.02 ± 0.00
2	0.39 ± 0.12	0.50 ± 0.08	0.10 ± 0.09
3	2.10 ± 0.91	0.57 ± 0.16	0.82 ± 0.20
4	2.33 ± 0.60	1.44 ± 0.42	0.96 ± 0.12
5	1.06 ± 0.18	0.79 ± 0.12	0.75 ± 0.19
6	1.00 ± 0.13	1.38 ± 0.92	0.54 ± 0.20
7	0.87 ± 0.30	0.25 ± 0.09	0.64 ± 0.21
8	1.40 ± 0.42	1.07 ± 0.13	0.71 ± 0.15

Farwa Island has high fishery production, but this Island had been exposed for heavy pollution due to GCCI for more than 40 years. Farwa Island is the most important coastal and marine site in western Libya, in terms of its high marine and coastal biodiversity based on several surveys and studies during the last years. However, no information was recorded according to mercury pollution. This region is characterized by an exceptional importance in terms of fish and artisanal fisheries, aquaculture, sea birds, sea grass meadows, land/seascape features and, above all, as one of the few regions in the Mediterranean to experience active tidal movements. In addition to some endangered species which makes it an important area for larva and juvenile protection. In the term of biodiversity, Farwa has many economically important species and certain endangered species are recognized [18].

In the term of toxic pollutants in industrial wastewater and their environmental impact and health effect, the sea water around of GCCI should be treated to remove of Hg^{2+} ions. Variety of biological and physico-chemical methods for wastewater treatment has been developed. Among those technologies, reverse osmosis, activated carbon, advanced oxidation, alumina-coated carbon nanotubes, tire derived carbons, porous carbon, carbon nanotubes and fullerene and CNT/magnesium oxide composite have exhibited high efficiency for removal of heavy metals from different aqueous solution [25–33].

Table 5 Hg^{2+} concentrations in sediment samples collected from the west and east GCCI during the period January to August 2014 (±SD represent the standard division from the mean, $n = 3$ for each sample per month)

Sediments sample/month	Hg^{2+} Concentration ($\mu g\ g^{-1}$)								
	West of GCCI				East of GCCI				Control
	<100 m	500 m	1000 m	3000 m	100 m	500 m	1000 m	3000 m	Zwara city (20 km)
1	3.54 ± 1.10	1.38 ± 0.14	1.09 ± 0.04	0.64 ± 0.32	1.96 ± 1.01	0.55 ± 0.06	0.03 ± 0.0	0.01 ± 0.0	0.001 ± 0.0
2	6.74 ± 3.14	4.06 ± 1.81	1.07 ± 0.52	0.32 ± 0.19	1.55 ± 0.71	1.12 ± 0.24	0.75 ± 0.18	0.01 ± 0.0	0.001 ± 0.0
3	4.58 ± 1.43	3.04 ± 0.93	0.06 ± 0.09	0.02 ± 0.01	2.07 ± 0.91	0.75 ± 0.18	0.05 ± 0.01	0.001 ± 0.0	0.001 ± 0.0
4	11.14 ± 4.11	2.64 ± 0.83	1.95 ± 0.31	0.56 ± 0.08	3.65 ± 1.04	1.47 ± 0.91	0.01 ± 0.0	0.001 ± 0.0	0.001 ± 0.0
5	8.50 ± 2.84	5.07 ± 2.81	1.01 ± 0.41	0.75 ± 0.11	3.12 ± 1.11	0.06 ± 0.01	0.003 ± 0.0	0.001 ± 0.0	0.001 ± 0.0
6	2.46 ± 1.31	3.65 ± 1.71	0.95 ± 0.71	0.07 ± 0.22	4.67 ± 1.62	1.5 ± 0.46	0.001 ± 0.0	0.01 ± 0.0	0.003 ± 0.0
7	5.21 ± 2.28	4.06 ± 1.93	0.50 ± 0.01	0.43 ± 0.17	2.13 ± 0.98	0.04 ± 0.0	0.01 ± 0.0	0.002 ± 0.0	0.001 ± 0.0
8	1.56 ± 0.73	3.25 ± 0.88	0.36 ± 0.03	0.05 ± 0.0	3.17 ± 0.51	1.45 ± 0.29	0.003 ± 0.0	0.002 ± 0.0	0.001 ± 0.0

Conclusions

It can be concluded that the heavily contamination of fish, oysters as well as cuttlefish in marine environment around GCCI represent a main source for food poisoning among peoples living in this area. Therefore, the contaminated area should be treated to prevent health risk associated with mercury contamination.

Competing interests

The authors declared that they have no competing interest.

Authors' contributions

AA, RMS and AAS: conceived and planned the experiment. AA collected the samples and carried out the experiment. AAS: formulated the objectives, analysed the data, and drafted the manuscript. RMS has proofread and edited the Manuscript, provided guidance and improved the quality of the final manuscript. All authors read and approved the final manuscript. (AAB, RMSRM and A-GAAS).

Acknowledgments

The authors would like to thank Badu Society for Protection Marine Biology and Wild for allow us to use their laboratories. In addition, to express their appreciations to the Universiti Tun Hussein Onn Malaysia (UTHM), School of Civil and Environmental Engineering for Postdoctoral Fellowship to Adel Al-Gheethi.

Author details

[1]Environment Engineering Department, Subrata College, University of Zawia, Zawia, Libya. [2]Faculty of Civil & Environment Engineering, UTHM, Parit Raja, Malaysia. [3]High Institute of health sciences, Sana'a, Yemen.

References

1. Mittal A, Kaur D, Malviya A, Mittal J, Gupta VK. Adsorption studies on the removal of coloring agent phenol red from wastewater using waste materials as adsorbents. J Coll Interface Sci. 2009;337:345–54.
2. Mittal A, Mittal J, Malviya A, Kaur D, Gupta VK. Decoloration treatment of a hazardous triarylmethane dye, Light Green SF (Yellowish) by waste material adsorbents. J Coll Interface Sci. 2010;342:518–27.
3. Mittal A, Mittal J, Malviya A, Gupta VK. Removal and recovery of Chrysoidine Y from aqueous solutions by waste materials. J Coll Interface Sci. 2010;344:497–507.
4. SaleH TA, Gupta VK. Functionalization of tungsten oxide into MWCNT and its application for sunlight-induced degradation of rhodamine B. J Coll Interface Sci. 2010;362:337–44.
5. Saleh TA, Agarwal S, Gupta VK. Synthesis of MWCNT/MnO_2 and their application for simultaneous oxidation of arsenite and sorption of arsenate. Appl Catal B Environ. 2011;106:46–53.
6. Saleh TA, Gupta VK. Synthesis and characterization of alumina nano-particles polyamide membrane with enhanced flux rejection performance. Sep Pur Technol. 2012;89:245–51.
7. Vinod K, Gupa VK, Jain R, Nayak A, Agarwal S, Shrivastava M. Removal of the hazardous dye—Tartrazine by photodegradation on titanium dioxide surface. Mat Sci Eng: C. 2011;31:1062–7.
8. Gupta VK, Nayak A. Cadmium removal and recovery from aqueous solutions by novel adsorbents prepared from orange peel and Fe_2O_3 nanoparticles. Chem Eng J. 2012;180:81–90.
9. Gupta VK, Agarwal S, Saleh TA. Chromium removal by combining the magnetic properties of iron oxide with adsorption properties of carbon nanotubes. Water Res. 2011;45:2207–12.
10. Epstein E: Health issues related to beneficial use of biosolids. In: 16th Annual Residuals and Biosolids Management Conference of the Water Environment Federation, Texas. 2002, p. 9.
11. Clarkson TW. The toxicology of mercury. Crit Rev Clin Lab Sci. 1997;34:369–403.
12. Magos L. Physiology and toxicology of mercury. Metal Ions Biol Sys. 1997;34:321–70.
13. Langford N, Ferner R. Toxicity of mercury. J Hum Hypertens. 1999;13(10): 651–6.
14. Zaza S, de Balogh K, Palmery M, Pastorelli AA, Stacchini P. Human exposure in Italy to lead, cadmium and mercury through fish and seafood product consumption from Eastern Central Atlantic Fishing Area. J Food Comp Anal 2015, (Accepted). doi: 10.1016/j.jfca.2015.01.007.
15. Harada M. Minamata disease: methylmercury poisoning in Japan caused by environmental pollution. Crit Rev Toxicol. 1995;25:1–24.
16. Bernhard M. Manual of methods in aquatic environment research, part 3: sampling and analyses of biological material. Rome: FAO Fish Tech Paper No. 158, UNEP; 1976.
17. Öztürk M, Özözen G, Minareci O, Minareci E. Determination of heavy metals in fish, water and sediments of Avsar dam lake in Turkey, Iran. J Environ Health Sci Eng. 2009;6(2):73–80.
18. APHA. Standard methods for the examination of water and wastewater. 20th ed. Washington, DC: American Public Health Association; 1998.
19. Haddoud DA, Rawag AA. Marine protected areas along Libyan coast; In Report of the MedSudMed expert consultation on marine protected areas and fisheries management. MedSudMed Technical Documents No. 3 Rome (Italy), June 2007 GCP/RER/010/ITA/MSM-TD-03. 2007.
20. Pergent-Martini C. *Posidonia oceanica*: a biological indicator of past and present mercury contamination in the mediterranean sea. Marine Environ Res. 1998;45:101–11.
21. Hall RA, Zook EG, Meaburn GM. National Marine Fisheries Service. Survey of trace elements in the fishery resource. U.S. Department of Commerce National Oceanic and Atmospheric Administration National Marine Fisheries Service. 1978.
22. Voegborlo RB, Methnani AME, Abedin MZ. Mercury, cadmium and lead content of canned Tuna fish. Food Chem. 1999;67(4):341–5.

23. EPA US. Water quality criterion for the protection of human health-methylmercury. Office of Science and Technology, Office of Water, USEPA: U.S. Environmental Protection Agency; 2001.
24. Santos ECO, Camara VM, Jesus IM, Brabo ES, Loureiro ECB, Mascarenhas AFS, Fayal KF, Sa Filho GC, Sagica FES, Lima MO, Higuchi H, Silveira IM. A contribution to the establishment of reference values for total mercury levels in hair and fish in Amazonia. Environ Res. 2002;90:6–11.
25. Yasutake A, Matsumoto M, Yamaguchi M, Hachiya N. Current hair mercury levels in Japanese: survey in five districts. Tohoku J Exper Med. 2003;199:161–9.
26. Gupta VK VK, Srivastava SK, Mohan D, Sharma S. Design parameters for fixed bed reactors of activated carbon developed from fertilizer waste for the removal of some heavy metal ions. Waste Manag. 1997;17:517–22.
27. Gupta VK, Agarwal S, Saleh TA. Synthesis and characterization of alumina-coated carbon nanotubes and their application for lead removal. J Hazar Mat. 2011;185:17–23.
28. Saleh TA, Gupta VK. Photo-catalyzed degradation of hazardous dye methyl orange by use of acomposite catalyst consisting of multi-walled carbon nanotubes and titanium dioxide. J Colloid Interface Sci. 2012;371:101–6.
29. Saleh TA, Gupta VK. Processing methods, characteristics and adsorption behavior of tire derived carbons: A review. Adv Colloid Interface Sci. 2014;211:93–101.
30. Gupta VK, Kumar R, Nayak A, Saleh TA, Barakat MA. Adsorptive removal of dyes from aqueous solution onto carbon nanotubes: A review. Adv Colloid Interface Sci. 2013;193–194:24–34.
31. Gupta VK, Ali A, Saleh TA, Nayak A, Agarwal S. Chemical treatment technologies for waste-water recycling—an overview. RSC Adv. 2012;2:6380–8.
32. Gupta VK, Saleh TA. Sorption of pollutants by porous carbon, carbon nanotubes and fullerene- An overview. Environ Sci Poll Res. 2013;20:2828–43.
33. Saleh TA, Gupta VK. Column with CNT/magnesium oxide composite for lead(II) removal from water. Environ Sci Pollut Res Int. 2012;19:1224–8.

Hybrid heating systems optimization of residential environment to have thermal comfort conditions by numerical simulation

Nabi Jahantigh[1*], Ali Keshavarz[2] and Masoud Mirzaei[2]

Abstract

The aim of this study is to determine optimum hybrid heating systems parameters, such as temperature, surface area of a radiant heater and vent area to have thermal comfort conditions. DOE, Factorial design method is used to determine the optimum values for input parameters. A 3D model of a virtual standing thermal manikin with real dimensions is considered in this study. Continuity, momentum, energy, species equations for turbulent flow and physiological equation for thermal comfort are numerically solved to study heat, moisture and flow field. $K-\varepsilon RNG$ Model is used for turbulence modeling and *DO* method is used for radiation effects. Numerical results have a good agreement with the experimental data reported in the literature. The effect of various combinations of inlet parameters on thermal comfort is considered. According to Pareto graph, some of these combinations that have significant effect on the thermal comfort require no more energy can be used as useful tools. A better symmetrical velocity distribution around the manikin is also presented in the hybrid system.

Keywords: Virtual manikin, Thermal comfort, Radiant panels, Optimal conditions, Conventional heating

Introduction

The convectional air conditioning equipment used for heating and cooling environment systems consume a lot of energy. Hybrid heating systems consist of two types of heating systems, namely radiation and convection. They work together to provide an efficient thermal comfort within an environment. This type of system can supply continuous heating energy even when one of them is off. Therefore, this technique is a very promising method which can reduce the energy consumption without lowering the level of comfort conditions.

In general, the thermal comfort is affected by the air temperature, mean radiant temperature; air velocity and relative humidity are included in the environmental parameters whereas the activity level and metabolic rate are categorized as the personal ones. Hence, in the hybrid system, the radiant heater temperature, surfaces, location, the air flow field, and metabolism are the most important factors affecting the level of thermal comfort in an environment [1].

So far, researchers have proposed different models to obtain higher level of thermal comfort in an environment [2, 3]. Thermodynamic analysis of heat and mass of human body and its effects on thermal comfort were studied by Prek [4]. Jeet at el. [5] have evaluated the effect of high-temperature radiant heaters and windows on the thermal comfort. Despite Jeet's study, Myhern and Holmberg [6] have shown that low radiant panel temperature is more suitable for indoor environment. A combination of flow field around a human body was studied numerically by Murakumi, at el. [7]. A more complex model which includes the real body shape and physiology was considered by Kilic and Sevilgen [8]. They evaluated the heat transfer, mass, air flow and moisture around the human model.

As of now, the effects of flow and geometric parameters on thermal comfort have been studied in several papers individually. However, no detailed combinations of their interaction effects are seen in the literature. Therefore, in this study, the effects of input parameter such as temperature, surface area, and position of the radiant heaters along with their interactions on a hybrid heating system have been investigated. In addition, the

* Correspondence: njahantigh@uoz.ac.ir
[1]Mechanical Engineering Department, University of Zabol, Zabol, Iran
Full list of author information is available at the end of the article

Table 1 Range of input parameters

Effect Parameter	Min.	Max.
Inlet area of the convection flow(m)	0.025	1
Inlet flow velocity(m/s)	0.05	1
heater temperature(°C)	30	90
The position of heater along vertical direction (m)	0.0	3
The position of heater along Horizontal direction(m)	0.0	2
The heater area(m^2)	1	3.1

air flow parameters of the convection system were also considered. The main objective of this study is to achieve thermal comfort in an indoor environment. In this simulation, a 3D model of a virtual standing thermal manikin with real dimensions is used. A numerical method was used to solve the flow field around the manikin. Also an optimization toward thermal comfort conditions is done.

Governing equations and solutions

The governing equations, consisting of continuity, momentum, energy, and mass transfer in a room which includes a manikin, are solved here. The radiation and turbulence equations are also considered in this problem. In addition, the Factorial Design Method (FDM) is used to analyze and optimize the variable effective parameters.

The conservation of mass can be written as [9]:

$$\nabla.\left(\rho\,\vec{V}\right) = 0 \tag{1}$$

The conservation of momentum is described by [10].

$$\nabla.\left(\rho.\,\vec{V}\,.\,\vec{V}\right) = -\nabla p + \nabla.(\bar{\bar{\tau}}) + \rho\,\vec{g} \tag{2}$$

The stress tensor $\bar{\tau}$ is given by;

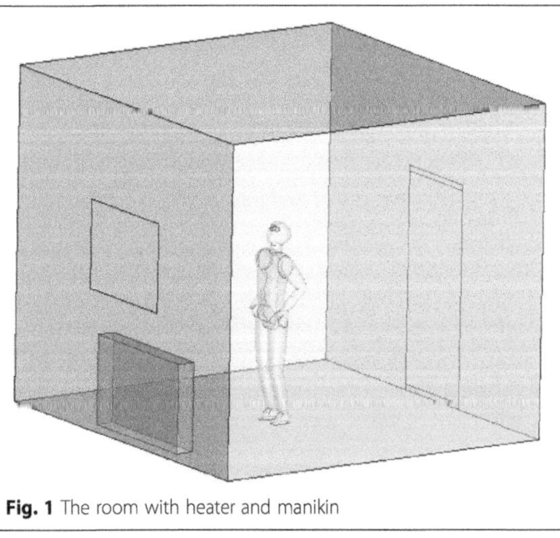

Fig. 1 The room with heater and manikin

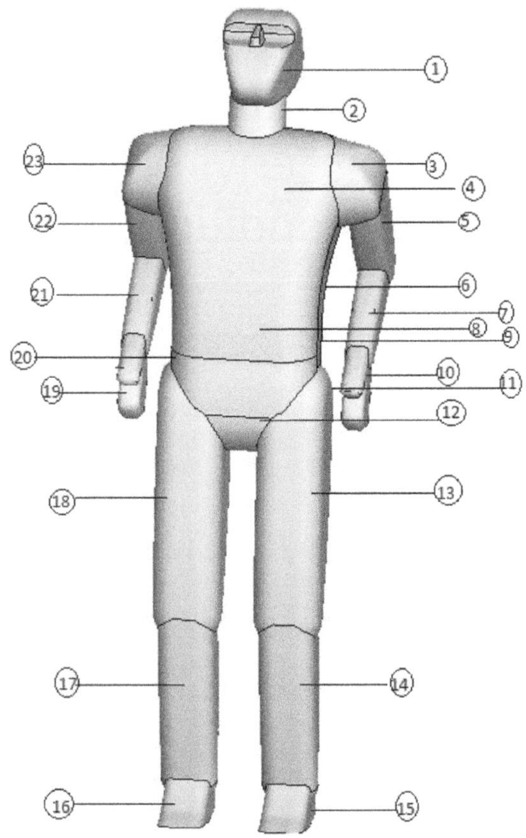

Fig. 2 The segment of the manikin model

Table 2 Segment of the manikin and their area

Number	Surface Name	Surface Area(m^2)
1	Head	0.15898
2	Neck	0.028926
3,23	Right & Left shoulder	0.048249
4	Brisket	0.234812
5,22	Right & Left arm	0.098026
6,20	Right & Left	0.021141
7,21	Right & Left forearm	0.068715
8	Bowl	0.038951
9	Waist	0.210502
10,19	Right & Left hand	0.052163
11	Basin	0.041288
12	Pelvis	0.027313
13,18	Right & Left tigh	0.287548
14,17	Right & Left leg	0.160346
15,16	Right & Left foot	0.051366

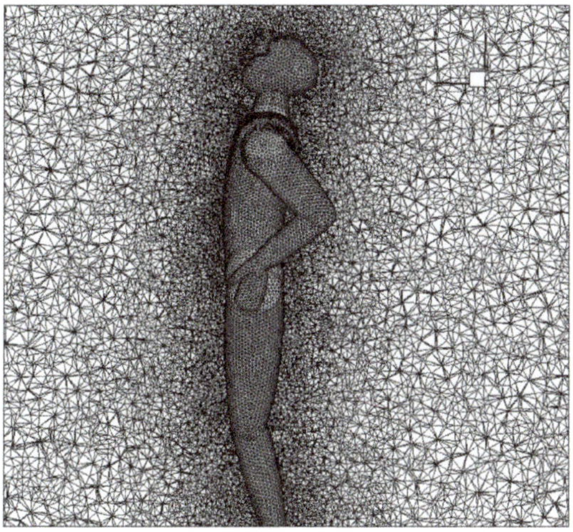

Fig. 3 The computational domain in the room

$$\bar{\bar{\tau}} = \mu\left[\left(\nabla \vec{V} + \nabla \vec{V}^{T}\right)\right] - \frac{2}{3}\nabla.\vec{V} I \tag{3}$$

The energy equation is:

$$\nabla.\left(\vec{V}(\rho E + p)\right) = \nabla.\left(k_{eff}\nabla T - \sum_j h_j \vec{J}_j + \left(\bar{\bar{\tau}}.\vec{V}\right)\right) \tag{4}$$

In Equation 4,

$$E = h - \frac{p}{\rho} + \frac{V^2}{2} \tag{5}$$

Where h is defined as

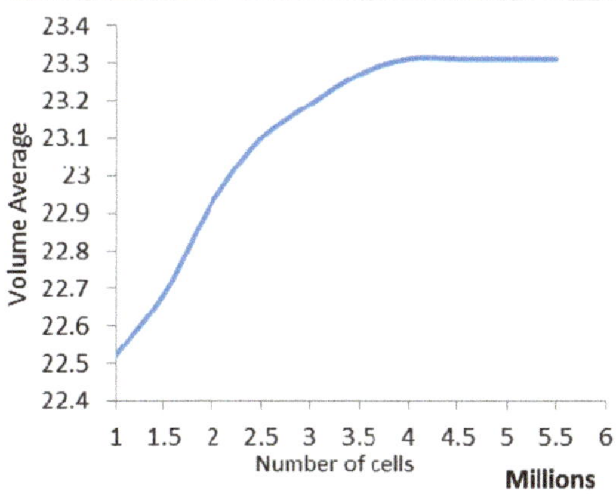

Fig. 4 The effects of the cell number on the volume-averaged temperature of room

Table 3 Boundary condition

zone	T °C	type	V m/s	Mass flow
inlet	10	velocity	0.15	9.5 $gH_2O/kgAir$
Out let		Pressure outlet		
body	33.1	covered		10 $gH_2O/kgAir$
	33.7	uncovered		
wall	25	No slip	0	

$$h = \sum_j Y_j h_j + \frac{p}{\rho} \tag{6}$$

Where, Y_j is the mass fraction of species j and

$$h_j = \int_{T_{ref}}^{T} C_{p,j} dT \tag{7}$$

Here T_{ref} is 298.15 K.

The conservation equation for the species transport in the general form is:

$$\frac{\partial}{\partial t}(\rho Y_j) + \nabla.\left(\vec{V} Y_j\right) = \nabla.\vec{J}_j \tag{8}$$

The mass diffusion $\vec{J}_j$ in turbulent flow is:

$$\vec{J}_j = -\left(\rho D_{j,m} + \frac{\mu_t}{sc_t}\right)\nabla Y_j - D_{T,j}\frac{\nabla T}{T} \tag{9}$$

Where, Sc_t is the turbulent Schmidt number.

The Predicted Mean Vote, PMV which is the response of large groups of people to the temperature sensitivity of an environment based on ASHRAE Standard is stated as the following equation [11].

$$PMV = (0.303\exp(-0.035M) + 0.028)L \tag{10}$$

The heat balance equation of a human body is given as;

$$S = M \mp W \mp R \mp C \mp K - E_{sk} - (C_{res} + E_{res}) \tag{11}$$

By solving the flow field, all terms in equation 11can be calculated.

Table 4 Physical characteristic of material [15]

	Door	Wall	Window
width	50	250	25
$\rho(kg/m^3)$	700	1940	840
$C_p(kj/kg.K)$	2.31	0.84	0.84
$K(w/m^2.K)$	0.173	0.06	0.2
ε	0.9	0.95	0.8

The emissivity coefficient value for the manikin has been considered as 0.98

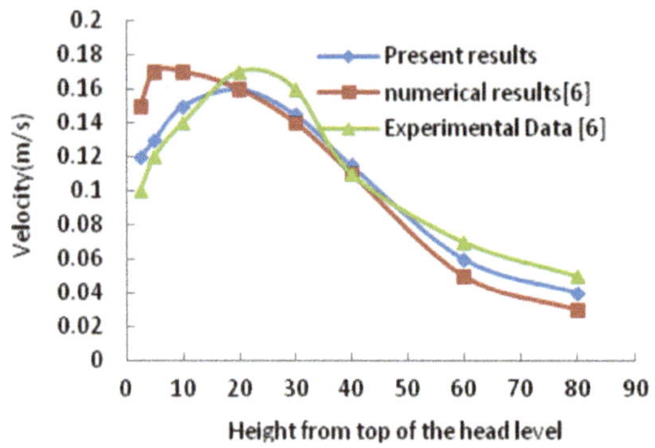

Fig. 5 Comparison the computed velocity with Numerical and experimental results of ref. [16]

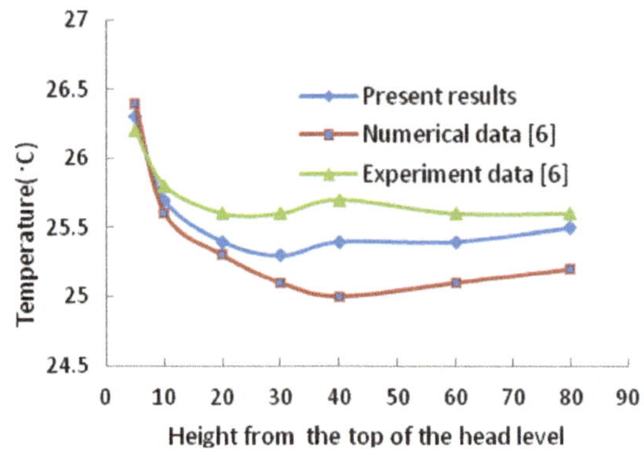

Fig. 6 Comparison the computed temperature with Numerical and experimental results of ref. [16]

When $S = 0$, the thermal equilibrium will be satisfied [6]. In equation 11 E_{sk}, C_{res} and E_{res} terms can be calculated as follows

$$E_{sk} = \frac{w(P-P_a)}{R_{cl}} \tag{12}$$

$$C_{res} = 0.0014M(34-T) \tag{13}$$

$$E_{res} = 1.72 \times 10^{-5}M(5867-P_a) \tag{14}$$

The Factorial Design Method (2^k) or two level design is used here for optimization [12]. The input and output parameters' range must also be specified. The input parameters are the area of convection flow, inlet flow rate, temperature, location, and the surface area of radiant heater. The output effective parameters are the radiation flux, convection flux, and PMV index. In this technique, the impact of the factor is defined as the difference between the high and low level of responses.

The values of input parameters based on some primary calculations are given in Table 1. The critical and major effects of parameters are defined in Pareto and normal probability graphs. Their effects can also be stated as a regression equation. Then, the model is optimized for the objective function with the method of least squares and logistic regression [13].

A 3D computational code was used to solve the flow field, energy, and mass equation. The PISO algorithm has been used [14]. In this approach, higher-order accuracy is achieved at cell faces. Pressure discretization is done by second order method. The $K - \varepsilon RNG$ is also suitable for low-Reynolds numbers and more accurate and reliable for a wider range of indoor environments and flows with heat transfer.

The *DO* radiation model is used to consider the radiation effects of heating surfaces and sources in the flow fluid simulation. It allows the solution of radiation at semi-transparent walls.

Geometry of the problem

As be shown in Fig. 1 the problem consists of a manikin model stand and a radiant heater located within a room. One window, a door, and two vents at the bottom and top of the door have been considered for the circulation of air flow. Room dimensions are 3 × 4 × 4 m. The manikin has a height of 1.75 m and weight of 75 kg. The dimension of the window and door is 1 × 1.2 m and 1 × 2 m, respectively. The size of the inlet, outlet and the heater are assumed to be variable for the optimization purpose.

The segments of the manikin model have been shown schematically in Fig. 2 and their values are tabulated in Table 2.

This problem was first modeled using Solid Work and, then, meshed by Hypermesh software. The problem is solved for several different heater locations to optimize its position in the room.

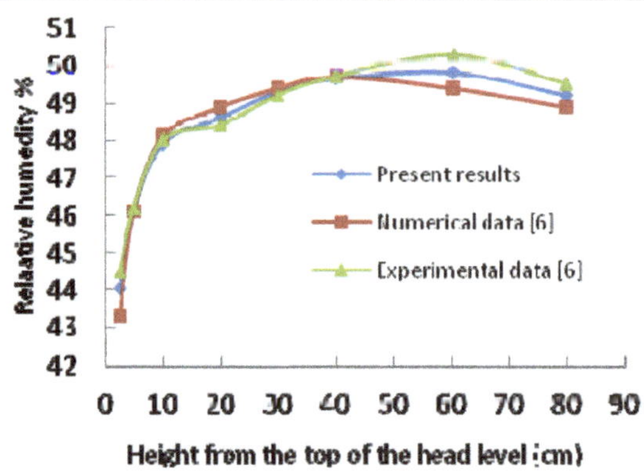

Fig. 7 Comparison the computed RH% with Numerical and experimental results of ref. [16]

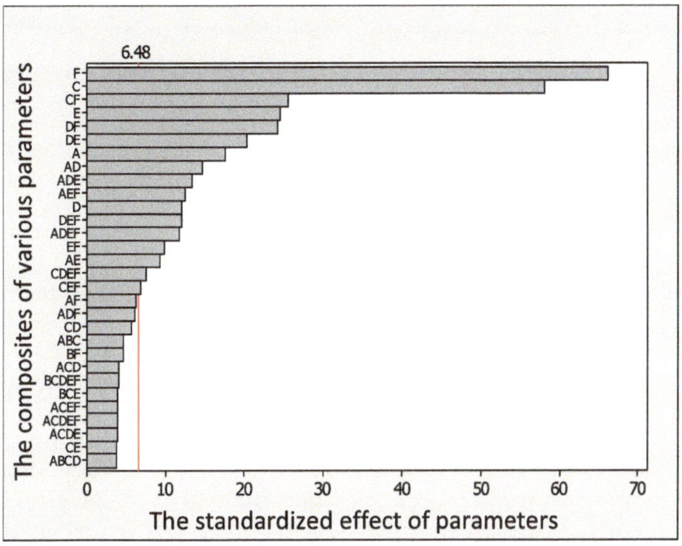

Fig. 8 The effect of the input parameter on the PMV index

Computational grid

Due to complex geometry and fine surfaces in this problem, generating structured grid for all sub regions is not an easy task. Therefore, a combination of unstructured-structured grid system is applied using Algorithm T-Grid. It has been shown in Fig. 3. Since the flow field around the manikin includes high gradients of flow parameters, an appropriate distribution function starts from the lower layer around the surface and continues to the maximum step. The problem was solved for several different grid sizes for its independency. As shown in Fig. 4 the final results are independent numbers of grids when it is selected as 3,900,000 [15].

Boundary conditions

The boundary conditions are given in Table 3. These values are taken based on ASHRAE standard [15]. The characteristics of building materials are given in Table 4.

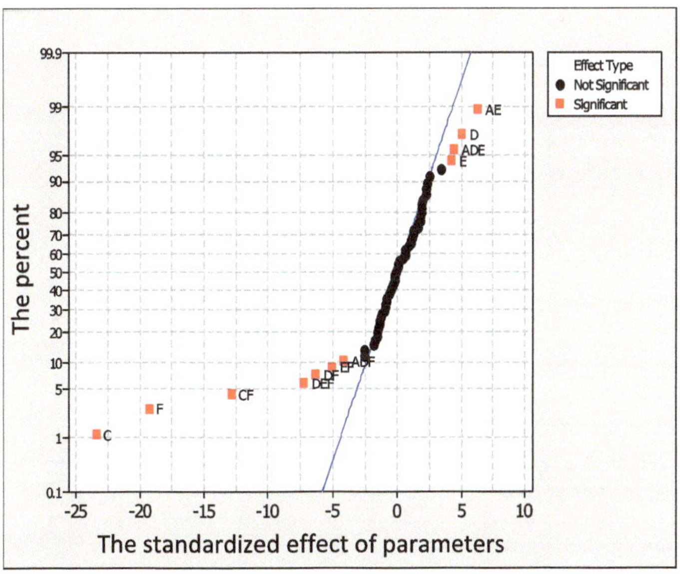

Fig. 9 The effect of the input parameter on the radiation flux

Table 5 Optimized value for objective parameter

Input parameter	Min.	Max.	Suggested value	Optimized value	Objective parameter	Target value	Computed value along the target
Inlet velocity(m/s)	0.025	1	0.2	0.1	PMV	0.001	−0.1
Inlet area(m^2)	0.05	1	0.4	0.12	Total flux	110	107.679
Radiation heater temperature(°C)	30	90	45	30.034	Radiation flux	40	39.778
The vertical position of heater (m)	0.0	3	.1	0.2	Relative humidity	50.	50.001
The horizontal position of heater (m)	0.0	2	2	1.85			
The heater area(m^2)	1.0	3.1	1.5	1.749			

Locating the heater opposite the person and under the window seems to be the best achievement for the above case. In this case, minimum heat losses are obtained while having optimum PMV value

Validation of results

For the validation of the present model, the calculated result was compared to the available experimental data in the literature [16]. The compression for the velocity, temperature and relative humidity are shown in Figs. 5, 6 and 7, respectively. As shown in these figures, the obtained values have a high agreement with the experimental data [16]. The maximum difference between the experimental and numerical velocity, temperature and relative humidity is 0.03 m/s, 0.4 °C and 0.5 %, respectively.

Results and discussion

The impact of input parameters on the objective functions

The effect of input parameters on the objective parameters using Pareto and normal charts are compared and discussed in Figs. 8 and 9 The Pareto chart presents the significant effect of the parameters whereas the normal chart indicates their percentage. The effect of input parameters on the total heat flux, PMV index, radiation heat flux, and relative humidity are shown in these Figures, respectively.

In these Figures, the letter A is the cross section area of the inlet vent, B is the input velocity, C is the heater temperature, D and E are the positions of heaters along the horizontal and vertical directions, and F is the surface area of the heater. The impacts of these parameters as well as their combinations are studied individually.

Hence, by glancing at all Figs. 8 and 9 it can be concluded that:F has the most effect on the object function and requires more energy C has the most effect on the objective function and needs no more energy. The combination of input parameters has different impacts on the objective function in comparison to their individual ones due to their interaction. Some of these combinations which can be used as useful tools have significant effect on thermal comfort and require no more energy

The optimization

The effect of input parameters on the objective parameters is determined in previous section and they are

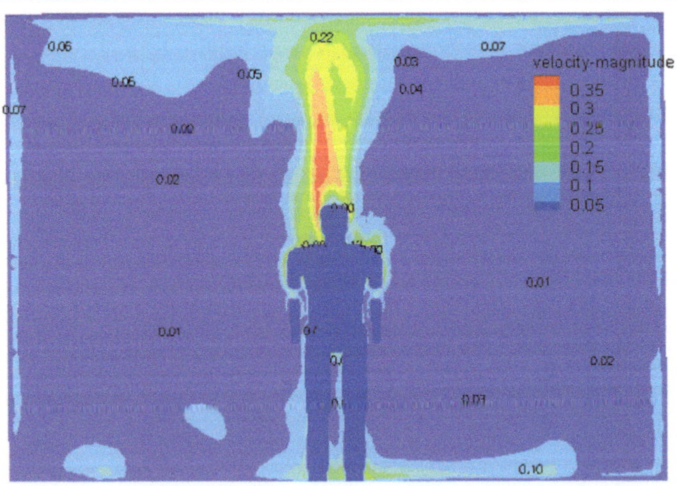

Fig. 10 The velocity contribution for optimum case

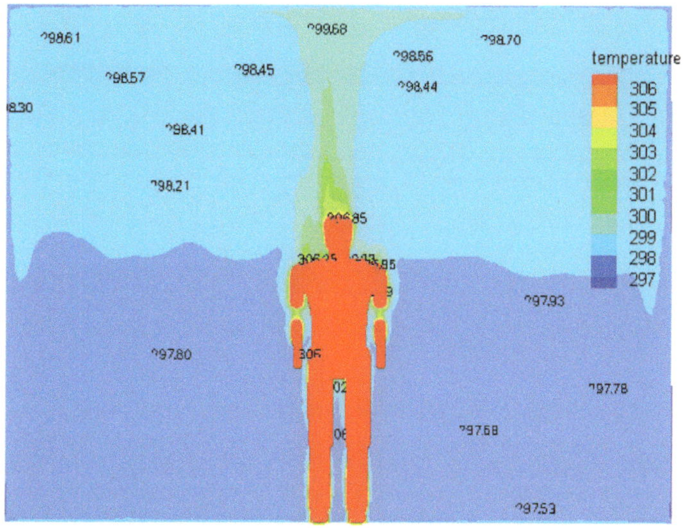

Fig. 11 The temperature contribution for optimum case

optimized here for different cases. In this case, the problem is optimized for the values of total flux 110w/m^2, radiation flux 40w/m^2, relative humidity 50 % and PMV 0.001. The optimized values are calculated and tabulated in Table 5.

Velocity, temperature and relative humidity distribution around the manikin

The Velocity, temperature, and humidity contours around the manikin surface are shown in Figs. 10, 11 and 12. A better symmetrical velocity distribution around the manikin is also presented in the hybrid system. The maximum velocity occurs near the head of the manikin due to larger temperature gradient. The all distribution values around the manikin are within the ASHRAE standard [15] and there is almost no stagnation zone which provides a proper thermal comfort for a person According to temperature contour in Fig. 11.

Thermal comfort

The fraction of convection and radiation heat flux in heating systems, convection and hybrid, for all segments of the manikin are tabulated in Table 6.

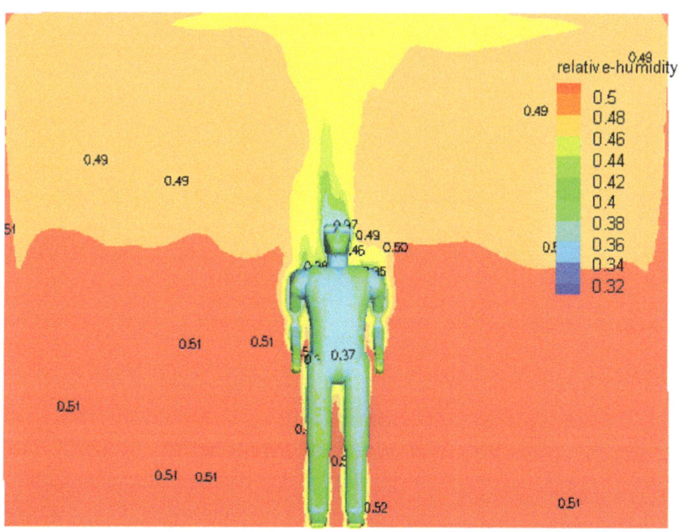

Fig. 12 The humidity contribution for optimum case

Table 6 Heat losses rate from body

Surface	Case-I		Case- II	
	Con. Flux(w/m^2)	Rad. Flux(w/m^2)	Conv. Flux(w/m^2)	Rad. Flux(w/m^2)
Head	43.14	38.61	39.65	41.53
Brisket	35.82	37.44	34.45	45.37
Bowl	33.73	35.90	31.92	46.03
Pelvis	31.73	32.27	30.68	39.85
Waist	33.32	31.76	32.57	38.32
Basin	33.84	34.79	31.91	40.23
Arm	37.1	32.47	36.54	41.39
Forearm	38.35	30.66	37.61	39.69
Shoulder	35.27	38.71	34.29	54.28
Thigh	34.44	31.69	33.73	48.37
Leg	41.34	36.10	40.69	43.84
Neck	33.36	35.23	38.62	45.78
foot	46.81	34.69	45.31	42.64
hand	41.69	29.24	40.15	38.69
Average	37.1	33.7	35.68	44.35

Table 7 presents the heat losses from the body and walls, and PMV values for both heating systems. As the values of PMV indicate, the heating hybrid systems can provide faster and better human thermal comfort in a residential room. The PMV value for the convection heating systems is −0.86 whereas for the hybrid system, it is 0.0034 which is almost near the ideal condition (PMV = 0) Despite the fact that the maximum velocity in this system is lower than the conventional heating system but it falls within the ASHRAE standard. This lower velocity makes lower heat losses through the walls and the manikin segments up to 25 %.

Conclusion

In this study, two heating systems, conventional and hybrid, are individually optimized and then compared with each other to have thermal comfort conditions. The Factorial Design Method (2^K) or two level designs has been used for optimization. The effect of input parameters and their interaction is investigated on the objective function, such as PMV index, relative humidity and heat fluxes. The effects of the input parameters in normal and Pareto charts are presented. Based on the present study, the individual and the interaction of input parameters effect are significant and different. Heater temperature has the most effect on the object function and requires more energy whereas C has the most effect on the objective function but needs no more energy thus some combination can be used as useful tools in designing heating systems. The thermal comfort can be obtained using less input energy by just increasing the surface area of the heater and its location. A better symmetrical velocity distribution around the manikin is also presented in the hybrid system. The lower velocity makes lower heat losses through the walls and the manikin segments up to 25 %. The heating hybrid systems can provide faster and better human thermal comfort in a residential room.

Table 7 Heat losses rate from body, room and PMV values in two cases

	Case 1	Case 2
T air	24.5	25.52
TMRT	24.03	25.23
Relative humidity	55.36	50.46
Convection flux	36.68	32.86
Radiation flux	33.61	45.23
losses	35.27	22.21
Total flux of the body	105.56	100.3
PMV	−0.89	0.0034
Total flux of the room	684.61	512.83

Thanksgiving

I would like to thank all those who have helped me in doing the research. Also, I want to thank you for giving us the opportunity to publish our paper in the Journal of Environmental Health Science and Engineering.

Nomenclature

C, Convective heat loss(w/m2)
C_{res}, Convection heat loss due to respiration(w/m2)
$D_{i,m}$, Mass diffusion coefficient for species
D_T, Turbulent diffusivity

E_{res}, Evaporative heat loss due to respiration(w/m2)
E, Total energy (J)
E_{sk}, Evaporative heat loss of skin
$\vec{g}$, Gravitational acceleration
h, Sensible enthalpy
I, Unit tensor
$\vec{J}_j$, Diffusion flux of species
k_{eff}, Effective conductivity
k_t, Turbulent thermal conductivity
L, The heat load of the body
M, Metabolic heat production(w/m^2)
P_α, ambient pressure air (kpa)
PMW, Predict mean vote
R_{cl}, Resistance of clothes
R, Radiative heat loss(w/m^2)
S, Heat storage(w\m^2)
$\vec{V}$, Velocity vector
W, External work(w/m^2)
Y_j, Mass fraction of species
μ, Molecular viscosity
ρ, Density
$\bar{\bar{\tau}}$, Stress tensor

Competing interests
The authors declare that they have no competing interests.

Authors' contribution
All authors read and approved the final manuscript.

Author details
[1]Mechanical Engineering Department, University of Zabol, Zabol, Iran.
[2]Mechanical Engineering Department, K. N. Toosi University of Technology, Tehran, Iran.

References
1. Bemani M., "Modern air conditioning practice", 3rd ed., ISBN-964-8142-31-9, Ketab Iran Publication.
2. Orosa JA. Research on general thermal comfort models. Eur J Sci Res. 2009;27(2):217–27. 1450-216X.
3. Van Hoof J, Hansen JLM. Quantifying the relevance of adaptive thermal comfort models in moderate thermal climate zones. Build Environ. 2007;42:156–70.
4. Prek M. Thermodynamic analysis of human heat and mass transfer and their impact on thermal comfort. Int J Heat Mass Transfer. 2005;48:731–9.
5. Jeet S, Chapman KS., Keshavarz A. "Window performance for human thermal comfort". 4765(RP)1126.
6. Myhern JA, Holmberg S. Flow: "Pattern and thermal comfort in a room with panel floor and wall heating". Energy and Building. 2008;40:524–6.
7. Muarkumi S, Zeng J, Hayashi T. "CFD analysis of wind environment around a human body". J Wind Eng Ind Aero. 1999;83:393–408.
8. Kilic M, Sevilgen G. "Modeling airflow, heat transfer and moisture transport around a standing human body by computational fluid dynamics". Int Communication in Heat and Mass transfer. 2008;35:1159–64.
9. White FM. "Viscous Fluid Flow", 2nd ed. omide enghelab publication, c2006.
10. Batchelor GK. "An Introduction to Fluid Dynamics". Cambridge, England: Cambridge Univ. Press; 1967.
11. Wyon DP, Fanger PO, Olesen BW, Pedersen CJK. "The mental performance of subjects clothed for comfort at two different air temperatures". Ergonomics. 1975;18:358–74.
12. Montgomery C. "Design and analysis of experiments". Douglas - 5th ed. ISBN 0-471-31649-0.
13. Jiju A. "Design of Experiments for Engineers and Scientists", ISBN: 0750647094 Publisher: Elsevier Science & Technology Books, Pub. Date: October; 2003.
14. Barth TJ, Jespersen D. "The design and application of upwind schemes on unstructured meshes". Reno, Nevada: Technical Report. AIAA –89-0366. AIAA 27th Aerospace Sciences Meeting; 1989.
15. ASHRAE. Hand Book-Fundamental Refrigeration and Air-Conditioning Engineers, Atlanta: American Society of Heating; 2001 (chapter 8).
16. Kilic M, Sevilgen G. Numerical analysis of air flow, heat transfer, moisture transport and thermal comfort in a room heated by two-panel radiators. Energy and Buildings. 2011;43:137–46.

Determination of hydrogen cyanide concentration in mainstream smoke of tobacco products by polarography

Shabnam Mahernia, Arash Amanlou, Gita kiaee and Massoud Amanlou*

Abstract

Background: There has been a worldwide concern for the health risks of cigarette smoking and hydrogen cyanide (HCN) considered as one of the hazardous tobacco compounds which is needed to be determined in order to reduce the dose related to smoke disease risk.

In this study, we prepare the experimental procedure to entrap the HCN from mainstream smoke of different brands of Tehran cigarette, through simulating human inhalation and determine its concentration applying polarography.

Results: The HCN level of the 50 commonly consumed tobacco products (47 cigarettes and 3 cigars) obtained from local store is ranged between 17.56 ± 1.02 and 1553.98 ± 0.56 μg per stick, this acquired amount is more than FDA approval (10 μg per stick), so the harmful effects of smoking is indicative.

Conclusions: The comparative study of the results shows that the price and the weight of each product do not indicate HCN level. As can be seen, R^2 value which is a statistical measure of how close the data are to the fitted regression line is low ($R^2 < 0.2$). So it should not be deceived by names such as ultra light or infinite gravity to suck, because this names or the price haven't effect on the amount of HCN and its destructive effects.

Keywords: Tobacco products, Cigarette, Hydrogen cyanide, Polarography

Background

Smoking is the major risk factor of mortality in the world according to the statistical information; the cigarette consumption during one century has increased over 100 times, which increases the concern over the safety of tobacco products [1, 2].

Tobacco smoke contains more than 5000 chemical compounds which 150 of these substances have been proved to be toxicants [3, 4]. Hydrogen cyanide is one of the tobaccos smoke poisonous substances which are formed from the combustion of the protein and nitrate compounds existed in tobacco at high temperatures in the oxygen deficient condition [5, 6] which it's chronic and low exposure causes neurological, respiratory, cardiovascular and thyroid effect [7–9].

The tobacco smoke pathway includes the part directly entered the mouth called mainstream and the part diffused in the surrounding, called side stream, which hazardous for nonsmoker. The level of HCN in mainstream smoke is ranged from 10 to 400 μg per cigarette (US Brands) which 0.6 to 27 % of these amounts exist in side stream smoke [10]. In the previous study the level of HCN in the non-filtered cigarette was between 400 to 500 μg per stick [11] and in another study the amount of HCN in the mainstream smoke of cigar, non-filtered cigarette and filtered cigarette was 1035, 59 and 448 μg per 1 g of tobacco, respectively and in small cigars it was between 510 to 780 μg per 1 g of tobacco [12].

There are different reported methods determine HCN in different samples including voltammetry [13], fluorometry [14, 15] gas chromatography [16], LC-MS-MS [17], HPLC-MS [18], potentiometry [19], spectrophotometry [20] and colorimetry [21]. Among them, polarography the subclass of voltammetry is the most precise and

* Correspondence: amanlou@tums.ac.ir
Department of Medicinal Chemistry, Faculty of Pharmacy and Pharmaceutical Sciences Research Center, Tehran University of Medical Sciences, Tehran, Iran

Table 1 Hydrogen cyanide concentration and price of different brands of cigars

No.	Brand	Cyanide concentration (μg/cig.)	Number of cig. per pocket	The price of each pocket($)	Weight of each cig. (mg)	The price of each cig. ($)
1	Bahman	368.067	20	0.58	828.4	0.02
2	Bahman	574.358	20	0.50	587.7	0.02
3	Bahman	57.655	20	0.50	547.8	0.02
4	Bistoon	227.491	20	0.41	943.7	0.02
5	CAFÉ CRÈME	791.067	10	2.08	921.6	0.20
6	CAFÉ CRÈME (AROME)	1464.900	10	2.08	1053.2	0.20
7	CAFÉ CRÈME (BLUE)	406.722	10	1.83	746.6	0.18
8	CAMEL Lights	184.825	20	1.62	810.1	0.08
9	Cima	237.400	20	0.66	863.9	0.03
10	Cima classic	120.720	20	0.60	687.6	0.03
11	Dunhill	300.717	20	2.25	781.9	0.11
12	Eclipse	740.235	20	12.50	1243.6	0.62
13	ESSE Lights	131.012	20	0.80	515.2	0.04
14	ESSE Special Gold	29.622	20	0.66	530.2	0.03
15	Jewels sweet	1553.584	20	1.62	6165.5	0.08
16	Kent	297.693	20	1.33	793.7	0.06
17	Kent	190.745	20	1.25	436.9	0.06
18	Kent (Blue7)	345.930	20	1.25	915.8	0.06
19	Kent (White1)	188.220	20	1.25	776.2	0.06
20	King Edward	598.518	5	1.41	3384.2	0.28
21	Magna	232.889	20	0.79	822.4	0.03
22	Magna	145.228	20	1.79	763.8	0.08
23	Magna	212.310	20	0.79	813.3	0.04
24	Marlboro Gold (Germany)	165.871	20	3.75	800.3	0.18
25	Marlboro (Extra) (USA)	164.309	20	4.16	900.2	0.20
26	Marlboro (Switzerland)	17.561	20	2.66	849.1	0.13
27	Marlboro (Switzerland)	47.892	20	2.91	969.7	0.14
28	Marlboro Lights	267.804	20	2.50	858.9	0.12
29	Marlboro Lights (USA)	42.916	20	2.91	776.4	0.14
30	Marlboro Lights (Switzerland)	74.536	20	2.91	786.5	0.14
31	Marlboro Lights (Switzerland)	69.344	20	1.83	816.5	0.09
32	Marlboro Ultra Lights (Switzerland)	127.336	20	2.66	835.1	0.13
33	Montana	332.493	20	0.50	855.6	0.02
34	Pall Mall	161.785	20	0.83	905.1	0.04
35	Pall Mall (Blue)	86.956	20	0.83	881.3	0.04
36	PHILLIES BLUNT	203.178	5	1.62	6974.5	0.32
37	Pine (Blue)	238.561	20	0.66	860.2	0.03
38	Pine (supper slims)	94.813	20	0.45	547.2	0.02
39	Winston	43.187	20	1.25	785.9	0.06
40	Winston	214.325	20	1.50	816.7	0.07
41	Winston	106.176	20	1.50	831.0	0.07

Table 1 Hydrogen cyanide concentration and price of different brands of cigars *(Continued)*

42	Winston Blue (Europe)	99.244	20	1.83	537.3	0.09
43	Winston Lights	66.326	20	2.50	943.1	0.12
44	Winston Lights (Imported)	209.294	20	4.58	814.0	0.22
45	Winston Lights (USA)	102.132	20	2.08	808.7	0.10
46	Winston Ultra Lights (USA)	42.634	20	2.25	794.1	0.11
47	Winston Ultra Lights (USA)	25.554	20	2.25	818.4	0.11
48	Winston Ultra Lights (Switzerland)	254.322	20	2.25	812.0	0.67
49	Zest Lights	150.623	20	0.66	829.9	0.03
50	Zika	288.120	20	2.91	924.0	0.14

inexpensive method based on the oxidation and reduction mechanism [22].

The aim of this study is focused on the determination of the HCN in mainstream smock of different brands of cigarette consumed in Tehran using polarography method.

Materials and methods

Collection of samples

A total of 50 types of different brands of the most consumed or available cigarettes (47) and cigars (3) were collected from local stores at September 2012. The 20 % of the samples were from Winston company, 18 % from Marlboro, 6 % from Magna, 8 % from KENT and 8 % from local or officially imported companies and the rest, 40 % are from a different companies (as shown in Table 1).

Reagents and chemicals

All chemicals used were of analytical reagent grade from Merck (Germany). Buffer solutions were prepared by dissolving boric acid (0.2 M) and potassium hydroxide (0.17 M) in 1000 ml ultrapure water and adjusting the solution to pH 10.2. Cyanide standard solution (1 g/L) was prepared by dissolving 0.2503 g KCN in 100 ml KOH 0.01 M in ultrapure water.

Apparatus

Analysis was conducted by the Metrohm Polarography device 797 VA Computrace, three electrode systems consisting of a dropping mercury electrode (DME) as the working electrode, an Ag/AgCl reference electrode and platinum counter electrode. The device outfitted in the following conditions: stirrer speed 2000 rpm, mode DP, purge time 300 s, equilibration time 5 s, pulse amplitude 50 mV, start potential 0 V, end potential 500 mV, voltage step 8 mV, voltage step time 0.8 s, sweep rate 10 mV/s, peak potential CN −240 mV. All instrumental settings were those recommended in the manufacturer's manual book and the instrumental conditions with the method of AB110-Det of cyanide [23]. All potentials quoted were measured against an Ag/AgCl reference electrode and the polarographic cell volume was 20 ml.

Method of analysis

The HCN in each cigarette and cigar mainstream smoke were collected using mainstream apparatus (Fig. 1) [24, 25]. The cigarette was applied to the entrance station and suction force obtained by the vacuum pump simulate the human inhalation and extract the tobacco smoke, the flow of smoke were passed through the glass tube filled with 100 ml NaOH (0.1 M) solution to entrap HCN as CN^- ion.

Subsequently, the mixture of above mentioned solution contain cigarette smoke (10 ml) and buffer solution (10 ml) was added to the polarographic vessel and deoxygenated for 10 min with high-purity nitrogen and achieved the peak of CN^- in the range of −0.5-0 V. To determine the CN^- concentration by standard addition method, 50 μl cyanide standard solution was added (two times) and the polarogram was obtained (Fig. 2).

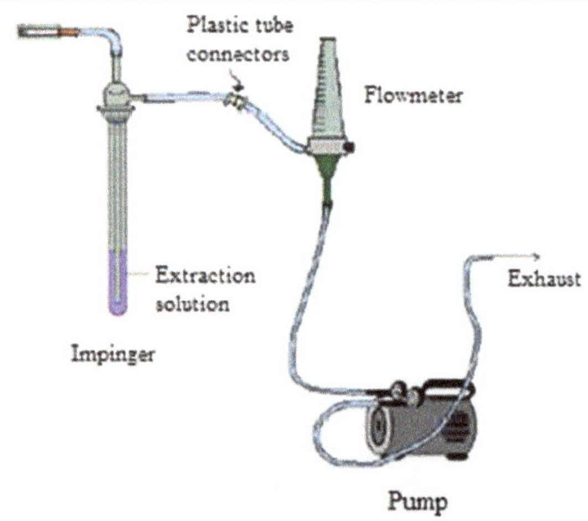

Fig. 1 Cigarette mainstream collecting apparatus

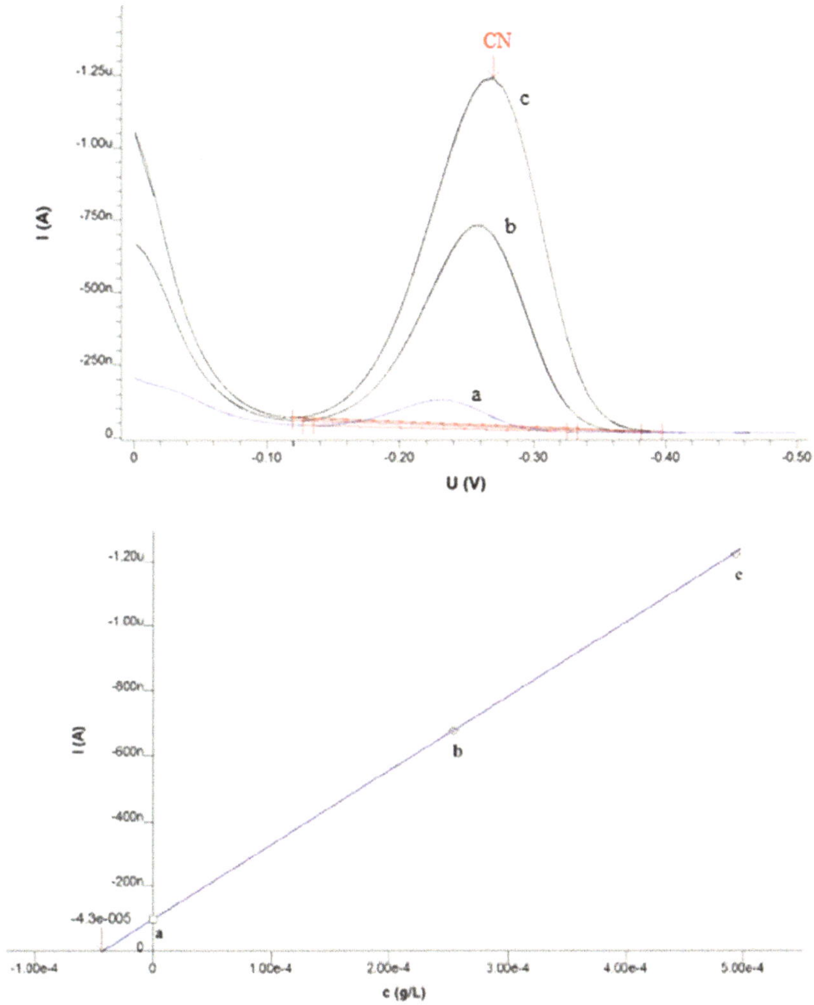

Fig. 2 The differential pulse polarogram of cyanide ion in cigarette smoke sample. **a** the peak of sample solution **b** the peak of first dilution of standard addition **c** the peak of second dilution of standard addition

Statistical analysis

All statistical analyses were performed using the statistical software for social sciences (SPSS Inc. Chicago, IL, Version 21). Statistical analyses of each sample were characterized by mean ± standard deviation. The mean levels of cyanide were compared across categories of price, and weight of each cigarette or cigars. The significance level was defined at 0.05 for the regression equations.

Result and discussion

The result of mainstream smoke HCN determination by polarography (Table 1) showed that among 50 samples the average amount of HCN was 184.825 µg per stick which the highest level of HCN pertain to Jewel sweet cigar, 1553.98 ± 0.56 µg per cigar, and the lowest was Swiss Marlboro with 17.56 ± 1.02 µg per cigarette. Moreover, the average amount of HCN in cigarettes and cigar were 218 µg and 785.09 µg, respectively, In addition the average weight of cigarette and cigar samples was 800 mg and 5500 mg, respectively, and the average weight of whole samples was 1084.24 mg.

The changes in the HCN levels are dependent on the preparation procedure of tobacco, which lead to the diverse amount of proteins and nitrate compounds of cigarette which render the conversion of HCN level emission. In addition it may be possible to assess the quality of cigarette especially ultralight by determining the amount of HCN as it is increased in the unfeigned products.

Furthermore, based on our study there is no connection between price, weight and appearance of cigarette,

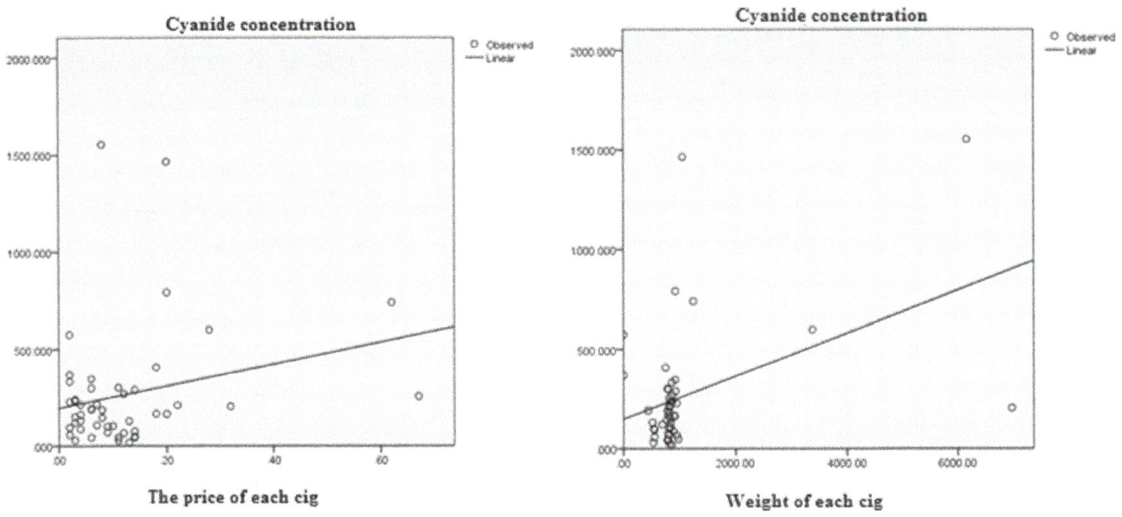

Fig. 3 The relationship between cyanide, weight and price each of cigarettes

cigar and HCN level. For instance, Jewels sweet and PHILLIES BLUNT cigars have the same price, but different level of HCN doesn't necessarily cause the higher HCN level emission. The regression method was applied for the development of the mentioned model. Validation of the method was conducted by analyzing the different set of independent data from the same source. As can be seen the R^2 which is a statistical measure of how close the data are to the fitted regression line is low (0.20) (Fig. 3). So it means the model is useless for prediction based on cigar and cigarette weight and its price.

In addition, previous studies demonstrated that even exposure to lower concentrations of cyanide may result in a range of non-specific features include headache, dizziness, throat discomfort, chest tightness and eye irritation which these symptoms would grow by more

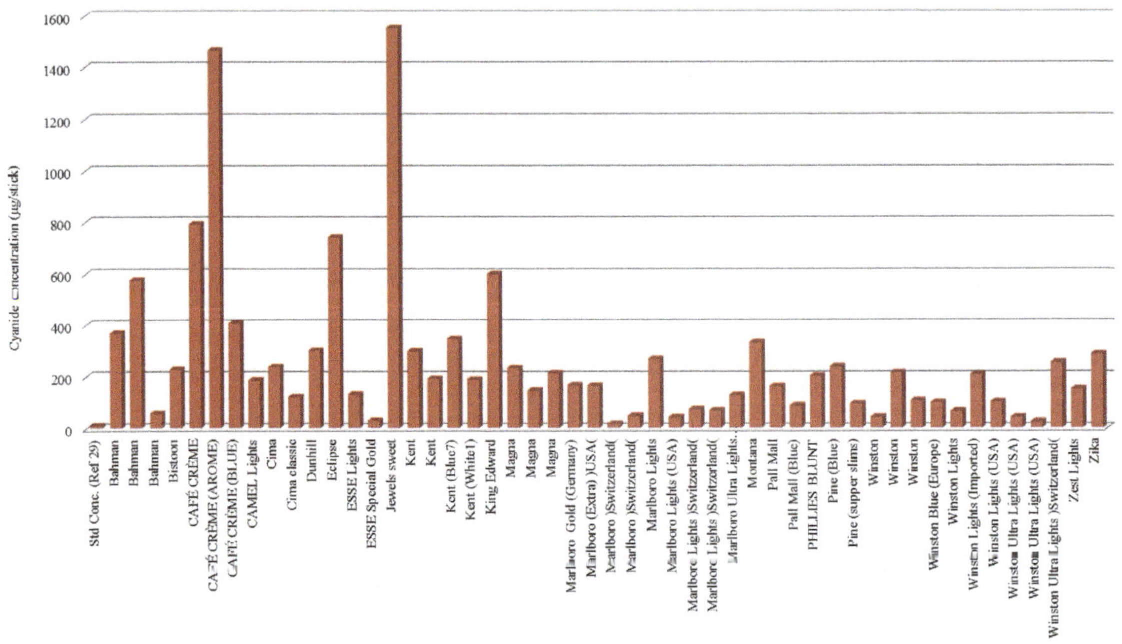

Fig. 4 Cyanide concentrations in different kind of Cig

substantial exposure [26–28]. Moreover the results of our study indicate that cyanide concentration of all samples, even light cigarette is above established levels for chronic toxic doses [9] (Fig. 4).

Conclusions

In this study, HCN of the toxic components of the tobacco smoke was determined by polarographic method. The results shows that the ranges of HCN level of 50 samples were varied between 17.56 ± 1.02 - 1553.98 ± 0.56 µg per stick. This acquired amount is more than FDA approval (10 µg per stick).

Competing interests

The authors declare that they have no competing interests.

Authors' contributions

All authors contributed to the concept and design, providing and analysis of data, drafting, revising and final approval. MA is responsible for the study registration. AA is responsible for collection. SM is responsible for experiments performing, assembly of data, data analysis, interpretation, SM and GK are responsible for writing the manuscript and correcting. All authors read and approved the final manuscript.

Acknowledgment

We gratefully acknowledge the financial support from Tehran University of Medical Sciences.

References

1. General S. Reducing the health consequences of smoking. 25 years of progress. US Department of Health and Human Services. 1989.
2. Shafey O, Eriksen M, Ross H, Mackay J. The Tobacco Atlas. 3rd ed. Atlanta, GA: Am Cancer Soc; 2009.
3. Fowles J, Dybing E. Application of toxicological risk assessment principles to the chemical constituents of cigarette smoke. Tob Control. 2003;12:424–30.
4. Green CR, Schumacher JN, Llovd RA, Rodgman A. Comparisons of the composition of tobacco smoke and the smokes from various tobacco substitutes. Beit Tabakforsch Intl. 2007;22:257–89.
5. Norman V, Ihrig A, Larson T, Moss B. The effect of some nitrogenous blend components on NO/NOx and HCN levels in mainstream and sidestream smoke. Beitr Tabakforsch. 1983;12:55–62.
6. Baker R. Smoke Chemistry, Tobacco production. Blackwell Publishing Ltd: Chemistry and technology; 1999. p. 398–439.
7. Blanc P, Hogan M, Mallin K, Hryhorczuk D, Hessl S, Bernard B. Cyanide intoxication among silver-reclaiming workers. JAMA. 1985;253:367–71.
8. Chandra H, Gupta B, Bhargava S, Clerk S, Mahendra P. Chronic cyanide exposure biochemical and industrial hygiene study. J Anal Toxicol. 1980;4:161–5.
9. El Ghawabi SH, Gaafar MA, El-Saharti AA, Ahmed SH, Malash KK, Fares R. Chronic cyanide exposure. a clinical, radioisotope, and laboratory study. Br J Ind Med. 1975;32:215–9.
10. Fiksel J, Slimak MW, Little AD. An Exposure and Risk Assessment for Cyanide. Monitoring and Data Support Division, Office of Water Regulations and Standards. US: Environmental Protection Agency; 1981.
11. Hoffmann D, Hoffmann I. Risks of tobacco smoke exposure are similar for all sources of tobacco smoke, and the magnitude of the risks experienced by cigar smokers is proportionate to the nature and intensity of their exposure. Chem and Toxicol. 1998;55.
12. Adams PI. Combustion temperatures in cigars and cigarettes, A comparative study. Tobacco Sci. 1968;12:144–50.
13. Safavi A, Maleki N, Shahbaazi H. Indirect determination of cyanide ion and hydrogen cyanide by adsorptive stripping voltammetry at a mercury electrode. Anal Chim Acta. 2004;503:213–21.
14. Lundquist P, Rosling H, Sörbo B, Tibbling L. Cyanide concentrations in blood after cigarette smoking, as determined by a sensitive fluorimetric method. Clin Chem. 1987;33:1228–30.
15. Chen D, Castro M, Valcarcel M. Flow-through sensor for the fluorimetric determination of cyanide. Talanta. 1990;37:1049–55.
16. Brunnemann KD, Yu L, Hoffmann D. Chemical studies on tobacco smoke. XLIX. Gas chromatographic determination of hydrogen cyanide and cyanogen in tobacco smoke. J Anal Toxicol. 1977;1:38–42.
17. Lacroix C, Saussereau E, Boulanger F, Goulle J. Online liquid chromatography-tandem mass spectrometry cyanide determination in blood. J Anal Toxicol. 2011;35:143–7.
18. Tracqui A, Raul J, Geraut A, Berthelon L, Ludes B. Determination of blood cyanide by HPLC-MS. J Anal Toxicol. 2002;26:144–8.
19. Bark L, Higson H. A review of the methods available for the detection and determination of small amounts of cyanide. Analyst. 1963;88:751–60.
20. Surleva AR, Visualizing DG, Hazard S. A simple spectrophotometric determination of hydrogen cyanide in cigarette smoke and filters. J Chem Edu. 2013;90:1654–7.
21. Fowler E, Steele TW. The determination of anionic surface-active agents in dilute aqueous solution. Johannesburg: National Institute for Metallurgy; 1968.
22. Surleva A. Recent achievements in toxic cyanide monitoring: review. Revue electronique internationale pour la science et la technologie. Numéro. 2009. p. 3.
23. Polarographic determination of free cyanide No, 110/2 e. In: Metrohm application bulletin
24. Determination of Hydrogen Cyanide in Sidestream Tobacco Smoke. Health Canada. 1999.
25. Diekmann J, Biefel C, Rustemeier K. Analysis of cigarette mainstream smoke for 1,1-dimethylhydrazine and vinyl acetate by gas chromatography–mass spectrometry. J Chromatogr Sci. 2002;40:509–14.
26. National Poisons Information Service (NPIS) Hydrogen cyanide. Toxbase®. 2000.
27. Lam KK, Lau FL. An incident of hydrogen cyanide poisning. Am J Emerg Med. 2000;18:172–5.
28. Agency for Toxic Substances and Disease Registry (ATSDR). Draft Toxicological Profile for Cyanide. Atlanta. US: US Department of Health and Human Services; 2004.

23

Pretreatment of garden biomass using Fenton's reagent: influence of Fe^{2+} and H_2O_2 concentrations on lignocellulose degradation

Vivek P Bhange[1], SPM Prince William[2*], Abhinav Sharma[2], Jagdish Gabhane[2], Atul N Vaidya[2] and Satish R Wate[2]

Abstract

Garden biomass (GB) is defined as low density and heterogeneous waste fraction of garden rubbish like grass clippings, pruning, flowers, branches, weeds; roots. GB is generally different from other types of biomass. GB is mostly generated through maintenance of green areas. GB can be processed for bio energy production as it contains considerably good amount of cellulose and hemicellulose. However, pretreatment is necessary to delignify and facilitate disruption of cellulosic moiety. The aim of the present investigation was to pretreat GB using Fenton's reagent and to study the influence of Fe^{2+} and H_2O_2 concentrations on degradation of lignin and cellulose. The data were statistically analyzed using ANOVA and numerical point prediction tool of MINITAB RELEASE 14 to optimize different process variables such as temperature, concentration of Fe^{2+} and H_2O_2. The results of the present investigation showed that Fenton's reagent was effective on GB, however, concentration of Fe^{2+} and H_2O_2 play crucial role in determining the efficiency of pretreatment. An increase in H_2O_2 concentration in Fenton's reagent significantly increased the rate of cellulose and lignin degradation in contrast to increasing concentration of Fe^{2+} ion which led to a decrease in lignocellulosic degradation.

Keywords: Fenton's reagent, Pretreatment, Lignin, Cellulose, Garden biomass

Introduction

Biomass, in general, fourth largest energy source in the world, provides about 13% of world energy consumption [1]. Globally, biomass has an annual primary production of 220 billion oven dry ton [2]. Many cities, large or small, have developed gardens and recreational parks. The number of parks and other recreational centers, home gardens etc. contribute to the sizable quantum of garden biomass (GB) generation. Maintenance of green areas produces significant amount of waste in the form of GB [3]. GB is generally different from other types of biomass, and it is defined as low density and heterogeneous waste fraction of garden rubbish like grass clippings, pruning, flowers, branches, weeds, roots. The disposal of garden biomass is mainly through open burning, dumping and composting in India. Although these methods of disposal are universally applicable they neither recover energy nor eco-friendly except for composting.

GB contains recalcitrant or complex compounds such as cellulose and lignin, and relatively small amounts of saccharides, amino acids, proteins, aliphatic compounds and carbohydrates [3,4]. As GB is rich in cellulose, it can be used as a raw material for bio energy production after suitable pretreatment. Pretreatment is necessary to delignify and facilitate the disruption of lignocellulosic moiety. Pretreatment alters the structure of cellulose and making it more accessible to the enzyme that convert carbohydrate polymer into fermentable sugar [5,6].

There are different methods of pretreatment available for various substrates. However, it is necessary to evaluate every pretreatment process as the efficiency of pretreatment differs from substrate to substrate. Generally, pretreatment methods are either physical or chemical. Some methods incorporate both effects [7]. However, it is necessary to evaluate pretreatment processes for different substrates. Fenton's reagent defined as a mixture of hydrogen peroxide and

* Correspondence: spmp_william@neeri.res.in
[2]Solid and Hazardous Waste Management Division, National Environmental Engineering Research Institute, Nehru Marg, Nagpur-20, Maharashtra, India
Full list of author information is available at the end of the article

ferrous ion is one of the most effective methods for the oxidation of organic compounds.

Fenton process is a reaction between hydrogen peroxide (H_2O_2) and ferrous ion (Fe^{2+}), producing the hydroxyl radical (•OH). •OH radical is a strong oxidant capable of oxidization and degradation of various organic compounds into carbon dioxide and water. Thus, the degradation process could be increased with increasing •OH concentration and vice versa [8-12].

$$Fe^{2+} + H_2O_2 \rightarrow Fe^{3+} + OH^- + {}^{\bullet}OH$$

The ferric ions produced during the reaction further react with hydrogen peroxide regenerating ferrous ions, thus continuing the process [13].

$$Fe^{3+} + H_2O_2 \rightarrow Fe^{2+} + HOO\bullet + H^+$$

However, the efficiency of Fenton's reaction depends mainly on H_2O_2 concentration, Fe^{2+}/H_2O_2 ratio, pH and reaction time [14].

In the present study we aimed at evaluating the effectiveness of Fenton's reaction for pretreatment with a major emphasis on the influence of Fe^{2+} and H_2O_2 concentrations on degradation of lignin and cellulose.

Materials and methods

Preparation of the feedstock

Garden biomass (GB) consisting of grass cuttings, fallen leaves, flowers, roots, twigs etc. were collected from the garden area of National Environmental Engineering Research Institute (NEERI). After initial screening, GB was air-dried for24 hours followed by 3 days of sun drying. The dried material was pulverized using a pulveriser to the size of 1 to 5 mm for further experiments and stored in an air tight container.

Pretreatment by Fenton's reagent

Fenton's reagent was prepared by mixing $FeSO_4.7H_2O$ and H_2O_2 in distilled water in different proportions. The $FeSO_4.7H_2O$ concentration varied from 250 ppm to 1000 ppm and H_2O_2 concentration varied from 1000 ppm to 10000 ppm. Every time Fenton's reagent was prepared fresh and used in the experiment. All the experiments were carried out with 5 g of GB and 100 mL of Fenton's reagent of different composition. All the reactions were initially carried out at 30°C and repeated at 50 and 80°C. The reaction was carried out in a shaker and reaction time was varied from 60 min to 180 min. The reaction mixture was filtered and then the treated GB was thoroughly washed and dried at 60°C for 2 days. The concentration of lignin and cellulose was estimated as described in section 2.3.

Analytical methods

The dried sample of GB was ground to powder for chemical analysis. The organic carbon content of GB was estimated by combustion method according to Nelson & Sommers, 1982 [15]. Known quantity (mg) of substrate (GB) and its hydrolysed residue after pretreatment was taken and analyzed for cellulose by HNO_3-ethanol method. Lignin content of samples was estimated by 72% (w/w) H_2SO_4 method and hemicellulose by Liu method [16]. The total nitrogen (TN) content of the sample was estimated using LECO Protein-Nitrogen Analyzer (Model FP528).

Evaluation of cellulose and lignin degradation

Degradation of cellulose and lignin was evaluated on the basis of solid recovery [17,18] and actual degradation was calculated on the basis of residual concentration after pretreatment.

Cellulose recovery

Actual degradation (g) and actual degradation (%) of cellulose and solid recovery was calculated according to following formula:

$$\text{Solid recovery } (\%) = \frac{\text{Dry weight of sample after pretreatment}}{\text{Initial weight of sample (g)}} \times 100$$

$$\text{Recovered cellulose (g)} = \frac{\text{Conc. } (\%) \text{ of cellulose after pretreatment} \times \text{Solid recovery}}{\text{Material taken for pretreatment}}$$

Actual degradation (g) and Actual degradation percentage (%) of cellulose was calculated by following formula:

$$\text{Actual degradation (g) of cellulose} = \text{Initial conc. of cellulose} - \text{Recovered cellulose}$$

$$\text{Actual degradation } (\%) \text{ of cellulose} = \frac{100 \times \text{Actual degradation (g) of cellulose}}{\text{Initial conc. of cellulose}}$$

Lignin recovery

Actual degradation (g), actual degradation (%) of lignin and solid recovery was calculated according to following formula:

$$\text{Solid recovery } (\%) = \frac{\text{Dry weight of sample after pretreatment}}{\text{Initial weight of sample (g)}} \times 100$$

$$\text{Recovered lignin (g)} = \frac{\text{Conc. } (\%) \text{ of lignin after pretreatment} \times \text{Solid recovery}}{\text{Material taken for pretreatment}}$$

Actual degradation (g) and Actual degradation percentage (%) of lignin was calculated by following formula:

$$\text{Actual degradation (g) of lignin} = \text{Initial conc. of cellulose} - \text{Recovered cellulose}$$

$$\text{Actual degradation (\%) of lignin} = \frac{100 \times \text{Actual degradation (g) of lignin}}{\text{Initial conc. of lignin}}$$

Statistical guided experimental design and procedure

The Fenton's pretreatment was statistically evaluated by applying statistical methodology viz. analysis of variance (ANOVA) followed by response surface methodology for process optimization [19,20]. The experimental runs were designed to cover variables that assess impact of pretreatment on cellulose and lignin degradation. The effects of Fe^{2+} concentration (X1), Hydrogen peroxide concentration (X2) and Temperature (X3) on lignin and cellulose degradation were described statistically. The regression analysis was performed to estimate the response function as a second-order polynomial:

$$Y = \beta_0 + \sum_{i=1}^{K}\beta_i X_i^2 + \sum_{i=1}^{K}\beta_{ij} X_i^2 + \sum_{i=1}^{k-1} \times \sum_{j=2}^{k}\beta_{ij} X_i X_j \tag{1}$$

Where Y is the predicted response, β_i, β_j, β_{ij} are coefficients estimated from regression, they represent the linear, quadratic and cross-products of X_1,X_2,X_3 on response.

A statistical program package MINITAB RELEASE 14, was used for regression analysis of the data obtained and to estimate the coefficient of regression equation. The equations were validated by analysis of variance (ANOVA) analysis. The significance of each term in the equation is to estimate the goodness of fit in each case. Response surfaces were drawn to determine the individual and interactive effects of test variable on degradation of respective components.

Table 1 Initial characterization of garden biomass

Parameter	Concentration (%)
Total organic matter	94.10
Organic carbon	49.12
Cellulose	30.54
Hemicellulose	26.24
Lignin	25.68
Nitrogen	1.65

Table 2 Levels of process variables in un-coded form for Fenton pre-treatment

Process variables	Levels of process variables		
Fe^{2+} concentration ppm (X_1)	250	500	1000
Hydrogen Peroxide concentration (ppm) (X_2)	1000	5000	10000
Reaction temperature (°C) (X_3)	30	50	80

Results & discussion

Initial characterization of GB

GB was analyzed to find out concentration of various constituents such as lignin, cellulose, hemicellulose, organic matter, organic carbon etc. (Table 1).

Table 3 Design matrix along with predicted and experimental values for cellulose degradation (%) by Fenton's pretreatment

Runs	Fe^{2+} (ppm)	H_2O_2 (ppm)	Reaction temperature (°C)	Cellulose degradation (%)	
				Observed value	Predicted value
	250	1000	30	26.433	24.591
	250	1000	50	27.337	28.535
	250	1000	80	20.000	19.662
	250	5000	30	30.767	30.552
	250	5000	50	31.340	34.495
	250	5000	80	27.000	25.622
	250	10000	30	43.067	41.901
	250	10000	50	47.230	45.844
	250	10000	80	35.000	36.971
	500	1000	30	13.367	16.098
	500	1000	50	*	*
	500	1000	80	10.000	11.168
	500	5000	30	24.267	22.058
	500	5000	50	*	*
	500	5000	80	20.000	17.129
	500	10000	30	31.267	33.408
	500	10000	50	40.790	37.351
	500	10000	80	26.000	28.478
	1000	1000	30	16.933	15.496
	1000	1000	50	17.487	19.440
	1000	1000	80	14.000	10.567
	1000	5000	30	19.467	21.457
	1000	5000	50	*	*
	1000	5000	80	15.000	16.527
	1000	10000	30	32.800	32.806
	1000	10000	50	38.230	36.749
	1000	10000	80	27.000	27.876

*Outliers removed.

A perusal of results showed that GB contained 94.10% of total organic matter, 49.12% of organic carbon, 38.54% of cellulose, 25.68% of lignin and 26.24% of hemicellulose. The total nitrogen content of GB was found to be 1.65%.

Model fitting

The Levels of process variables, design of experiment along with experimental and predicted responses is given in Table 2, 3 and 4, respectively.

Full quadratic multiple regression analysis of experimental data yielded the following regression equations for the degradation of cellulose and lignin achieved through Fenton's pretreatment:

Table 4 Design matrix along with predicted and experimental values for lignin degradation (%) by Fenton's pretreatment

Runs	Fe^{2+} (ppm)	H_2O_2 (ppm)	Reaction temperature (°C)	Lignin degradation (%)	
				Observed value	Predicted value
1	250	1000	30	43.000	41.940
2	250	1000	50	52.000	52.634
3	250	1000	80	39.800	36.885
4	250	5000	30	46.500	45.032
5	250	5000	50	55.113	55.725
6	250	5000	80	39.340	39.976
7	250	10000	30	47.630	48.821
8	250	10000	50	57.390	59.515
9	250	10000	80	43.520	43.766
10	500	1000	30	33.580	36.155
11	500	1000	50	45.210	46.848
12	500	1000	80	28.660	31.099
13	500	5000	30	41.563	39.246
14	500	5000	50	48.560	49.940
15	500	5000	80	36.220	34.190
16	500	10000	30	42.900	43.036
17	500	10000	50	55.230	53.729
18	500	10000	80	40.300	37.980
19	1000	1000	30	35.940	32.680
20	1000	1000	50	44.317	43.374
21	1000	1000	80	26.733	27.625
22	1000	5000	30	33.580	35.772
23	1000	5000	50	47.437	46.466
24	1000	5000	80	28.750	30.716
25	1000	10000	30	37.550	39.562
26	1000	10000	50	53.230	50.255
27	1000	10000	80	33.420	34.506

Cellulose degradation

$$\begin{aligned} Y_1 = 16.7866 - 0.0667432 * X_1 + 0.000970293 * X_2 \\ + 0.985852 * X_3 + 0.0000436 * X_1 * X_1 \\ + 0.0000000866 * X_2 * X_2 - 0.00985 * X_3 * X_3 \end{aligned} \quad (2)$$

Lignin degradation

$$\begin{aligned} Y_2 = 1.81315 - 0.0393363 * X_1 + 0.000782833 * X_2 \\ + 2.23014 * X_3 + 0.0000216 * X_1 * X_1 \\ - 0.00000000166 * X_2 * X_2 - 0.02119 * X_3 * X_3 \end{aligned} \quad (3)$$

Where Y_1 is the % cellulose degradation achieved by Fenton's pretreatment, Y_2 is % lignin degradation by Fenton's pretreatment, X_1 is Fe^{2+} concentration, X_2 and X_3 are hydrogen peroxide concentration (ppm) and reaction temperature, respectively.

Tables 3 and 4 show degradation of cellulose and lignin at different concentrations of Fe^{2+} and H_2O_2 in Fenton reagent. A perusal of results indicated that Fenton's reagent is effective on GB. The degradation of cellulose and lignin responded positively to the concentration of H_2O_2 and reaction temperature. Whereas increasing concentration of Fe^{2+}decreased the rates of

Table 5 Analysis of variance (ANOVA) of model parameters

Terms	Coefficient	F	P
Cellulose degradation (%)			
Constant	16.7866		
Fe (X_1)	−0.0667432	61.47	0.000
H_2O_2 (X_2)	0.000970293	222.65	0.000
Reaction temperature (X_3)	0.985852	19.48	0.000
Fe * Fe (X_1* X_1)	4.36930E-05	24.77	0.000
H_2O_2* H_2O_2 (X_2 * X_2)	8.66348E-08	2.55	0.129
Reaction temperature * Reaction temperature (X_3 * X_3)	−0.00985858	25.89	0.000
R-Sq = 95.79% R-Sq(pred) = 91.36% R-Sq(adj) = 94.31%			
Lignin degradation (%)			
Constant	1.81315		
Fe (X_1)	−0.0393363	86.45	0.000
H_2O_2 (X_2)	0.000782833	47.74	0.000
Reaction temperature (X_3)	2.23014	25.77	0.000
Fe * Fe (X_1* X_1)	2.15921E-05	0.006	0.006
H_2O_2* H_2O_2 (X_2 *X_2)	−1.66049E-09	0.970	0.970
Reaction temperature * Reaction temperature (X_3 * X_3)	−0.0211932	0.000	0.000
R-Sq = 95.20% R-Sq(pred) = 91.26% R-Sq(adj) = 93.76%			

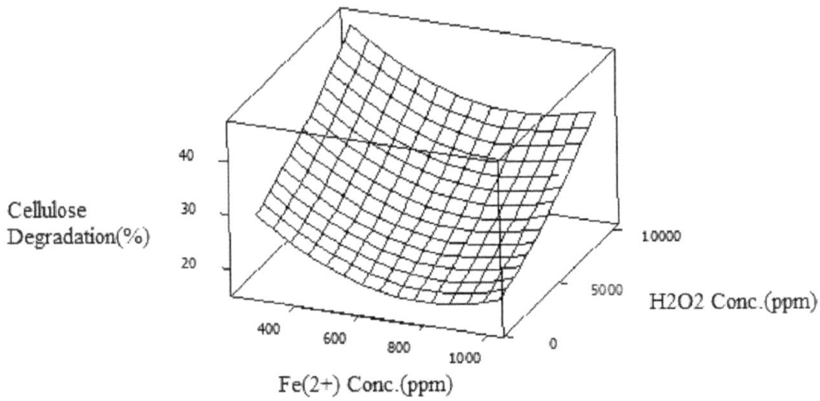

Figure 1 Cellulose degradation (% w/w) as a function of Fe^{2+} concentration (ppm) and H_2O_2 concentration (ppm).

lignin and cellulose degradation. The best effective concentration (BEC) of Fe^{2+} and H_2O_2 was found to be 250 ppm and 10000 ppm, respectively at a temperature of 50°C. Though the degradation of lignin and cellulose was significant at this BEC, compared to the other conventional methods such as alkali or H_2O_2 oxidation tried on other lignocellulosic biomass, Fenton's pretreatment pronounced only a low level of delignification [21,22]. However, there is no such report to our search which exclusively deals with the effects of Fenton's reagent on lignin and cellulose degradation in GB. The cellulose reduction rates as observed (47.23%) in the present investigation are slightly higher than that of Liu and Cheng [23] who reported maximum of 20.28% removal of cellulose and 20.09% of lignin using acid pretreatment on herbal residue. However, Ayeni et al. [24] reported 17% lignin removal by alkaline peroxide assisted wet air oxidation with no loss of cellulose. The effect of H_2O_2 alone on wood waste was also studied by Ayeni et al. [24] who reported 11% lignin removal without loss of cellulose.

The regression coefficients values for Fenton pretreatment with respect to cellulose and lignin removal is close to one ($R^2 > 95\%$), indicating the aptness of second order polynomial in predicating the response in terms of the chosen independent values, moreover the predicted values were found to be in close agreement with the experimental results (Table 2). The adjusted R^2 value (94.31% and 93.76% respectively) obtained by correcting the R^2 value for sample size and number of terms for cellulose removal is indicative of high significance of the model. The ANOVA model for the degradation of lignin and cellulose is shown in Table 5.

The ANOVA demonstrates that the model is more significant. This is evident from the calculated *F*-values 64 and 66 for effect of Fenton's pretreatment on cellulose and lignin removal respectively ($P = <0.05$). The ANOVA results also Indicate that the coefficients for linear

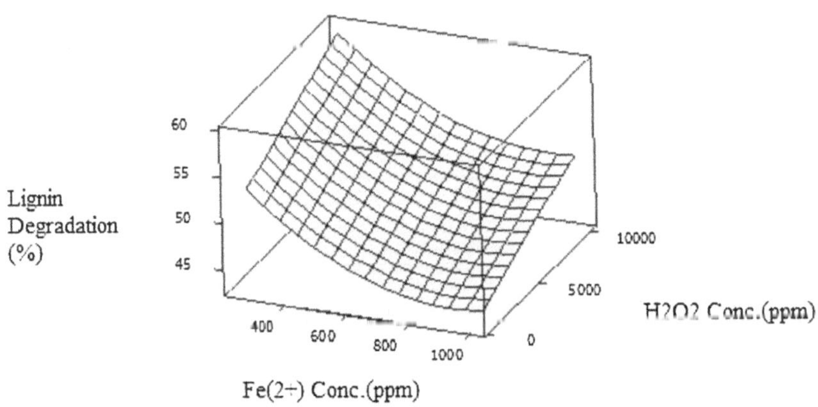

Figure 2 Lignin degradation (% w/w) as a function of $Fe2^{+}$ concentration (ppm) and H_2O_2 concentration (ppm).

effects are significant ($P = <0.01$) for cellulose degradation and for lignin removal. The positive linear effect for H_2O_2 concentration and temperature indicate an increase in cellulose and lignin removal with increase in peroxide concentration and temperature in contrast to the observed negative linear effect for Fe^{2+} concentration. The concentration of Fe^{2+} ions present in the pretreatment solution should be in catalytic amounts as over dosage leads to adsorption on the substrate which may lead to subdued processing activity after treatment.

Many studies reported in literature have revealed that the use of a much higher concentration of Fe^{2+} could lead to the self-scavenging of •OH radical by Fe^{2+} and induce the decrease in degradation rates [25-27]. According to Neyens & Baeyens, 2003, when the amount of Fe^{2+}employed exceeds that of H_2O_2, the treatment tends to have the effect of chemical coagulation. When the two amounts are reversed, the treatment tends to have the effect of chemical oxidation [28].

The effects of Fe^{2+} ion and H_2O_2 concentration on lignin and cellulose degradation when temperature was set at their centre point are shown in Figures 1 and 2. An increase in H_2O_2 concentration during pretreatment lead to considerable increase in lignin and cellulose degradation in contrast to increasing Fe^{2+} ion concentrations which lead to a decrease in cellulose removed from biomass. For example the cellulose and lignin removal increased from 13% to 31% & from 33% to 42% respectively at 500 ppm Fe^{2+} ion concentration when the H_2O_2 concentration was increased from 1000 to 10000 ppm.

The interactive effect of reaction time was however insignificant in Fenton pretreatment for lignin and cellulose removal and hence omitted from the regression analysis.

Overall, there is a predominance of the linear effects over the quadratic and interactive effects for both lignin and cellulose removal from the biomass. Higher peroxide concentrations lower Fe^{2+} concentrations higher reaction temperatures favour cellulose and lignin removal from the biomass.

Conclusion

Effect of Fenton's pretreatment on lignin and cellulose degradation of GB was studied. The results showed that Fenton's reagent was effective on GB, however, concentration of Fe^{2+} and H_2O_2 play crucial role in determining the effectiveness of lignin and cellulose degradation. An increase in H_2O_2 concentration in Fenton's reagent significantly increased the rates of cellulose and lignin degradation in contrast to increasing Fe^{2+} ion concentrations which led to a decrease in lignin and cellulose degradation. Further studies are necessary to compare and contrast Fenton's pretreatment with other pretreatments and to understand the compatibility of Fenton's pre-treated biomass for bioenergy production.

Competing interests

The authors declare that they have no competing interests.

Authors' contributions

VB and SPMPW are the main investigators, performed all experimental work and paper writing, JG carried out data analysis, AS carried out statistical analysis, ANV and SRW provided all essential supports. All authors read and approved the final manuscript.

Authors' information

Department of Biotechnology, Priyadarshini Institute of Engineering and Technology, Nagpur-19, Maharashtra, India.
Solid and Hazardous Waste Management Division, National Environmental Engineering Research Institute, Nehru Marg, Nagpur-20, Maharashtra, India.

Acknowledgement

The encouragement and support provided by the Principal and Management of Priyadarshini Institute of Engineering and Technology, Nagpur to Mr. Vivek P. Bhange is greatly acknowledged.

Author details

[1]Department of Biotechnology, Priyadarshini Institute of Engineering and Technology, Nagpur-19, Maharashtra, India. [2]Solid and Hazardous Waste Management Division, National Environmental Engineering Research Institute, Nehru Marg, Nagpur-20, Maharashtra, India.

References

1. Hall DO, House J, Scrase I. Overview of biomass energy, in industrial uses of biomass Energy-The example of Brazil. In: Rosill Calle F, Bajay S, Rothman H, editors. Taylor & Francis, London;2000. p26.
2. Hall DO, Rosill CF. Biomass Resources other than wood. London: World Energy Council; 1998.
3. Tai H-S, He W-H. A novel composting process for plant wastes in Taiwan military barracks. Resour Conserv Recycl. 2007;51:408–17.
4. Cofie Olufunke. Adams Bradford A. Organic Waste Reuse for Urban Agriculture, Case study of Ouagadougou city in Burkina Faso. 2006.
5. Bak JS, Ko JK, Han YH, Lee BC, Choi IG, Kim KH. Improved enzymatic hydrolysis yield of rice straw using electron beam irradiation. J Ferment Technol. 2009;62:377–84.
6. Mosier N, Wyman C, Dale B, Elander R, Lee YY, Holtzapple M, et al. Features of promising technologies for pretreatment of lignocellulosic biomass. Bioresour Technol. 2005;96:673–86.
7. Hsu TA. Pretreatment of Biomass, Handbook of Bioethanol, production and utilization. Washington, DC: Taylor and Francis; 1996.
8. Lin SH, Lo CC. Fenton process for treatment desizing wastewater. Water Res. 1997;31:2050–6.
9. Tang WZ, Huang CP. 2,4-Dichlorophenol oxidation kinetics by Fenton's reagent. Environ Technol. 1996;17:1371–7.
10. KangYW HKY. Effect of reaction conditions on the oxidation efficiency in the Fenton process. Water Res. 2000;34:2786–90.
11. Hsueh CL, Huang YH, Wang CC, Chen CY. Degradation of azo dyes using low iron concentration of Fenton and Fenton-like system. Chemosphere. 2005;58:409–1414.
12. Muruganandham M, Swaminathan M. Decolourisation of reactive orange by Fenton and photo-Fenton oxidation technology. Dyes Pigments. 2004;63:315–21.
13. Prateek J, Nadanathangam V. Effect of Fenton's pretreatment on cotton cellulosic substrates to enhance its enzymatic hydrolysis response. Bioresour Technol. 2012;103:219–26.
14. Barbusiński K. Fenton reaction-controversy concerning the chemistry. Ecol Chem Eng. 2009;16:3.
15. Nelson DW, Sommers LE. Total carbon, organic carbon and organic matter. In: Page AL, editor. Methods of Soil Analysis Part II. Madison: American Society of agronomers; 1982. p. 539–79.
16. Liu S. Analysis and Measurement in Papermaking Industry. Beijing, China: Chemical Industry Press; 2004.

17. Sluiter A, Ruiz R, Scarlata C, Sluiter J, Templeton D. Determination of Extractives in Biomass, National Renewable Energy Laboratory, Midwest Research Institute, Golden, CO. NREL/TP-510-42619. 2008.
18. Sluiter JB, Ruiz RO, Scarlata CJ, Sluiter AD, Templeton DW. Compositional analysis of lignocellulosic feedstocks. 1. Review and description of methods. J Agric Food Chem. 2010;58:9043–53.
19. Montgomery DC, Anderson W, Russell S, Aiello E. Design and Analysis of Experiments. New York: John Wiley, and sons Publishers; 2001. p. 427–92.
20. Mathews P. Design of experiments with MINITAB. India: Pearson Education (Singapore) Pte. Ltd; 2005. p. 437–74.
21. Kumar P, Barrett DM, Delwiche MJ, Stroeve P. Methods for pretreatment of lignocellulosic biomass for efficient hydrolysis and biofuel production. Ind Eng Chem Res. 2009;48:3713–29.
22. Mosier N, Hendrickson R, Ho N, Sedlak N, Ladish MR. Optimization of pH controlled liquid hot water pretreatment of corn stover. Bioresour Technol. 2005;96:1986–93.
23. Liu C-Z, Cheng X-Y. Microwave-assisted acid pretreatment for enhancing biogas production from herbal-extraction process residue. Energy Fuels. 2009;23:6152–5.
24. Ayeni AO, Hymore FK, Mudliar SN, Deshmukh SC, Satpute DB, Omoleye JA, et al. Hydrogen peroxide and lime based oxidative pretreatment of wood waste to enhance enzymatic hydrolysis for a biorefinery: Process parameters optimization using response surface methodology. Fuel. 2013;106:187–94.
25. Chen R, Pignatello JJ. Role of quinone intermediates as electron shuttles in Fenton and photo assisted Fenton oxidations of aromatic compounds. Environ Sci Technol. 1997;31:2399–406.
26. Joseph JM, Destaillats H, Hung HM, Hoffmann MR. The sonochemical degradation of azobenzene and related azo dyes: rate enhancements via Fenton's reactions. J Phys Chem A. 2000;104:301–7.
27. Hameed BH, Lee TW. Degradation of malachite green in aqueous solution by Fenton process. J Hazard Mater. 2009;164:468–72.
28. Neyens E, Baeyens J. A review of classic Fenton's peroxidation as an advanced oxidation technique. J Hazard Mater. 2003;98:33–50.

PERMISSIONS

All chapters in this book were first published in JEHSE, by BioMed Central; hereby published with permission under the Creative Commons Attribution License or equivalent. Every chapter published in this book has been scrutinized by our experts. Their significance has been extensively debated. The topics covered herein carry significant findings which will fuel the growth of the discipline. They may even be implemented as practical applications or may be referred to as a beginning point for another development.

The contributors of this book come from diverse backgrounds, making this book a truly international effort. This book will bring forth new frontiers with its revolutionizing research information and detailed analysis of the nascent developments around the world.

We would like to thank all the contributing authors for lending their expertise to make the book truly unique. They have played a crucial role in the development of this book. Without their invaluable contributions this book wouldn't have been possible. They have made vital efforts to compile up to date information on the varied aspects of this subject to make this book a valuable addition to the collection of many professionals and students.

This book was conceptualized with the vision of imparting up-to-date information and advanced data in this field. To ensure the same, a matchless editorial board was set up. Every individual on the board went through rigorous rounds of assessment to prove their worth. After which they invested a large part of their time researching and compiling the most relevant data for our readers.

The editorial board has been involved in producing this book since its inception. They have spent rigorous hours researching and exploring the diverse topics which have resulted in the successful publishing of this book. They have passed on their knowledge of decades through this book. To expedite this challenging task, the publisher supported the team at every step. A small team of assistant editors was also appointed to further simplify the editing procedure and attain best results for the readers.

Apart from the editorial board, the designing team has also invested a significant amount of their time in understanding the subject and creating the most relevant covers. They scrutinized every image to scout for the most suitable representation of the subject and create an appropriate cover for the book.

The publishing team has been an ardent support to the editorial, designing and production team. Their endless efforts to recruit the best for this project, has resulted in the accomplishment of this book. They are a veteran in the field of academics and their pool of knowledge is as vast as their experience in printing. Their expertise and guidance has proved useful at every step. Their uncompromising quality standards have made this book an exceptional effort. Their encouragement from time to time has been an inspiration for everyone.

The publisher and the editorial board hope that this book will prove to be a valuable piece of knowledge for researchers, students, practitioners and scholars across the globe.

LIST OF CONTRIBUTORS

Biljana Balabanova
Faculty of Agriculture, Goce Delčev University, Krste Misirkov bb, 2000 Štip, Macedonia

Trajče Stafilov and Katerina Bačeva
Institute of Chemistry, Faculty of Science, Ss. Cyril and Methodius University, Arhimedova 5, 1000 Skopje, Macedonia
Research Center for Environment and Materials, Macedonian Academy of Sciences and Arts, Krste Misirkov 2, 1000 Skopje, Republic of Macedonia

Mohammad Fadhil Abid, Amir Aziz Abdulrahman and Noor Hussein Hamza
Chemical Engineering Department, University of Technology, Baghdad, Iraq

Soheila Hamidzadeh
Payam Noor University of Varamin, Qarchak, Varamin, Tehran, Iran

Marzieh Torabbeigi
Faculty of Health, Safety and Environment, Shahid Beheshti University of Medical sciences, P. O. Box 16858-116, Tehran, Iran

Seyed Jamaleddin Shahtaheri
Department of Occupational Health Engineering, School of Public Health, Institute for Environmental Research, Tehran University of Medical Sciences, Tehran 14155-6446, Iran

Turgay Dindaroğlu
Faculty of Forestry, Department of Forest Engineering, Kahramanmaras Sutcu imam University, 46100 Kahramanmaras, Turkey

Shengmou Huang and Gan Lin
School of chemical engineering and food science, Hubei University of Arts and Science, Xiangyang 441053, China

Selçuk Erkaya
Engineering Faculty, Mechatronics Engineering Department, Erciyes University, Kayseri 38039, Turkey

Abdurrahman Geymen and Bülent Bostancı
Engineering Faculty, Geomatics Engineering Department, Erciyes University, Kayseri 38039, Turkey

Ceyda Yaman and Gönül Gündüz
Chemical Engineering Department, Ege University, 35100 Bornova, İzmir, Turkey

Mohammad Reza Fadaei Tehrani and Abolfazl Shamsai
Department of Civil Engineering, Sharif University of Technology, Tehran, Iran

Manoochehr Vossughi
Institute of Biotechnology and Environment (IBE), Department of Chemical Engineering, Sharif University of Technology, Tehran, Iran

Karina Bustos-Ramírez
Centro Conjunto de Investigación en Química Sustentable, UAEM-UNAM. Km.12 de la carretera Toluca-Atlacomulco, San Cayetano 50200, Estado de México, México
División de Estudios de Posgrado e Investigación, Instituto Tecnológico de Querétaro, Av. Tecnológico s/n Esq. M. Escobedo, Col. Centro Histórico, 76000 Querétaro, México
Centro de Física Aplicada y Tecnología Avanzada, Universidad Nacional Autónoma de México, Boulevard Juriquilla 3001, 76230 Querétaro, México

Carlos Eduardo Barrera-Díaz and Reyna Natividad-Rangel
Centro Conjunto de Investigación en Química Sustentable, UAEM-UNAM. Km.12 de la carretera Toluca-Atlacomulco, San Cayetano 50200, Estado de México, México

Miguel De Icaza-Herrera
Centro de Física Aplicada y Tecnología Avanzada, Universidad Nacional Autónoma de México, Boulevard Juriquilla 3001, 76230 Querétaro, México

Ana Laura Martínez-Hernández and Carlos Velasco-Santos
División de Estudios de Posgrado e Investigación, Instituto Tecnológico de Querétaro, Av. Tecnológico s/n Esq. M. Escobedo, Col. Centro Histórico, 76000 Querétaro, México
Centro de Física Aplicada y Tecnología Avanzada, Universidad Nacional Autónoma de México, Boulevard Juriquilla 3001, 76230 Querétaro, México

Seyed Kamran Foad Marashi and Hamid-Reza Kariminia
Department of Chemical and Petroleum Engineering, Sharif University of Technology, P.O. Box 11155-9465, Azadi Ave., Tehran, Iran

Brahmi Mounaouer and Hassen Abdennaceur
Water Research and Technology Center, University Tunis Cartage, Borj Cédria Science and Technology Park, P.O. Box 273, Soliman 8020, Tunisia

K. Thirugnanasambandham and V. Sivakumar
Department of Chemical Engineering, AC Tech Campus, Anna University, Chennai 600 025TN, India

Akbar Gholampour
Center for Air Pollution Research, Institute for Environmental Research, Tehran University of Medical Sciences, Tehran, Iran
School of Public Health, Tabriz University of Medical Sciences, Tabriz, Iran

Ramin Nabizadeh, Mohammad Sadegh Hassanvand and Hasan Taghipour
Center for Air Pollution Research, Institute for Environmental Research, Tehran University of Medical Sciences, Tehran, Iran

Shahrokh Nazmara
School of Public Health, Tehran University of Medical Sciences, Tehran, Iran

Amir Hossein Mahvi
School of Public Health, Tehran University of Medical Sciences, Tehran, Iran
Center for Solid Waste Research, Institute for Environmental Research, Tehran University of Medical Sciences, Tehran, Iran
National Institute of Health Research, Tehran University of Medical Sciences, Tehran, Iran

Kambiz Tahvildari, Yasaman Naghavi Anaraki and Sogol Mirpanji
Department of chemistry, Islamic Azad University, North Tehran Branch, Tehran, Iran

Reza Fazaeli
Modeling and Optimization Research Center in Science and Engineering, Islamic Azad University, South Tehran Branch, Tehran, Iran

Elham Delrish
Nano-ophthalmology Department, Stem Cells Preparation Unit, Eye Research Center, Farabi Eye Hospital, Tehran University of Medical Sciences, Tehran, Iran

Mohammad Hassan Ehrampoush, Mohammad Miria and Mohammad Hossien Salmani
Department of Environmental Health, School of Public Health, Shahid Sadoughi University of Medical Science, Yazd, Iran

Amir Hossein Mahvi
Center for solid Waste Research, Institute for Environmental Research, Tehran University of Medical Science, Tehran, Iran

Kamaleddin Abedi, Farshid Ghorbani-Shahna and Abdolrahman Bahrami
Department of occupational health engineering, Research center for health services, Hamedan University of Medical Sciences, Hamedan, Iran

Babak Jaleh
Department of physics, Bu-Ali Sina University, Hamedan, Iran

Rasoul Yarahmadi
Department of occupational health, Occupational health research center, School of public health, Iran University of Medical Sciences, Tehran, Iran

Mohammad Khazaei, Shahrokh Nazmara and Ramin Nabizadeh
Department of Environmental Health Engineering, School of Public Health, Tehran University of Medical Sciences, Tehran, Iran

Simin Nasseri
Department of Environmental Health Engineering, School of Public Health, Tehran University of Medical Sciences, Tehran, Iran
Center for Water Quality Research, Institute for Environmental Research, Tehran University of Medical Sciences, Tehran, Iran

Mohammad Reza Ganjali
Center of Excellence in Electrochemistry, Faculty of Chemistry, University of Tehran, Tehran, Iran
Biosensor Research Center, Endocrinology & Metabolism Molecular-Cellular Sciences Institute, Tehran University of Medical Sciences, Tehran, Iran

Mehdi Khoobi
Department of Medicinal Chemistry, Faculty of Pharmacy and Pharmaceutical Sciences Research Center, Tehran University of Medical Sciences, Tehran 14176, Iran

Amir Hossein Mahvi
Department of Environmental Health Engineering, School of Public Health, Tehran University of Medical Sciences, Tehran, Iran
Center for Water Quality Research, Institute for Environmental Research, Tehran University of Medical Sciences, Tehran, Iran
Center for Solid Waste Research, Institute for Environmental Research, Tehran University of Medical Sciences, Tehran, Iran

Elham Gholibegloo
Department of Chemistry, Faculty of Science, University of Zanjan, Zanjan, Iran

Dalel Daâssi
Laboratory of Enzyme Engineering and Microbiology, Ecole Nationale d'Ingénieurs de Sfax, University of Sfax, Route de Soukra Km 4.5, BP 1173, Sfax 3038, Tunisia
Department of Biology, Faculty of Sciences and Arts, Khulais, University of Jeddah, Jeddah, Saudi Arabia

Hela Zouari-Mechichi , Moncef Nasri and Tahar Mechichi
Laboratory of Enzyme Engineering and Microbiology, Ecole Nationale d'Ingénieurs de Sfax, University of Sfax, Route de Soukra Km 4.5, BP 1173, Sfax 3038, Tunisia

Fakher Frikha
Faculty of Sciences, University of Sfax, Route de Soukra Km 4,5, Sfax 3000, Tunisia

Susana Rodríguez-Couto
CEIT, Unit of Environmental Engineering, Paseo Manuel de Lardizábal 15, 20018 San Sebastian, Spain
5IKERBASQUE, Basque Foundation for Science, Alameda de Urquijo 36, 48011 Bilbao, Spain

Hamid Shirkhanloo
Occupational and Environmental Health Research Center (OEHRC), Iranian Petroleum Industry Health Research Institute (IPIHRI-PIHO), Tehran 1485733111, Iran
Research Institute of Petroleum Industry (RIPI), Tehran 14665-1137, Iran

Aisan Khaligh
Department of Chemistry, Semnan University, Semnan 35131-1911, Iran

Farideh Golbabae
Occupational Health Engineering Department, School of Public Health, Tehran University of Medical Sciences, Tehran 6446-14155, Iran

Zargham Sadeghi
Occupational and Environmental Health Research Center (OEHRC), Iranian Petroleum Industry Health Research Institute (IPIHRI-PIHO), Tehran 1485733111, Iran

Amir Vahid and Alimorad Rashidi
Research Institute of Petroleum Industry (RIPI), Tehran 14665-1137, Iran

Adel A.S. Banana
Environment Engineering Department, Subrata College, University of Zawia, Zawia, Libya

R. M. S. Radin Mohamed
Faculty of Civil & Environment Engineering, UTHM, Parit Raja, Malaysia

A. A. S. Al-Gheethi
Faculty of Civil & Environment Engineering, UTHM, Parit Raja, Malaysia
High Institute of health sciences, Sana'a, Yemen

Nabi Jahantigh
Mechanical Engineering Department, University of Zabol, Zabol, Iran

Ali Keshavarz and Masoud Mirzaei
Mechanical Engineering Department, K. N. Toosi University of Technology, Tehran, Iran

Shabnam Mahernia, Arash Amanlou, Gita kiaee and Massoud Amanlou
Department of Medicinal Chemistry, Faculty of Pharmacy and Pharmaceutical Sciences Research Center, Tehran University of Medical Sciences, Tehran, Iran

Vivek P Bhange
Department of Biotechnology, Priyadarshini Institute of Engineering and Technology, Nagpur-19, Maharashtra, India

SPM Prince William, Abhinav Sharma, Jagdish Gabhane, Atul N Vaidya and Satish R Wate
Solid and Hazardous Waste Management Division, National Environmental Engineering Research Institute, Nehru Marg, Nagpur-20, Maharashtra, India

Index